Veterinary Clinical Pathology

A Case-Based Approach

Veterinary Clinical Pathology
A Case-Based Approach

Kathleen P. Freeman

DVM, BS, MS, PhD, DipECVCP, FRCPath, MRCVS
RCVS Specialist in Veterinary Pathology (Clinical Pathology)
European Veterinary Specialist in Clinical Pathology
IDEXX Laboratories Ltd., Wetherby, West Yorkshire, United Kingdom

Stefanie Klenner

Dr.med.vet., DipECVCP
European Veterinary Specialist in Clinical Pathology
scil animal care company GmbH
Viernheim, Germany

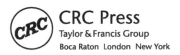

CRC Press
Taylor & Francis Group
Boca Raton London New York

CRC Press is an imprint of the
Taylor & Francis Group, an **informa** business

CRC Press
Taylor & Francis Group
6000 Broken Sound Parkway NW, Suite 300
Boca Raton, FL 33487-2742

© 2015 by Taylor & Francis Group, LLC
CRC Press is an imprint of Taylor & Francis Group, an Informa business

No claim to original U.S. Government works

Printed on acid-free paper
Version Date: 20150302

International Standard Book Number-13: 978-1-4822-2587-7 (Paperback)

Visit the Taylor & Francis Web site at
http://www.taylorandfrancis.com

and the CRC Press Web site at
http://www.crcpress.com

Contents

Preface

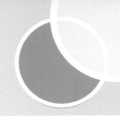

This book aims to provide a variety of clinical pathology cases covering multiple species and submitted by a selection of clinical pathologists and clinicians. It is not meant to cover all possible clinical pathology diagnoses, but offers a compilation of cases with clinical pathological results encountered by the contributors. The book was inspired by examples provided to the authors by their teachers and mentors when discussing cases and their thought processes in order to encourage the development of their own clinicopathological skills during training. We were further motivated by the need expressed by many veterinary students and trainees in general veterinary medicine, clinical pathology and internal medicine with whom we have interacted to have wider experience of the thought processes of experienced clinical pathologists and clinicians with regard to interpretation of laboratory data.

It was fascinating to see the systematic approaches that each contributor has taken with the cases they have elected to submit. Although the order of consideration and the terminology and phrases used by each contributor may differ slightly, there are many common threads that will be recognised as you read through these cases. You may find that you have 'favourite' contributors whose thought process and approach you admire, and you may seek to incorporate their style, phrases and approach into your own clinical repertoire.

The role of clinicians and clinical pathologists in today's environment lies in providing context, 'telling the story' and giving meaning in order to tie together the clinical presentation and laboratory data and assure the best possible patient care. By providing 'meaning' for ourselves, the owners and our colleagues we are establishing the basis for ongoing learning and a way to approach cases that will help all of us to become better practitioners of the art and science of veterinary medicine and to better communicate with our clients, owners and colleagues.

We hope these cases will provide an opportunity for students, residents, general practitioners and all veterinarians who would like to challenge or improve their skills in veterinary clinical pathology to see various presentations of cases and the ways that the contributors of these cases approach the analysis and interpretation of the data. The format, with general assessment of the laboratory data and questions to be answered regarding its interpretation, pathological mechanisms and clinical significance, should be of benefit in tying together the clinical pathology results, the pathophysiological base for these results, their interpretation, and further testing or information that may be of benefit for diagnosis, monitoring and/or prognosis. When a contributor uses laboratory results to skilfully 'tell the story' of the patient and explain the 'detective work' of the clinician and its interpretation, it is a joy to read!

We therefore present a collection of cases with a wide variety of clinical pathological abnormalities. Topics include haematology, clinical chemistry, endocrinology, acid–base and blood gas analysis, haemostasis, urinalysis, biological variation and quality control. The cases about quality control are unique for such a book and reflect our deep belief that this is an issue of huge importance for all of us. Every laboratory result represents a result with some degree of 'probability' associated with it, since all laboratory results contain some degree of inherent error. Knowledge of the nature of such variation (errors) and how they may influence our laboratory results helps all of us to become better pathologists and clinicians.

The level of difficulty of the various cases is wide, giving beginners the possibility to start improving their clinicopathological skills, providing more complicated cases or cases treating unfamiliar topics (e.g. biological variation) for the more experienced reader and increasing learning opportunities for the less experienced.

We hope that these cases will be of interest to a wide audience and provide a resource for continuing development of expertise in interpretation of laboratory data. We have endeavoured to ensure that the approaches and information are accurate and that recommendations for Further Reading are provided for many of the topics. We hope that you will enjoy these cases and the expertise of the contributors in presenting them for you.

Kathleen P. Freeman
Stefanie Klenner

Contributors

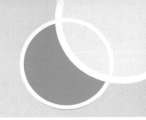

Natali Bauer, PD Dr. (habil.) DipECVCP
Justus-Liebig-Universität Gießen
Gießen, Germany

Andrea Di Bella, DVM, DipECVIM-CA,
    CertSAM, MRCVS
East Grinstead, West Sussex, England

Carola Campora, MVB, DipECVCP, MRCVS
IDEXX Laboratories Ltd.
Wetherby, West Yorkshire, England

Francesco Cian, DVM, DipECVCP, FRCPath, MRCVS
European Veterinary Specialist in Clinical Pathology
Animal Health Trust, Newmarket, England

Rick L. Cowell, DVM, MS, MRCVS, DipACVP
    (Clinical Pathology)
IDEXX Laboratories, Inc.
Stillwater, Oklahoma, USA

Myriam Defontis, DVM, DipECVCP
Frank Duncombe Laboratory
Caen, France

Joan Duncan, BVMS, PhD, FRCPath, MRCVS
NationWide Laboratories
Poulton-le-Fylde, Lancashire, England

Marco Duz, MedVet, MVM, DipECEIM, MRCVS
European Specialist in Equine Internal Medicine
University of Glasgow
Glasgow, Scotland

Jean F. Feldman, DVM
Hamburg, New York, USA

Kathleen P. Freeman, DVM, BS, MS, PhD,
    DipECVCP, FRCPath, MRCVS
RCVS Specialist in Veterinary Pathology
    (Clinical Pathology)
European Veterinary Specialist in Clinical Pathology
IDEXX Laboratories Ltd.
Wetherby, West Yorkshire, England

Lisle George, DVM, PhD, DipACVIM
University of California Davis School of Veterinary
    Medicine
Davis, California, USA

Karen Gerber, BVSc, Hons BVSc, DipACVP
    (Clinical Pathology), GCertEd
Registered Specialist Veterinary Clinical Pathologist
James Cook University
Townsville, Queensland, Australia

Tim Jagger, BVM&S, MSc, FRCPath, MRCVS
IDEXX Laboratories Ltd.
Wetherby, West Yorkshire, England

Mads Kjelgaard-Hansen, DVM, PhD
University of Copenhagen
Frederiksberg, Copenhagen, Denmark

Stefanie Klenner, Dr.med.vet., DipECVCP
European Veterinary Specialist in Clinical Pathology
scil animal care company GmbH
Viernheim, Germany

Annemarie T. Kristensen, DVM, PhD, DACVIM-SA,
    DECVIM-CA & Oncology
University of Copenhagen
Frederiksberg, Copenhagen, Denmark

Ernst Leidinger, DVM, DipECVCP
Invitro Veterinary Laboratories
Vienna, Austria

Judith Leidinger, DVM
Specialist in Veterinary Clinical Pathology
Invitro Veterinary Laboratories
Vienna, Austria

Carlo Masserdotti, DVM, DipECVCP
Specialist in Clinical Biochemistry
Laboratorio Veterinario San Marco
Padua, Italy

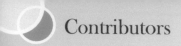

Contributors

Elspeth Milne, BVM&S, PhD, DipECVCP,
    FRCPath, FRCVS
European and RCVS Recognised Specialist
    in Veterinary Clinical Pathology
University of Edinburgh
Easter Bush Campus, Roslin, Scotland

Paola Monti, DVM, MSc, FRCPath, DipAVCP
    (Clinical Pathology)
DWR Diagnostics
Six Mile Bottom, Cambridgeshire, England

Eleonora Piseddu, DVM
IDEXX Laboratories - Novara Day Lab
Novara, Italy

Dawn Seddon, BVSc, MSc VetPath, DipACVP
    (Clinical Pathology)
New Zealand Veterinary Pathology
Hamilton, New Zealand

Bo Wiinberg, DVM, PhD
University of Copenhagen
Frederiksberg, Copenhagen, Denmark

Broad Classification of Cases

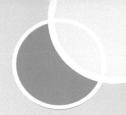

Note: There may be considerable overlapping between topics in the various cases. For example, cases concerning general clinical chemistry may also contain information about urinalysis, haemostasis, acid–base and quality control to a higher or lower amount.

Blood gas analysis
4, 17, 30, 50, 69, 89, 106, 156

Clinical chemistry
1, 2, 5, 7, 9, 12, 14, 15, 18, 19, 23, 24, 28, 31, 32, 34, 37, 39, 42, 43, 45, 47, 51, 53, 58, 59, 60, 61, 68, 74, 75, 78, 81, 82, 84, 86, 90, 96, 101, 102, 105, 107, 108, 113, 114, 116, 119, 121, 123, 126, 129, 141, 142, 150, 152, 155, 164, 170, 172, 173, 179, 180, 182, 184, 186, 192, 195, 196, 198, 200

Endocrinology
3, 16, 26, 38, 56, 63, 67, 76, 92, 97, 100, 110, 118, 124, 127, 135, 144, 147, 154, 161, 177, 190

Haematology
8, 21, 27, 40, 41, 46, 49, 54, 66, 70, 71, 79, 83, 87, 88, 94, 99, 115, 130, 136, 138, 139, 153, 158, 162, 167, 169, 176, 181, 187

Haemostasis
10, 35, 57, 91, 103, 133, 134, 143, 194

Infectious disease
6, 20, 25, 36, 52, 55, 65, 73, 85, 95, 104, 112, 120, 125, 131, 137, 145, 149, 151, 159, 166, 171, 188, 174, 185, 193, 197, 199

Protein electrophoresis
13, 33, 48, 80, 109, 122, 165, 191

Quality control
22, 64, 72, 98, 111, 128, 140, 148, 157, 168, 175, 178, 189

Urinalysis
11, 29, 44, 62, 77, 93, 117, 132, 146, 160, 163, 183

Abbreviations

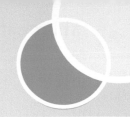

α-1-AGP	alpha-1-acid-glycoprotein
ACTH	adrenocorticotropic hormone
ACVP	American College of Veterinary Pathologists
ADH	antidiuretic hormone
AID	anaemia of inflammatory disease
AKI	acute kidney injury
ALP	alkaline phosphatase
ALT	alanine aminotransferase
ANP	atrial natriuretic peptide
APPs	acute phase proteins
aPTT	activated partial thromboplastin time
AST	aspartate aminotransferase
ASVCP	American Society for Veterinary Clinical Pathology
BCS	body condition score
BJP	Bence-Jones protein
BMBT	buccal mucosal bleeding time
BNP	B-type natriuretic peptide
bpm	beats per minute/breaths per minute
BUN	blood urea nitrogen
C-BNP	carboxy-terminal fragment of BNP, active form
CFU	colony-forming unit
CK	creatine kinase
CLL	chronic lymphocytic leukaemia
CNS	central nervous system
cPLI	canine pancreatic lipase
CRP	C-reactive protein
CRT	capillary refill time
CSF	cerebrospinal fluid
cTLI	canine trypsin-like immunoreactivity
CV_A	analytical coefficient of variation
CV_G	inter-individual coefficient of variation
CV_I	intra-individual coefficient of variation
DHNS	diabetic hyperosmolar non-ketotic syndrome
DIC	disseminated intravascular coagulation
DKA	diabetic ketoacidosis
DM	diabetes mellitus
DSH	domestic shorthair (cat)
ECG	electrocardiogram

ECVCP	European College of Veterinary Clinical Pathologists
EG	ethylene glycol
ELISA	enzyme-linked immunosorbent assay
EMS	equine metabolic syndrome
FBC	full (complete) blood count
FDPs	fibrin/fibrinogen degradation products
FE-K	urinary fractional excretion of potassium
FeLV	feline leukaemia virus
FE-Na	urinary fractional excretion of sodium
FIP	feline infectious peritonitis
FIV	feline immunodeficiency virus
fPLI	feline pancreatic lipase
FT4	free T4
FT4D or FT4ED	free T4 measured by equilibrium dialysis
GFR	glomerular filtration rate
GGT	gamma glutamyl transferase
GI	gastrointestinal
G:I ratio	glucose:insulin ratio
GLDH	glutamate dehydrogenase
GnRH	gonadotropin releasing hormone
HAC	hyperadrenocorticism, Cushing's disease
hCG	human chorionic gonadotropin
HCO_3	bicarbonate concentration
Hct	haematocrit
HDDST	high-dose dexamethasone suppression test
Hgb	haemoglobin
HMWK	high molecular weight kininogen
hpf	high-power field
HR	heart rate
HUS	haemolytic-uraemic syndrome
IFAT	indirect immunofluorescent antibody test
IL	interleukin
IM	intramuscular
IMHA	immune-mediated haemolytic anaemia
IoI	index of individuality
IRIS	International Renal Interest Society
IV	intravenously
IVFT	intravenous fluid therapy

LDDST	low-dose dexamethasone suppression test	QGI	quality goal index
LDH	lactate dehydrogenase	RAAS	renin–angiotensin–aldosterone system
LDL	low-density lipoprotein	RBC	red blood cell
lpf	low-power field	RCV	reference change value
LUC	large unstained cell	RDW	red cell distribution width
		RI	reference interval
MAA	SAA produced in the mammary gland	RIA	radioimmunoassay
MAP	mitogen-activated protein (kinase)	RISQI	reciprocal of the square root of insulin
MCH	mean corpuscular haemoglobin		
MCHC	mean corpuscular haemoglobin concentration	RR	respiratory rate
MCV	mean corpuscular volume	SAA	serum amyloid A
MHC	major histocompatibility complex	SG	specific gravity
MIRG	modified insulin:glucose ratio	SIADH	syndrome of inappropriate ADH secretion
n.d.	not done	SPE	serum protein electrophoresis
NPR-A	renal A-type natriuretic peptide receptor	SSA	sulphosalicylic acid
NPR-C	C-type natriuretic peptide receptor	T	temperature
NRBC	nucleated red blood cell	T3	tri-iodo-thyronine
NSAID	non-steroidal anti-inflammatory drug	T4	thyroxine
NT-proBNP	N-terminal of the prohormone brain natriuretic peptide	TE_a	total allowable error
		TEG	thromboelastography, thromboelastogram
OspA	outer surface protein A	TF	tissue factor
		TgAA	thyroglobulin autoantibody
PA	plasma or serum aldosterone	TIBC	total iron binding capacity
PCO_2	partial pressure of carbon dioxide	TLI	trypsin-like immunoreactivity
$PaCO_2$	arterial carbon dioxide pressure	TNF	tumour necrosis factor
PCR	polymerase chain reaction	TRH	thyroid-releasing hormone
PCV	packed cell volume	TSH	thyroid-stimulating hormone (thyrotropin)
PLE	protein-losing enteropathy		
PLN	protein-losing nephropathy	TT4	total thyroxine
PMSG	pregnant mare serum gonadotropin		
PO_2	partial pressure of oxygen	UPCR	urine protein:creatinine ratio
PaO_2	arterial oxygen pressure	USG	urine specific gravity
PP	psychogenic polydipsia		
PPID	pars pituitary intermedia dysfunction	VLDL	very low-density lipoprotein
PRA	plasma renin activity	VlsE	variable major protein-like sequence expression
PT	prothrombin time		
PTH	parathyroid hormone	vWD	von Willebrand's disease
PTHrP	parathyroid hormone related protein	vWF	von Willebrand factor
PTT	partial thromboplastin time		
PU/PD	polyuria/polydipsia	WBC	white blood cell

Approach to Analysis of Cases

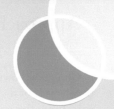

For those readers less experienced in analysis of case data, we thought it may be of benefit to present a bit of the 'thinking' that goes into the approach to case analysis and interpretation. This represents the thoughts of the editors based on their combined experience and their exposure to case data over a number of years and at various institutions and situations.

Philosophy

There is always discussion about the use of comprehensive profiles versus profiles selected based on clinical signs and clinical examination findings. At this time, a good general 'comprehensive' minimum database with a complete blood count, urinalysis and multisystem biochemistry profile is considered the standard for laboratory work up of cases in which a clinical diagnosis is not of high certainty based on the clinical examination or other ancillary tests. The benefit of assessing multiple systems lies in determining whether multiple problems are present and whether the findings are compatible with the known aetiopathogenesis and pathophysiology associated with various conditions. Use of the problem-oriented approach helps in the mental organisation and 'sifting' of data with mental designation and documentation of 'highly significant', 'significant', 'lesser significance' or 'unremarkable' findings.

The last few decades have seen a rapid rise in the volume of laboratory testing, with the development of many new technologies. A reliance on laboratory testing and on the clinical pathologist or clinician as the 'story teller' and 'translator of meaning' for laboratory testing appears likely to continue for the foreseeable future.

When reading case write ups written by trainees practicing for learning and for examination preparation, it is a joy to see them develop so that they are able to extract the 'story' from the laboratory data, tie it together in a way that presents good evidence-based conclusions, and point out those items that are part of known patterns and those that are harder or impossible to explain based on the single or multiple problems that have been identified. Such aberrant data may eventually be explained based on further clinical developments, effects of treatment and/or further laboratory testing.

The literature indicates that much laboratory data is likely to be ignored or is not acted upon in a manner that is timely and in keeping with providing the best possible patient care. Some clinicians try to use laboratory testing to confirm their clinical suspicions and some may ignore abnormal data that do not 'fit in' with their clinical findings. The 'best practice' orientation is to determine what findings fit together and to identify those that are unexpected based on the current understanding of disease mechanisms and aetiopathogenesis and pathophysiology, perhaps indicating the presence of additional contributing or causal conditions or a need for further investigation and understanding of the condition.

Other clinicians may claim that they use laboratory testing to identify subclinical conditions or conditions that may be difficult or impossible to identify based on clinical findings alone, but then also claim to dismiss 'abnormal' findings as 'irrelevant' or 'laboratory error' if an explanation for their presence is not apparent or understood. This is the 'clinician laboratory testing paradox' well known to many laboratorians, and it is our mission to be the 'detectives' of the clinical world and an important bridge between the clinics and the world of pathology and anatomy, which are the foundation for veterinary medicine and laboratory medicine.

The clinical pathologist brings unique expertise in knowledge of laboratory instruments, methods and statistical analyses (such as uncertainty associated with the measurements) to the discussion of laboratory findings. As recent discussions with clinicians regarding guideline development for the ASVCP Quality Assurance and Laboratory Standards Committee and the ECVCP Laboratory Standards Committee have shown, clinicians expectations for instrument/method capability (accuracy and precision) may exceed that attainable with current state-of-the-art instruments and methods. In this book some cases are addressing newer applications, such as biological variation and use of the reference change value (critical difference), which provide opportunities for a new understanding of changes in serial data for monitoring the health of veterinary patients and the progression of a disease and its response to treatment.

Purpose

The purpose of case evaluation is to arrive at an interpretation − that is, the synthesis of clinical and laboratory findings in order to reach a clinical diagnosis, with indication of the certainty of such an interpretation and other possible differential diagnoses. Based on the probabilities associated with various findings, further recommendations regarding additional testing, monitoring or prognosis may be possible.

Clinicians, owners and clinical pathologists all desire an 'answer' or a clinical diagnosis from which to proceed. Sometimes this will be based on a highly confident anchor, while other times it will be less firmly based, but still within a 'sea of probability' that has wider boundaries but has a sound basis for its definition. Occasionally, there are challenging cases that resemble 'navigation by starlight across the open ocean' with few or no landmarks. These are the ones that you hope to continue to learn from and, by the journey's end, have clinical or postmortem evidence to unravel the threads and reveal the eventual conclusion to the mystery. That is why dedication to undertaking the 'correct steps' in clinicopathological investigation, whenever possible, and obtaining follow-up information about clinical progress should be instilled in every clinician and clinical pathologist. Only by acquiring continual knowledge about the results and the ongoing clinical and laboratory findings can we know if the interpretations we provide are correct and continue to learn.

Process

Case evaluation is about *pattern recognition*. Patterns of findings help steer you toward or away from various general categories of disease. Then, a good foundation knowledge of diseases and conditions seen in the species of interest and across many species may allow further refinement as to the underlying cause. Finally, expert species knowledge and experience in the laboratory diagnosis of specific conditions may allow a highly specific interpretation and clinical diagnosis to be made.

The order in which individuals look at laboratory tests and their groupings is often remarkably similar amongst experienced pathologists and this has influenced the order in which laboratory data are presented in this book.

Approach

Regardless of your experience with laboratory data, expertise can be obtained by exposure to the thought processes and discussions presented by experienced pathologists. There is a body of literature looking at 'expert thought processes' and how they differ from those of the novice in a variety of vocations, but particularly in medicine, where the development of the synthetic processes needed for interpretation helps separate those with 'more gifted' and 'less gifted' medical expertise. It is our hope that by being exposed to the numerous clinicians who have contributed to this book you will reap the benefits of exposure to multiple expressions, turns of phrase and patterns of 'telling the story' in a way that will help you continue to learn about clinical laboratory medicine and its applications.

Questions

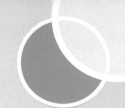

CASE 1

A 6-week-old Clydesdale filly was found collapsed in the field the day after it had been seen galloping round with its mother.

EXAMINATION FINDINGS

The filly was conscious but recumbent, dyspnoeic and poorly responsive to stimuli.

BIOCHEMISTRY

Analyte (units)	Result	Reference Interval (adult horses)	Reference Interval (3–6-week-old foals)
Total protein (g/l)	45.2	58–75	42–66
Albumin (g/l)	**17.7**	23–35	26–37
Globulins (g/l)	27.5	30–50	15–33
GGT (U/l)	**263**	13–44	13–30
ALP (U/l)	**365**	84–180	1,195–2,513
GLDH (U/l)	**311**	1–12	8–31
AST (U/l)	**210,000**	258–554	329–337
CK (U/l)	**335,400**	150–385	204–263
Bile acids (µmol/l)	**47.2**	1–15	0–8
Urea (mmol/l)	**57.3**	2.5–8.3	2.8–4.1
Creatinine (µmol/l)	**1,121**	40–150	97–138
Calcium (mmol/l)	**1.8**	2.6–3.3	2.9–3.1
Phosphorus (mmol/l)	**3.4**	0.8–1.8	2.2–2.7
Sodium (mmol/l)	**100**	134–150	135–145
Potassium (mmol/l)	**2.9**	2.7–5.9	4.1–5.0
Chloride (mmol/l)	**69**	98–118	96–102

HAEMATOLOGY

No significant abnormalities.

URINALYSIS

Item	Result	Reference Interval
Appearance	**Red–brown**	Yellow
USG	1.025	>1.025
Sediment analysis		
Erythrocytes	**6/hpf**	<5
Leucocytes	None	<5
Epithelial cells	15/lpf	None to few
Crystals	None	None
Casts	**Many red–brown, finely granular casts**	None
Bacteria	None	None
Dipstick evaluation		
pH	7.3	7.5–8.5
Protein	**4+**	Negative
Bilirubin	**1+**	Negative
Glucose	Negative	Negative
Ketone bodies	Negative	Negative
Blood	**4+**	Negative

QUESTIONS

1 What is your analysis of these results?
2 What are your differential diagnoses?
3 What additional testing would you recommend?

CASE 2

A 1-year-old female Havana cat was referred with a history of recent anaemia (PCV = 14%) documented 2 weeks previously. The cat was living with four other oriental cats, mainly indoors. Vaccination against calicivirus, herpesvirus, panleucopaenia and feline leukaemia virus and deworming was up to date.

EXAMINATION FINDINGS

Unremarkable. T = 39.1°C (102.4°F); HR = 160 bpm; RR = 30 bpm; BCS = 4/9; weight = 3.8 kg (8.3 lb).

HAEMATOLOGY

Measurand (units)	Result	Reference Interval
RBC count (10^9/l)	**4.8**	5.0–10.0
Haemoglobin (g/l)	**79**	80–150
Haematocrit (l/l)	**0.25**	0.30–0.45
MCV (fl)	52	39–55
MCH (pg)	16.4	12.5–17.5
MCHC (g/l)	**316**	320–360
RDW (%)	**24.1**	17.3–22.0
Aggregate reticulocytes (10^9/l)	**177**	0–60
Platelet count (10^9/l)	213	190–400
WBC count (10^9/l)	**26.9**	5.5–19.5
Neutrophils (10^9/l)	**19.9**	2.5–12.5
Band neutrophils (10^9/l)	0	0.0–0.3
Lymphocytes (10^9/l)	3.0	1.5–7.0
Eosinophils (10^9/l)	1.5	0.0–1.5
Monocytes (10^9/l)	**1.0**	0.0–0.85
Basophils (10^9/l)	0	Rare
NRBC (10^9/l)	**0.5**	Rare

No peripheral blood smear examination was done.

COOMBS TEST

Test	Result
Polyvalent Coombs reagent	Negative at 4°C (29.2°F) and 37°C (98.6°F)
Anti-cat IgG	Negative at 4°C (29.2°F) and 37°C (98.6°F)
Anti-cat IgM	Negative at 4°C (29.2°F) and 37°C (98.6°F)
Cold autoagglutination	Negative

BIOCHEMISTRY

Analyte (units)	Result	Reference Interval
Total protein (g/l)	84	57–89
Albumin (g/l)	34	22–40
Globulins (g/l)	49	28–51
ALT (U/l)	**451**	12–130
ALP (U/l)	51	14–111
Glucose (mmol/l)	**9.02**	4.11–8.83
Cholesterol (mmol/l)	5.56	1.68–5.81
Bilirubin (µmol/l)	<2	0–15
Bile acids (fasting) (µmol/l)	**15**	0–10
Bile acids (post-prandial) (µmol/l)	**35**	0–25
BUN (mmol/l)	10.2	5.7–12.9
Creatinine (µmol/l)	136	71–212
Sodium (mmol/l)	160	144–160
Potassium (mmol/l)	4.3	3.5–5.8
Chloride (mmol/l)	122	109–122
Phosphorus (mmol/l)	1.64	1.00–2.42
Calcium (mmol/l)	2.83	1.95–2.83

URINALYSIS

Item	Result	Reference Interval
Colour	Yellow	Yellow
Turbidity	Clear	Clear
USG	1.034	>1.035
Dipstick evaluation		
pH	6.5	Acidic
Glucose	Negative	Negative
Ketone bodies	Negative	Negative
Bilirubin	Negative	Negative
Protein	Negative	Negative
Blood	Negative	Negative
Sediment analysis		
Erythrocytes	0	<5
Leucocytes	0	<5
Casts	0	None
Crystals	0	None
Epithelial cells	0	None to few

INFECTIOUS DISEASES

Test	Result
FIV antibodies (ELISA)	Negative
FeLV antigen (ELISA)	Negative
FCoV antibodies (IFAT)	**Positive (titre >1,280)**
Mycoplasma haemofelis (PCR)	Negative
Mycoplasma haemominutum (PCR)	Negative
Candidatus mycoplasma turincensis (PCR)	Negative

COAGULATION PROFILE

Analyte (units)	Patient	Reference Interval
PT (seconds)	11.2	8–13
aPTT (seconds)	22.7	10–25
D-dimer (ng/ml)	250	0–250

IMAGING RESULTS

Thoracic radiographs were unremarkable. Abdominal ultrasound revealed abnormal hepatic parenchyma with patchy, mixed echodensity and hyperechoic sparkling areas and hyperechoic foci 1–2 cm in diameter. The hepatic lymph nodes were slightly enlarged (0.5 1 cm in diameter). A small quantity of free peritoneal fluid was detected.

A few attempts to retrieve the abdominal fluid were made but only a small quantity of blood (0.1 ml) was collected. It was thought to be iatrogenic as it clotted.

A fine needle aspirate (FNA) of the liver was performed (**Fig. 2.1**). There were some clusters of hepatocytes with

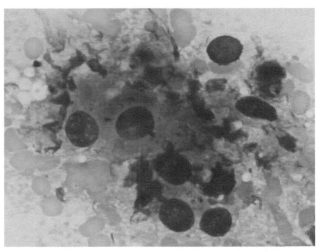

FIG. 2.1 Hepatic aspirate from this Havana cat. Wright–Giemsa, ×100 (oil).

some extracellular purple-staining material. A few non-degenerate neutrophils were also detected.

QUESTIONS

1 What is your evaluation of the laboratory data?
2 What is your diagnosis/interpretation for this case?
3 What pathophysiology is likely underlying the findings in this case?
4 What other tests would you recommend performing, and why?

CASE 3

A 15-month-old male Border Collie presented with a history of occasional vomiting over the preceding 5 days.

EXAMINATION FINDINGS

No abnormalities were detected on clinical examination and the patient was treated with maropitant citrate monohydrate. The following day the dog was anorexic. On day 2 the dog was dehydrated (7%); T = 35.1°C (95°F); HR = 48 bpm.

HAEMATOLOGY

Measurand (units)	Result (Day 2)	Reference Interval
RBC count (10¹²/l)	**8.93**	5.4–8.5
Haemoglobin (g/l)	**217**	120–180

Measurand (units)	Result (Day 2)	Reference Interval
Haematocrit (l/l)	**0.63**	0.37–0.56
MCV (fl)	70	67–75
MCHC (g/l)	340	310–350
Platelet count (10⁹/l)	304	200–900
WBC count (10⁹/l)	10.4	5–18
Neutrophils (10⁹/l)	6.34	3.7–13.32
Lymphocytes (10⁹/l)	2.7	1.00–3.60
Monocytes (10⁹/l)	0.31	0.00–0.72
Eosinophils (10⁹/l)	1.04	0.00–1.25
Blood film examination	No abnormalities noted	

BIOCHEMISTRY

Analyte (units)	Result (Day 2)	Reference Interval
Total protein (g/l)	60	55–75
Albumin (g/l)	31	29–35
Globulins (g/l)	29	18–38
ALP (U/l)	73	0–135 (Adult)
ALT (U/l)	**57**	0–40
GGT (U/l)	3	0–14
Total bilirubin (µmol/l)	1.0	0–5.0
Glucose (mmol/l)	3.2	3.0–5.5
Urea (mmol/l)	**41.8**	3.5–7.0
Creatinine (µmol/l)	**389**	0–130
Phosphorus (mmol/l)	**3.1**	0.9–1.6
Calcium (mmol/l)	**3.19**	2.3–3.0
Chloride (mmol/l)	95	95–117
Sodium (mmol/l)	**128**	135–150
Potassium (mmol/l)	**8**	3.5–5.6
Sodium:potassium ratio	**16:1**	>27:1

OTHER INVESTIGATIONS

Item	Result	Reference Interval
USG	**1.021**	>1.030
ECG	No P waves identified	

ACTH STIMULATION TEST

Analyte (units)	Result	Reference Interval
Basal cortisol (nmol/l)	**<28**	28–125
Cortisol post ACTH* (nmol/l)	**<28**	125–520

* Sample collected 60 minutes after an IV injection of 250 µg of tetracosactide, a synthetic analogue of ACTH.

QUESTIONS

1 What is your evaluation of the laboratory data?
2 How might prior therapy affect confirmation of the diagnosis?
3 Briefly outline the pathophysiology underlying these laboratory abnormalities.

CASE 4

A 7-year-old female neutered mixed-breed dog presented because she had diarrhoea for the past several days.

EXAMINATION FINDINGS

There was mild discomfort in the abdomen as well as dry mucous membranes.

ACID–BASE AND BLOOD GAS DATA

Analyte (units)	Result	Reference Interval
Arterial pH	**7.24**	7.36–7.44
PaCO$_2$ (mmHg)	**24**	36–44
PaO$_2$ (mmHg)	95	85–95
Plasma HCO$_3^-$ (mmol/l)	**10**	18–26
Serum Na$^+$ (mmol/l)	145	145–155
Serum K$^+$ (mmol/l)	**6.5**	4–5
Serum Cl$^-$ (mmol/l)	**124**	105–115
Anion gap	?	15–25

QUESTIONS

1 What is the anion gap (AG) in this case?
2 What is your assessment of the arterial pH?
3 What is your assessment of the likely underlying aetiology?
4 Is there appropriate compensation for this condition?
5 Why is the K$^+$ increased in this case?
6 Why is the Cl$^-$ increased in this case?
7 What is a likely underlying aetiological mechanism for metabolic acidosis?

CASE 5
A 14-year-old female neutered mixed-breed dog presented with vomiting and anorexia of 2 days' duration.

EXAMINATION FINDINGS

The dog was lethargic and demonstrated markedly icteric sclerae (**Fig. 5.1**), mucous membranes and skin. Rectal examination revealed pale mud-coloured faeces.

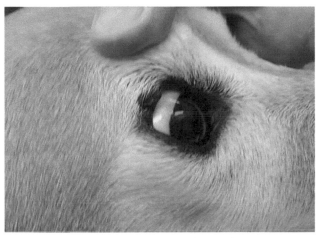

FIG. 5.1 Note the markedly icteric sclera of this dog.

BIOCHEMISTRY

Analyte (units)	Result	Reference Interval
Total protein (g/l)	69.5	55–70
Albumin (g/l)	31.4	30–37
Globulins (g/l)	**38.1**	23–36
Glucose (mmol/l)	4.66	3.3–6.5
Bilirubin (µmol/l)	**156.82**	<3.6
Cholesterol (mmol/l)	**19.11**	3.3–8.6
Triglycerides (mmol/l)	**1.39**	<0.75
ALP (U/l)	**3,674**	<131
ALT (U/l)	**5,833**	<85
GLDH (U/l)	**1,010**	<10
Urea (mmol/l)	3.3	3.03–9.82
Creatinine (µmol/l)	110	53–123
Sodium (mmol/l)	**144**	147–152
Chloride (mmol/l)	**99**	102–110
Potassium (mmol/l)	3.6	3.35–4.37
Ionised calcium (mmol/l)	1.29	1.23–1.43
Phosphate (mmol/l)	1.56	0.79–2.1

HAEMATOLOGY

Unremarkable.

QUESTIONS

1 Describe and discuss the significant biochemistry findings, and give the most likely cause of the icterus.
2 What further examinations are recommended to determine the aetiology of the disease in this dog?

CASE 6
An 11-year-old male neutered DSH cat has a history of vaccination against calicivirus, herpesvirus, panleukopaenia and feline leukaemia virus and deworming being up to date. The owner says the cat is acting a little strange and is foaming at the mouth. The owner wants to leave the cat at the clinic for the day for observation. The cat has a previous history of cardiomyopathy and is being treated with diltiazem extended release (30 mg daily).

EXAMINATION FINDINGS

T = 38.3°C (101°F); weight = 4.65 kg (10 lb); HR = 200 bpm; RR = 34 bpm; mucous membranes pale; grade IV/VI heart murmur.

HAEMATOLOGY

Measurand (units)	Result	Reference Interval
RBC count (10^{12}/l)	**1.83**	5–10
Haemoglobin (g/l)	**32.5**	80–150
Haematocrit (l/l)	**0.11**	0.30–0.45
MCV (fl)	**60.6**	39–55
MCH (pg)	**17.7**	12.5–17.5
MCHC (g/l)	**293**	320–360
Aggregated reticulocytes (10^9/l)	90	0–60
Platelet count (10^9/l)	**100 (clumped)**	190–400
WBC count (10^9/l)	13.1	5.5–19.5
Neutrophils (10^9/l)	10.03	2.5–12.5
Lymphocytes (10^9/l)	**0.826**	1.5–7.0
Eosinophils (10^9/l)	0	0–1.5
Monocytes (10^9/l)	**0.944**	0.0–0.85
Basophils (10^9/l)	0	Rare
NRBCs (per 100 WBCs)	**3**	Rare

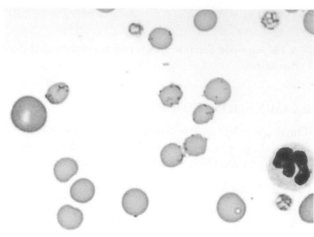

FIG. 6.1 Photomicrograph of the blood smear. Wright–Giemsa, ×100 (oil).

BLOOD SMEAR EVALUATION

3+ polychromasia; 2+ anisocytosis; 1+ autoagglutination.

INFECTIOUS DISEASES TESTS

Test	Result
FIV antibodies (ELISA)	Negative
FeLV antigen (ELISA)	Negative
FCoV antibodies (IFA)	Negative

QUESTIONS

1 Does the anaemia appear regenerative?
2 What is the significance of the blood smear picture?

CASE 7

A 9-year-old female cat was recently diagnosed with lymphoma. She is now presented for a regular check before treatment is instituted. A blood smear is prepared from the cat (Fig. 7.1).

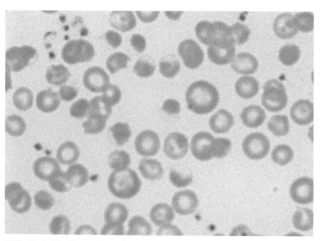

FIG. 7.1 Erythrocytes shown on a blood smear from a cat. May–Grünwald–Giemsa, ×100 (oil).

QUESTIONS

1 Name the abnormality visible in the blood smear.
2 List possible reasons for this finding for dogs, cats, and horses. What is the reason in this case?
3 Describe the underlying pathological mechanism leading to this finding.

CASE 8
A 12-year-old male neutered DSH cat presented for a routine annual health check.

HAEMATOLOGY

Measurand (units)	Result	Reference Interval
RBC count (10¹²/l)	**4.7**	5–10
Haemoglobin (g/l)	**127**	49–93
Haematocrit (l/l)	**0.18**	0.24–0.45
MCV (fl)	**39.6**	40–55
MCH (pg)	**27.02**	19.5–27.0
MCHC (g/l)	**705**	184–220
Platelet count (10⁹/l)	198	180–550
WBC count (10⁹/l)	14.8	6–18
Neutrophils (10⁹/l)	**13.59**	2.5–12.5
Lymphocytes (10⁹/l)	0.84	1.5–7.0
Monocytes (10⁹/l)	0.31	0.0–0.9
Eosinophils (10⁹/l)	0.07	0.0–1.5
Basophils (10⁹/l)	0.01	0.0–0.4

BIOCHEMISTRY

Analyte (units)	Result	Reference Interval
Total protein (g/l)	74.5	54.7–78.0
Albumin (g/l)	29.7	21–33
Globulins (g/l)	49.9	26–51
Glucose (mmol/l)	**31.2**	3.89–6.11
ALP (U/l)	37.3	0–39.7
ALT (U/l)	55	0–70
Urea (mmol/l)	9.65	7.14–10.7
Creatinine (µmol/l)	152	0–168
Sodium (mmol/l)	149	147–156
Chloride (mmol/l)	117	115–130
Potassium (mmol/l)	4.2	3.6–4.8
Ionised calcium (mmol/l)	1.21	1.17–1.32
Phosphate (mmol/l)	**5.1**	0.8–1.9

BLOOD SMEAR EVALUATION

Shows slight anisocytosis of the RBCs. Neutrophils occasionally display small Döhle bodies. Rare platelet clumps are detected in the feathered edge.

QUESTIONS

1 What is the most likely explanation for the laboratory abnormalities?
2 State and explain the causes for an increased MCHC.
3 How do you explain the biochemistry changes in light of the abnormalities discussed in the first two questions?

CASE 9
A 5-year-old male neutered cross-breed dog had accidental access to the psoriasis cream used by his owner. He now has PU/PD.

HAEMATOLOGY

Unremarkable.

BIOCHEMISTRY

Analyte (units)	Result	Reference Interval
Total protein (g/l)	**77**	55–75
Albumin (g/l)	**45**	25–40
Globulins (g/l)	32	23–35
Glucose (mmol/l)	6	3.3–6.5
ALP (U/l)	112	0–130
ALT (U/l)	69	0–85
Urea (mmol/l)	**12.2**	3.3–8.0

Analyte (units)	Result	Reference Interval
Creatinine (µmol/l)	**158**	45–150
Sodium (mmol/l)	148	135–155
Chloride (mmol/l)	113	105–120
Potassium (mmol/l)	4	3.35–4.37
Total calcium (mmol/l)	**3.55**	2.30–2.80
Ionised calcium (mmol/l)	**1.86**	1.18–1.40
Phosphate (mmol/l)	**1.52**	0.78–1.41

URINALYSIS

Item	Result	Reference Interval
Colour	Straw colour	Yellow
Turbidity	Slightly cloudy	Clear
USG	**1.006**	>1.030
Dipstick evaluation		
pH	5.5	
Protein	Trace	Negative to trace
Glucose	Negative	Negative
Ketone bodies	Negative	Negative
Bilirubin	Negative	Negative
Blood	Negative	Negative

QUESTIONS

1 Is this azotaemia likely to be pre-renal, renal or post-renal? Why?
2 How would you explain the low USG?
3 Explain the possible cause of the reported hypercalcaemia.
4 What is your diagnosis?

CASE 10

A 3-year-old male West Highland White Terrier was admitted to the hospital 2 days ago.

EXAMINATION FINDINGS

At admission the dog was lethargic, with clinical signs of systemic inflammatory response (febrile, increased HR and RR). Pancreatitis was diagnosed and treatment initiated. Forty-eight hours later dog had not clinically improved significantly, he was bleeding from venipuncture sites and development of a consumptive coagulopathy (DIC) was suspected.

SELECTED LABORATORY TEST RESULTS

At admission

Measurand (units)	Result	Reference Interval
RBC count (10^{12}/l)	**4.2**	4.6–8.4
Haemoglobin (l/l)	120	119–190
Haematocrit (l/l)	**0.35**	0.39–0.59
Platelet count (10^9/l)	**105**	200–500
WBC count (10^9/l)	**27.2**	6.5–18.1
Neutrophils (10^9/l)	**20.5**	3.2–12.1
Band neutrophils (10^9/l)	**1.0**	<0.3
Lymphocytes (10^9/l)	4.5	1–4.8
Monocytes (10^9/l)	0.6	0–1.2
Eosinophils (10^9/l)	0.6	0–1.2
Basophils (10^9/l)	0	0–0.05
C-reactive protein (mg/l)	**135**	<35
Fibrinogen (g/l)	1.2	1–4

Present (48 hours)

Measurand (units)	Result	Reference Interval
RBC count (10^{12}/l)	**4.4**	4.6–8.4
Haemoglobin (l/l)	**101**	119–190
Haematocrit (l/l)	**0.34**	0.39–0.59
Platelet count (10^9/l)	**87**	200–500
WBC count (10^9/l)	**25.2**	6.5–18.1
Neutrophils (10^9/l)	**18.4**	3.2–12.1
Band neutrophils (10^9/l)	**1.2**	<0.3
Lymphocytes (10^9/l)	4.1	1–4.8
Monocytes (10^9/l)	0.6	0–1.2
Eosinophils (10^9/l)	0.9	0–1.2
Basophils (10^9/l)	0	0–0.05
C-reactive protein (mg/l)	**140**	<35
Fibrinogen (g/l)	**0.8**	1–4
aPTT (seconds)	**14**	10–13
PT (seconds)	**10**	7–9
D-dimer (mg/l)	**4.2**	<0.5

To confirm suspicion of DIC, the presence of (a) activation of coagulation, (b) inhibitor consumption and (c) increased fibrinolytic activity has to be demonstrated along with an obvious clinical cause.

QUESTION

1 Are all these aspects demonstrated in the clinical history and laboratory tests to confirm suspicion of DIC?

CASE 11

A 5-year-old male neutered DSH cat presented because of a few episodes of feline lower urinary tract disease (FLUTD).

URINALYSIS

Item	Result	Reference Interval
Colour	Light yellow	Variable
Transparency	**Turbid**	Clear
USG	1.035	1.020–1.060
Dipstick evaluation		
pH	6.5	Acidic
Protein	Negative	Traces
Ketone bodies	Negative	Negative
Bilirubin	Negative	Negative
Blood	**+**	Negative

Urine sediment analysis
See **Fig. 11.1**.

QUESTIONS

1 What crystals can be seen on the picture?
2 What is the most important differential diagnosis?
3 How can you differentiate between these two types of crystals?
4 What do the crystals shown indicate?

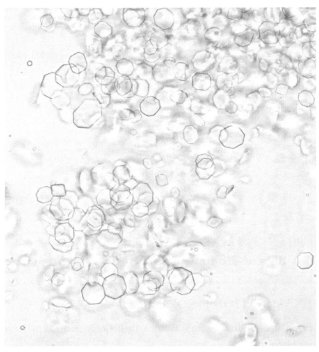

FIG. 11.1 Unstained urine sediment. ×40.
(Courtesy Dr Judith Leidinger)

CASE 12

A 1-year-old male Cocker Spaniel presents for lethargy and anorexia.

HAEMATOLOGY

The MCV, MCH, MCHC and platelet count are within normal limits.

Measurand (units)	Result	Reference Interval
RBC count (10¹²/l)	**4.62**	5.5–8.5
Haemoglobin (g/l)	**94**	130–195
Haematocrit (l/l)	**0.31**	0.37–0.55
WBC count (10⁹/l)	**28.5**	6–17
Neutrophils (10⁹/l)	**21.38**	3.0–11.5
Band neutrophils (10⁹/l)	**0.57**	0–0.5
Lymphocytes (10⁹/l)	**4.28**	1.0–3.6
Monocytes (10⁹/l)	0.86	0.04–1.35
Basophils (10⁹/l)	0	0.0–0.4
Eosinophils (10⁹/l)	**1.43**	0.0–1.25

BIOCHEMISTRY

Analyte (units)	Result	Reference Interval
Total protein (g/l)	**51.3**	54–71
Albumin (g/l)	**20.8**	26–33
Globulins (g/l)	30.4	27–44
Glucose (mmol/l)	6.29	3.66–6.31
Total bilirubin (μmol/l)	0.5	0–3.4
Cholesterol (mmol/l)	**7.98**	3.5–7.0
Triglycerides (mmol/l)	0.56	0.29–3.88
ALP (U/l)	27	0–97
ALT (U/l)	33	0–55
GLDH (U/l)	8	0–12
Urea (mmol/l)	**14.97**	3.57–8.57
Creatinine (μmol/l)	**177**	35–106
Sodium (mmol/l)	150	141–152

Analyte (units)	Result	Reference Interval
Chloride (mmol/l)	113	100–120
Potassium (mmol/l)	4.2	3.6–5.35
Ionised calcium (mmol/l)	1.3	1.16–1.31
Phosphate (mmol/l)	**3.7**	0.7–1.6

URINALYSIS

Item	Result	Reference Interval
USG	**1.010**	>1.030
Urine protein (mg/l)	**2,164**	0–1,000
Dipstick evaluation		
pH	6.5	Acidic
Bilirubin	Negative	Negative to trace
Blood	Negative	Negative
Glucose	Negative	Negative

Item	Result	Reference Interval
Ketone bodies	Negative	Negative
Protein	**3+**	Negative
Protein:creatinine ratio	**9.8**	<0.2
Sediment analysis		
Erythrocytes	<5	0–5/hpf
Leucocytes	<5	0–5/hpf
Epithelial cells	None	Rare/lpf
Crystals	None	Variable/lpf
Casts	None	Variable/lpf
Bacteria	None	None

QUESTIONS

1 Describe and discuss the laboratory abnormalities. What is the most likely diagnosis?
2 How is this diagnosis defined?

CASE 13

A 10-year-old male neutered cross-breed dog presented for lethargy and weight loss.

EXAMINATION FINDINGS

No abnormalities other than a thin body condition were identified.

BIOCHEMISTRY

Analyte (units)	Result	Reference Interval
Total protein (g/l)	84	56–72
Albumin (g/l)	23	27–38
Globulins (g/l)	61	22–36

OTHER TESTS

Agarose gel serum protein electrophoresis was performed (**Figs. 13.1, 13.2**).

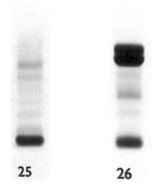

FIG. 13.1 Stained agarose gel electrophoresis. Albumin band is at the bottom of the gel. Left gel (25) is from a dog that is within normal limits. Right gel (26) is from this patient.

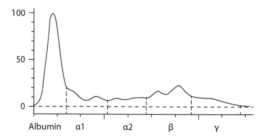
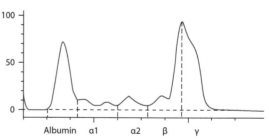

FIG. 13.2 Densitometry tracing of agarose gel. Top tracing is from a dog that is within normal limits. Bottom tracing is from this patient.

QUESTIONS

1 What is your interpretation of the agarose gel serum protein electrophoresis?
2 What are the differential diagnoses in this case?
3 What other type of serum protein electrophoresis may be helpful in confirming the finding suggested by the agarose gel electrophoresis?

CASE 14
A 10-year-old female neutered Siamese cat had been lethargic for several weeks and had a decreased appetite. Additionally, the owners noted mild weight loss.

EXAMINATION FINDINGS

Examination revealed a mild discomfort in the cranial abdominal region. A parasitological faecal examination was unremarkable.

HAEMATOLOGY

Unremarkable.

BIOCHEMISTRY

Analyte (units)	Result	Reference Interval
Total protein (g/l)	52.4	54.7–78.0
Albumin (g/l)	20.9	21–33
Globulins (g/l)	31.5	26–51
Glucose (mmol/l)	15.4	3.89–6.11
Total bilirubin (µmol/l)	8	<3.4
ALP (U/l)	42.3	0–39.7

Analyte (units)	Result	Reference Interval
ALT (U/l)	95	0–70
Urea (mmol/l)	12.3	7.14–10.7
Creatinine (µmol/l)	192	0–168
Sodium (mmol/l)	155	147–156
Chloride (mmol/l)	124	115–130
Potassium (mmol/l)	4.7	3.6–4.8
Ionised calcium (mmol/l)	1.22	1.17–1.32
Phosphate (mmol/l)	2.1	0.8–1.9
fPLI (µg/l)	249	2.0–6.1

QUESTIONS

1 What is the most likely explanation for the laboratory abnormalities? Describe the pathomechanism.
2 What further analyses would you recommend, and why?

CASE 15
The owner of a 17-year-old Cob gelding asked for a health check on his horse because it was losing weight and had an oculonasal discharge.

EXAMINATION FINDINGS

The rectal temperature was 40°C (104°F) and the submandibular and prescapular lymph nodes were moderately enlarged.

HAEMATOLOGY

Measurand (units)	Result	Reference Interval
RBC count (10¹²/l)	4.61	5.5–9.5
Haemoglobin (g/l)	83	80–140
Haematocrit (l/l)	0.23	0.24–0.45
MCV (fl)	50	40–56

Measurand (units)	Result	Reference Interval
MCHC (g/l)	363	340–380
WBC count (10⁹/l)	21.2	6–12
Neutrophils (10⁹/l)	12.29	3.0–6.3
Band neutrophils (10⁹/l)	0	0–0.17
Lymphocytes (10⁹/l)	7.21	1.3–4.3
Monocytes (10⁹/l)	1.7	0–1.0
Eosinophils (10⁹/l)	0	0–1.0
Basophils (10⁹/l)	0	0–0.3
Fibrinogen (g/l) (heat precipitation method)	4.2	2–4

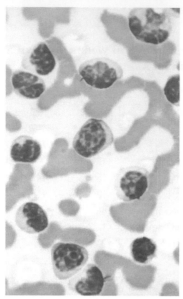

FIG. 15.1 Peripheral blood smear containing marked rouleaux of erythrocytes and a moderately increased number of atypical lymphoid cells. The platelet estimate is markedly decreased.

BIOCHEMISTRY

Analyte (units)	Result	Reference Interval
Total protein (g/l)	**84.9**	58–75
Albumin (g/l)	26.4	23–35
Globulins (g/l)	**58.5**	30–50
GGT (U/l)	19	13–44
GLDH (U/l)	2	1–12
AST (U/l)	210	258–554
CK (U/l)	**118**	150–385
Total bilirubin (µmol/l)	**55**	17–34
Urea (mmol/l)	5.2	2.5–8.3
Creatinine (µmol/l)	112	40–150
Calcium (mmol/l)	**3.6**	2.6–3.3
Phosphorus (mmol/l)	0.8	0.8–1.8

QUESTIONS

1 What is your analysis of these results?
2 What are your differential diagnoses?
3 What additional testing would you recommend?

CASE 16

A 4-year-old male Giant Schnauzer presented with a history of weight gain and exercise intolerance.

EXAMINATION FINDINGS

Unremarkable.

HAEMATOLOGY

Measurand (units)	Result	Reference Interval
RBC count (10¹²/l)	**4.51**	5.4–8.5
Haemoglobin (g/l)	**104**	120–180
Haematocrit (l/l)	**0.30**	0.37–0.56
MCV (fl)	67	67–75
MCHC (g/l)	350	310–350
Platelet count (10⁹/l)	460	200–900
WBC count (10⁹/l)	8.8	5–18
Neutrophils (10⁹/l)	5.9	3.7–13.32
Lymphocytes (10⁹/l)	2.11	1.00–3.60
Monocytes (10⁹/l)	0.53	0.00–0.72
Eosinophils (10⁹/l)	0.26	0.00–1.25

BLOOD FILM EVALUATION

Normocytic-normochromic erythrocytes. No morphological abnormalities detected.

BIOCHEMISTRY

Analyte (units)	Result	Reference Interval
Total protein (g/l)	68	55–75
Albumin (g/l)	32	29–35
Globulins (g/l)	35	18–38
ALP (U/l)	87	0–135
ALT (U/l)	23	0–40
Gamma GT (U/l)	7	0–14
Total bilirubin (µmol/l)	1.4	0–5.0
Cholesterol (mmol/l)	**9.4**	3.8–7.9
CK (U/l)	101	0–400
Urea (mmol/l)	4.5	3.5–7.0
Creatinine (µmol/l)	99	0–130
Calcium (mmol/l)	2.78	2.3–3.0
Phosphorus (mmol/l)	1.6	0.9–1.6
T4 (nmol/l)	**<6**	13–52
cTSH (ng/ml)	**1.51**	<0.41
TgAA (%)	**536**	<200% negative; >200% positive

QUESTIONS

1 What is your diagnosis?
2 Explain how the profile abnormalities relate to the diagnosis.

CASE 17
Grain was introduced to a group of dairy cows housed in a fixed feedlot a couple of days ago.

EXAMINATION FINDINGS

One 2-year-old cow showed clinical signs including a low body temperature (36.8°C [98.2°F]), RR = 70 bpm, HR = 99 bpm, profuse diarrhoea and absent primary contractions in the rumen. Undigested grain kernels were visible in the stool of the cow.

ACID–BASE AND BLOOD GAS DATA

Analyte (units)	Result	Reference Interval
Arterial pH	**7.29**	7.36–7.44
$PaCO_2$ (mmHg)	**25**	36–44
PaO_2 (mmHg)	94	85–95
Plasma HCO_3^- (mmol/l)	**12**	18–26
Serum Na^+ (mmol/l)	146	145–155
Serum K^+ (mmol/l)	**5.9**	4–5
Serum Cl^- (mmol/l)	108	105–115
Anion gap	?	15–25

QUESTIONS

1 What is your assessment of the arterial pH?
2 What is your assessment of the likely underlying aetiology?
3 What is the anion gap (AG) in this case?
4 Is there appropriate compensation for this condition?
5 What is a likely underlying aetiological mechanism for this condition?

CASE 18
A 9-year-old female neutered DSH cat presented with a history of obstipation that had not improved following an enema.

EXAMINATION FINDINGS

The cat was slightly sedated, hypothermic and hardly able to stand. A marked tachypnea was also noted.

HAEMATOLOGY

Measurand (units)	Result	Reference Interval
RBC count (10^{12}/l)	8.51	5–10
Haemoglobin (g/l)	155	79–150
Haematocrit (l/l)	0.44	0.24–0.45
MCV (fl)	51.5	40–55
Platelet count (10^9/l)	273	180–550
WBC count (10^9/l)	**1.7**	6–18
Neutrophils (10^9/l)	**0.37**	2.5–12.5
Lymphocytes (10^9/l)	**0.38**	1.5–7.0
Monocytes (10^9/l)	**0.92**	0.04–0.85
Eosinophils (10^9/l)	0.01	0.0–1.50
Basophils (10^9/l)	0.01	0.0–0.04
Large unstained cells (LUCs) (10^9/l)	0.00	0.0–0.58

LUCs: this variable is specific for the ADVIA® Haematology System used in this case and includes plasma cells, reactive lymphocytes and lymphatic blasts.

BIOCHEMISTRY

Analyte (units)	Result	Reference Interval
Total protein (g/l)	59.1	54.7–78.0
Albumin (g/l)	28.6	21–33
Globulins (g/l)	**30.5**	26–51
Glucose (mmol/l)	**16.8**	3.9–6.1
Bilirubin (μmol/l)	1	<3.4
Cholesterol (mmol/l)	3	2.46–3.37
Triglycerides (mmol/l)	0.58	<1.14
ALP (U/l)	21	<40
ALT (U/l)	**129**	<70
GLDH (U/l)	5	<11.3
Urea (mmol/l)	**12.67**	7.14–10.7
Creatinine (μmol/l)	140	<168
Sodium (mmol/l)	**164**	147–156
Chloride (mmol/l)	**111**	102–110
Potassium (mmol/l)	4.10	3.60–4.80
Calcium (mmol/l)	**0.5**	1.17–1.32
Phosphate (mmol/l)	**26.21**	0.8–1.9
Magnesium (mmol/l)	**0.29**	0.43–0.65

BLOOD GAS ANALYSIS

Analyte (units)	Result	Reference Interval
pH	**7.09**	7.32–7.44
PCO$_2$ (mmHg)	38.9	28–48
HCO$_3^-$ (mmol/l)	**9.1**	21–28

URINALYSIS (cystocentesis)

Item	Result	Reference Interval
USG	**1.025**	>1.035
Dipstick analysis		
pH	6	
Bilirubin	Negative	Negative
Blood	**++**	Negative
Glucose	Negative	Negative
Protein	**++**	Negative to trace
Sediment evaluation		
Erythrocytes	<5	0–5/hpf
Leucocytes	<5	0–5/hpf
Epithelial cells	<5	0–5/hpf
Crystals	0	Variable
Casts	0	None
Bacteria	0	None
hpf: ×40 magnification		

QUESTIONS

1 Describe and discuss the abnormalities of the haemogram, clinical biochemistry profile and blood gas analysis as well as the findings of the urinalysis. Calculate the anion gap (AG) (i.e. the difference between routinely measured cations and routinely measured anions) using the formula:

$$AG = ([Na^+] + [Ca^{2+}]) - ([Cl^-] + [HCO_3^-])$$
(reference interval <20 mmol/l)

What anion is most likely responsible for the abnormal AG in this cat?
2 What is the most likely aetiology of the abnormalities in this cat?
3 What is the prognosis in this patient?

CASE 19

An 11-year-old female mixed-breed dog presented because it was lethargic, had a decreased appetite and was occasionally vomiting.

HAEMATOLOGY

Measurand (units)	Result	Reference Interval
RBC parameters and platelets	Within normal limits	
WBC count (10⁹/l)	**23.6**	6–17
Neutrophils (10⁹/l)	**22.26**	3.0–11.5
Lymphocytes (10⁹/l)	**0.6**	1.0–3.6
Monocytes (10⁹/l)	0.44	0.04–1.35
Eosinophils (10⁹/l)	0.2	0.0–1.25
Basophils (10⁹/l)	0.1	0.0–0.04

QUESTIONS

1 Describe and discuss the laboratory abnormalities present.
2 Which analytes would you examine to assess the acute-phase response (APR) in this patient?
3 What actions does C-reactive protein (CRP) perform in the body?

CASE 20

A 6-year-old male cross-breed dog presented with a history of weight loss and exercise intolerance. There was evidence of a thyroid mass.

HAEMATOLOGY AND BIOCHEMISTRY

Unremarkable.

FURTHER TESTS

A fine needle aspirate of the thyroid mass was performed (**Fig. 20.1**). Thyroid neoplasia was diagnosed and histology was recommended in order to properly classify the lesion. Elongated parasites were observed in the aspirate from the thyroid mass, as a consequence of blood contamination. Elongated organisms were also observed in a thick blood smear (**Fig. 20.2**).

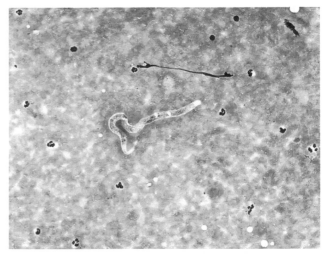

FIG. 20.2 Thick blood smear. Note the elongated parasite. ×10.

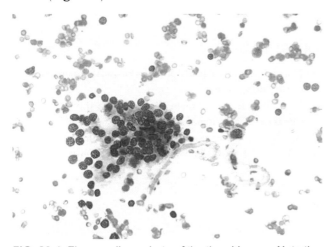

FIG. 20.1 Fine needle aspirate of the thyroid mass. Note the cluster of well-differentiated thyroid epithelial cells. Two elongated parasites are visible. Wright–Giemsa, ×10.

QUESTIONS

1 What is the parasite in the thyroid aspirate and blood smear?
2 What haematological and serum abnormalities might you expect related to this parasitic infection?

CASE 21
A 14-year-old female neutered DSH cat is eating not as well as before, is occasionally vomiting and has a markedly increased body condition score.

HAEMATOLOGY

Unremarkable. A routine blood smear evaluation revealed RBCs of abnormal shape (**Fig. 21.1**).

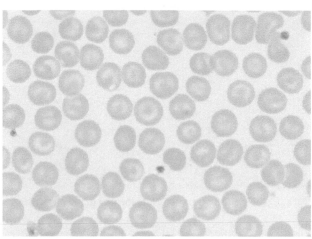

FIG. 21.1 Erythrocytes shown on a blood smear. May–Grünwald–Giemsa, ×100 (oil).

BIOCHEMISTRY

Analyte (units)	Result	Reference Interval
Total protein (g/l)	60.5	54.7–78.0
Albumin (g/l)	27.4	21–33
Globulins (g/l)	32.6	26–51

Analyte (units)	Result	Reference Interval
Glucose (mmol/l)	5.9	3.89–6.11
GGT (U/l)	**20**	0–5
ALP (U/l)	**168**	0–39.7
ALT (U/l)	**130**	0–70
Urea (mmol/l)	8.65	7.14–10.7
Creatinine (µmol/l)	143	0–168
Sodium (mmol/l)	**133**	147–156
Chloride (mmol/l)	121	115–130
Potassium (mmol/l)	3.8	3.6–4.8
Ionised calcium (mmol/l)	1.26	1.17–1.32
Phosphate (mmol/l)	1.5	0.8–1.9

QUESTIONS

1 Name the type of poikilocytosis of erythrocytes present in the blood smear.
2 Describe the mechanism that leads to the presence of this type of abnormal RBC shape.
3 In which diseases does this type of poikilocytosis occur? What is the most likely cause in this patient?

CASE 22
You have to explain to a veterinary surgeon why variations in serial laboratory results occur even when the patient is healthy.

QUESTIONS

1 Briefly discuss the factors that can lead to variation in laboratory test results. Define the index of individuality (IoI) and how it is calculated.

2 Why is it important to know the degree of biological variation in a patient?

CASE 23

A 9.5-year-old llama gelding presented for progressive weight loss despite an increase in the quality of hay being fed. It was dewormed with fenbendazole, but weight loss continued. The llama was current on vaccinations against rabies, clostridial diseases and tetanus.

HAEMATOLOGY

Measurand (units)	Results		Reference Interval
	Day 1	Day 14	
RBC count (10⁹/l)	**8.74**	**8.23**	10.5–17.2
Haemoglobin (g/l)	**108**	**102**	12–192
Haematocrit (l/l)	0.27	**0.25**	0.27–0.45
MCV (fl)	**30.4**	29.8	22.8–29.9
MCH (pg)	12.3	12.3	10.1–12.7
MCHC (g/l)	405	415	93–468
PCV (spun Hct) (%)	**26**	**26**	27–45
WBC count (10⁹/l)	8.4	11.7	8.0–21.4
Neutrophils (10⁹/l)	7.14	9.71	4.71–14.86
Band neutrophils (10⁹/l)	**0.92**	**1.05**	0–0.15
Eosinophils (10⁹/l)	**0.17**	**0.12**	0.65–4.87
Monocytes (10⁹/l)	0.17	0.59	0–1.00
Plasma protein (g/l) (refractometer)	n.d.	52	51–79

BLOOD SMEAR EVALUATION

Day 1

RBC morphology – within normal limits; WBC morphology – moderate indented nuclear membranes, occasional ruptured WBCs, few neutrophils with lacy cytoplasm; platelet morphology – occasional platelet clumps.

Day 14

RBC morphology – within normal limits; WBC morphology – few indented nuclear membranes, few to moderate ruptured WBCs, moderate neutrophils with lacy cytoplasm, few neutrophils with swollen nuclei; platelet morphology – estimate normal.

BIOCHEMISTRY

Analyte (units)	Result		Reference Interval
	Day 1	Day 14	
Total protein (g/l)	55	56	51–78
Albumin (g/l)	**28**	**16**	31–52
Globulins (g/l)	27	**40**	14–31
A:G ratio	n.d.	0.4	Unknown
ALT (U/l)	n.d.	12	10–135

Analyte (units)	Result		Reference Interval
	Day 1	Day 14	
ALP (U/l)	81	98	10–100
GGT (U/l)	21	n.d.	3–30
AST (U/l)	131	n.d.	10–280
CK (U/l)	35	35	10–200
Total bilirubin (µmol/l)	n.d.	1.71	1.7–5.13
Cholesterol (mmol/l)	n.d.	0.78	0–3.32
Triglycerides (mmol/l)	n.d.	**0.38**	0.26–0.37
Glucose (mmol/l)	n.d.	6.55	4.11–8.55
Amylase (U/l)	n.d.	857	Unknown
BUN (mmol/l)	5.36	5.71	3.21–12.14
Creatinine (µmol/l)	n.d.	129	106.7–244
Chloride (mmol/l)	n.d.	108	100–118
Sodium (mmol/l)	146	n.d.	140–155
Calcium (mmol/l)	1.9	**1.8**	1.85–2.60
Phosphorus (mmol/l)	**0.97**	1.58	1.45–2.36
Magnesium (mmol/l)	0.74	n.d.	0.62–1.23
Potassium (mmol/l)	**3.9**	n.d.	4.0–6.5

At further examination 2 weeks later, the oral mucous membranes were brick red. Examination of the teeth using a speculum demonstrated no abnormalities. A rectal examination was within normal limits. A faecal sample was collected for Johnes testing and a faecal egg count. Blood samples were obtained for selenium levels (a concern of the owner) and a repeat serum chemistry and FBC. Because of continued weight loss, 50 mg of moxidectin was given orally.

ADDITIONAL TESTING

Faecal egg count (sugar floatation)

- *Eimeria punoensis* 3 oocysts/gram
- Strongyles 41 eggs/gram
- *Trichuris* spp. 30 eggs/gram

Whole blood selenium

26.0 µg/dl (normal for llama 1 year or older is 7.0–35.1 µg/dl).

After discussing the case with colleagues, the laboratory was requested to perform protein electrophoresis to try and diagnose a possible tumour.

Electrophoresis (whole blood)

Analyte (units)	Result	Reference Interval
Total protein (g/l)	56	Normals not established
Albumin (g/l)	20.2	Normals not established
Total alpha globulin (g/l)	4.3	Normals not established
Total beta globulin (g/l)	11.7	Normals not established
Gamma globulins (g/l)	19.8	Normals not established
A:G ratio	0.56	Normals not established

Comment was made that according to published reference intervals the llama is mildly hypoalbuminaemic and may have a mild polyclonal gammopathy. These are nonspecific findings and could be related to underlying inflammation or antigenic stimulation.

Two days after the blood work had been drawn the llama was given an injection of a long-acting cefalosporin and vitamin E/selenium at the owner's request. Four days later he was re-examined because he was weak. His vital signs were normal, his mucous membranes were still red and there was a suspicion he was not drinking well. An attempt was made to pass a nasogastric tube, which produced copious amounts of saliva. It was unclear if the tube was able to be passed into the first stomach compartment. Other diagnostic options and euthanasia were discussed. The owner elected to continue symptomatic treatment. The gelding was eating minor amounts of grain on the following 2 days. He was found dead 3 days after the last examination.

QUESTION

1 What is your evaluation of the laboratory data?

CASE 24
A 13-year-old female neutered cross-breed dog presented because of chronic lethargy.

EXAMINATION FINDINGS

Examination revealed a patient in lateral recumbency, a mild tachycardia (140 bpm) and presence of a perianal mass (3 cm [1.18 in] in diameter).

HAEMATOLOGY

Results are unremarkable except for platelets of $13 \times 10^9/l$ (reference interval, 150–500).

BIOCHEMISTRY

Analyte (units)	Result	Reference Interval
Total protein (g/l)	**73.4**	55.3–69.84
Albumin (g/l)	32.6	29.6–37.01
Globulins (g/l)	**40.8**	22.9–35.6
Glucose (mmol/l)	7.29	3.3–6.53
Total bilirubin (µmol/l)	3.51	0–3.6
Cholesterol (mmol/l)	5.9	3.3–6.53
Triglycerides (mmol/l)	0.63	0.08–0.75
ALP (U/l)	56	0–130
ALT (U/l)	58	0–85

Analyte (units)	Result	Reference Interval
GLDH (U/l)	8	0–9.9
CK (U/l)	**164**	<143
Urea (mmol/l)	6.53	3.3–9.82
Creatinine (µmol/l)	68	53–122
Sodium (mmol/l)	**150**	141–146
Chloride (mmol/l)	111	104–112
Potassium (mmol/l)	3.45	3.35–4.37
Ionised calcium (mmol/l)	**3.04**	1.23–1.43
Phosphorus (mmol/l)	**0.67**	0.79–2.1
Ionised magnesium (mmol/l)	**0.28**	0.47–0.63
PT (seconds)	7.2	6.52–8.16
aPTT (seconds)	11.6	9.85–14.22
PTH (pg/ml)	**<2**	8–45
PTHrP (pmol/l)	**23**	<0.9

QUESTIONS

1 What are the principal causes of hypercalcaemia?
2 What are the principal causes of thrombocytopaenia?
3 What further tests are required?

CASE 25

A 2-year-old male mixed-breed dog that originated from Spain displays generalised lymphadenopathy.

HAEMATOLOGY

Measurand (units)	Result	Reference Interval
RBC count (10^{12}/l)	**5**	5.5–8.5
Haemoglobin (g/l)	**70**	74–112
Haematocrit (l/l)	**0.24**	0.37–0.55
MCHC (g/l)	202	196–221
MCV (fl)	75	60–77
Platelet count (10^9/l)	389	150–500
WBC count (10^9/l)	8.2	6–17
Neutrophils (10^9/l)	6	3.0–11.5
Lymphocytes (10^9/l)	1.2	1.0–3.6
Monocytes (10^9/l)	0.5	0.04–1.35
Eosinophils (10^9/l)	0.4	0.0–1.25
Basophils (10^9/l)	0.1	0.0–0.04

BLOOD FILM EVALUATION

Physiological anisocytosis, rare acanthocytes, rare echinocytes, leucocytes appear normal in their number and morphology. Platelet estimate adequate.

BIOCHEMISTRY

Analyte (units)	Result	Reference Interval
Total protein (g/l)	**81**	54–71
Albumin (g/l)	**23.9**	26–33
Globulins (g/l)	**57.1**	27–44
Glucose (mmol/l)	6	3.66–6.31
Total bilirubin (µmol/l)	0.1	0–3.4
Cholesterol (mmol/l)	6.4	3.5–7.0
Triglycerides (mmol/l)	2.7	0.29–3.88
ALP (U/l)	56	0–97
ALT (U/l)	22	0–55
GLDH (U/l)	7	0–12
Urea (mmol/l)	**13.5**	3.57–8.57
Creatinine (µmol/l)	**127**	35–106
Sodium (mmol/l)	146	141–152
Chloride (mmol/l)	100	100–120
Potassium (mmol/l)	3.9	3.6–5.35
Ionised calcium (mmol/l)	1.3	1.16–1.31
Phosphate (mmol/l)	**1.93**	0.7–1.6

CYTOLOGY

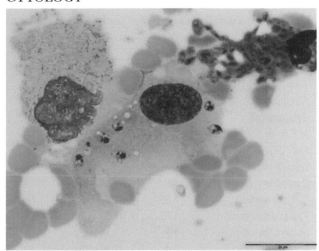

FIG. 25.1 Fine needle aspirate of a lymph node from the dog. May–Grünwald–Giemsa, ×100 (oil).

QUESTIONS

1 What abnormality do you detect in the cell on the cytological slide?
2 Describe the laboratory abnormalities present and discuss their association with the underlying cause of the disease present in this dog.
3 How is the disease transmitted?

CASE 26

A 10-year-old male neutered Lhasa Apso is showing PU/PD and urinating in the house with acute onset.

EXAMINATION FINDINGS

The dog has a pendulous abdomen and a hairless ventrum.

BIOCHEMISTRY

Analyte (units)	Result	Reference Interval
Total protein (g/l)	71	52–82
Albumin (g/l)	30	22–39
Globulins (g/l)	41	25–45
ALP (U/l)	**1,048**	23–212
ALT (U/l)	**310**	10–100
Urea (mmol/l)	7.3	2.5–9.6
Creatinine (µmol/l)	**42**	44–159
Calcium (mmol/l)	2.55	1.98–3.00
Phosphorus (mmol/l)	1.52	0.81–2.19
Sodium (mmol/l)	**156**	144–160
Potassium (mmol/l)	3.4	3.5–5.8

Haematological findings are within normal limits.

ACTH STIMULATION TEST

Analyte (units)	Result	Reference Interval
Basal cortisol (nmol/l)	90.5	25–125
Cortisol 1 hour post ACTH (nmol/l)	**>1,380**	125–520

QUESTIONS

1 What is your interpretation of these findings?
2 What is the pathophysiology associated with these findings?
3 What other tests for hyperadrenocorticism are routinely available, and how does their sensitivity and specificity compare with those of the ACTH stimulation test?

CASE 27

An 8-month-old female English Springer Spaniel presented in an acute crisis with lethargy, weakness, pale mucous membranes and fever of 41°C (105.8°F).

EXAMINATION FINDINGS

Examination revealed hepatosplenomegaly and muscle wasting.

HAEMATOLOGY

Measurand (units)	Result	Reference Interval
RBC count (10^{12}/l)	**3.5**	5.5–8.5
Haemoglobin (g/l)	**83**	74–112
Haematocrit (l/l)	**0.28**	0.37–0.55
MCV (fl)	**85**	60–77
MCH (pg)	**2.37**	1.2–1.51
MCHC (g/l)	**296**	196–221
NRBCs (%)	**30**	Rare
Platelet count (10^9/l)	355	150–500
WBC count (10^9/l)	16	6–17
Neutrophils (10^9/l)	10.5	3.0–11.5
Lymphocytes (10^9/l)	3.5	1.0–3.6
Monocytes (10^9/l)	1.2	0.04–1.35
Basophils (10^9/l)	0	0.0–0.4
Eosinophils (10^9/l)	0.8	0.0–1.25

Technical comment: plasma markedly haemolytic. Total WBC count corrected for NRBCs.

QUESTIONS

1 Describe the abnormalities that are present and indicate the most likely diagnosis based on the present findings.
2 Describe the underlying pathophysiology of the disease. How do haemolytic crises develop?
3 What further diagnostics would you perform to support your diagnosis?

CASE 28

A 27-year-old male gelded miniature donkey lived at the same farm as a 37-year-old pony that had been off its feed about 2 weeks prior to observation of illness in the donkey. The pony had responded to treatment for an apparent impaction colic. One week before examination, the donkey had been noticed to be slightly off feed. The donkey was current on West Nile virus, rabies, eastern equine encephalomyelitis, western equine encephalomyelitis, tetanus, equine influenza and equine herpesvirus-1 vaccinations. An equine infectious anaemia test 1 month ago was negative.

EXAMINATION FINDINGS

The donkey was clinically laminitic, with increased pulses in all four feet but no sensitivity to hoof testers on any foot. T = 37.8°C (100.2°F); HR = 60 bpm (within normal range over the years for this excitable animal); RR = 12 bpm; weight = 124 kg (273 lb).

HAEMATOLOGY

Measurand (units)	Result Day 1	Reference Interval
RBC count (10¹²/l)	**4.16**	6.30–9.20
Haemoglobin (g/l)	**90**	112–163
Haematocrit (l/l)	**0.27**	0.31–0.44
MCV (fl)	**63.8**	40.4–52.0
MCH (pg)	**21.6**	14.9–19.0
MCHC (g/l)	338	331–385
Plasma protein (g/l)	73	52–78
WBC count (10⁹/l)	**13.1**	5–12
Neutrophils (10⁹/l)	**10.9**	2.6–6.5
Eosinophils (10⁹/l)	0.131	0–0.2
Lymphocytes (10⁹/l)	2.62	1.6–6.2
Monocytes (10⁹/l)	0.262	0–0.4

BLOOD SMEAR EVALUATION

Measurand (units)	Result
RBC morphology	Normal
Crenation	1+
Haemolised RBCs	Few
WBC appearance	Abnormal
Swollen nucleus	Few
Ruptured WBCs	Few
Vacuolated neutrophils	Occasional
Platelet estimate	8–10/hpf

BIOCHEMISTRY

(Done on site with VetScan)

Analyte (units)	Day 1	Day 3	Day 14	Reference Interval
Total protein (g/l)	58	65	72	57–80
Albumin (g/l)	35	27	34	22–37
Globulins (g/l)	23	38	38	20–50
ALP (U/l)		243		50–170
AST (U/l)	n.d.	595	537	5–200
CK (U/l)	n.d.	**5,269**	**1,212**	120–470
GGT (U/l)	n.d.	222	289	5–24
Total bilirubin (µmol/l)	**1.71**	**3.42**	**3.42**	8.55–39.33
Urea (mmol/l)	**14.99**	**13.21**	7.85	2.5–8.92
Creatinine (µmol/l)	**424**	**406.64**	**335.92**	45.76–167.77
Phosphorus (mmol/l)	1.16			0.61–1.39
Calcium (mmol/l)	**3.85**	3.18	3.53	2.88–3.55
Sodium (mmol/l)	128			126–146
Potassium (mmol/l)	4.8			2.5–5.2
Glucose (mmol/l)	5.11	4.83	5.61	3.61–6.11

The following day the donkey was slightly better after being given 1 g phenylbutazone for pain. The owners forced oral fluids that day and the donkey was put on IV fluids the following day. A urine sample was obtained.

URINALYSIS

Item	Result	Reference Interval
USG	1.010	>1.030
Dipstick evaluation		
pH	7	
Bilirubin	**1+**	Negative to trace
Glucose	**2+**	Negative
Ketone bodies	Negative	Negative
Protein	**1+**	Negative
Blood	**1+**	Negative
Sediment analysis		
Erythrocytes	<5	0–5/hpf
Leucocytes	<5	0–5/hpf
Epithelial cells	Rare	None
Crystals	None	Variable/lpf
Urine casts	None	None
Bacteria	None	0/lpf

The donkey was maintained on approximately 16 litres of fluids per day. Sodium cetiofur (250 mg IV bid) was prescribed. Detomidine was given IM for pain control. Shortly after administration he would begin eating. Phenylbutazolidine was discontinued after the second dose. IV fluids were continued for 3 more days. The patient became slowly more uncomfortable and fentanyl patches were tried on the forelimbs in addition to topical diclofenac at the coronary bands. Fluid therapy was continued as was the sodium cetiofur. The donkey was noted to be off feed at 14 days and the serum biochemistry was repeated.

QUESTIONS

1 What is your evaluation of the laboratory data?
2 What is your diagnosis/interpretation of this case?
3 What other tests could be performed, and why?

CASE 29

A 7-year-old male German Shepherd Dog. The dog is currently resident in Austria, but originated in Greece. Mildly enlarged mandibular lymph nodes are noted.

HAEMATOLOGY

Measurand (units)	Result	Reference Interval
RBC count (10^{12}/l)	**4.3**	5.5–8.0
Haemoglobin (g/l)	**98.3**	120–180
Haematocrit (l/l)	**0.29**	0.37–0.55
Reticulocytes (10^9/l)	**15.0**	28–60
WBC count (10^9/l)	**29.1**	6–15
Neutrophils (10^9/l)	**14.7**	3.3–12.0
Monocytes (10^9/l)	**1.2**	<0.5

BIOCHEMISTRY

Analyte (units)	Result	Reference Interval
Total protein (g/l)	**77.4**	57–75
Urea (mmol/l)	5.5	3.3–8.9
Creatinine (µmol/l)	0.7	<1.2
Leishmania infantium antibodies (IFAT)	**1:1,280**	Borderline titre: 1:80

LYMPH NODE ASPIRATE

See **Fig. 29.1**.

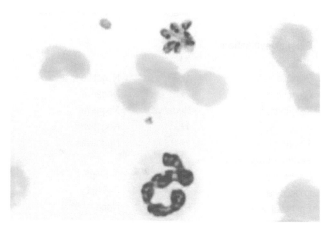

FIG. 29.1 Lymph node aspirate. Wright–Giemsa, ×100 (oil). Lymphoid cells are present in other fields. (Courtesy Dr Judith Leidinger)

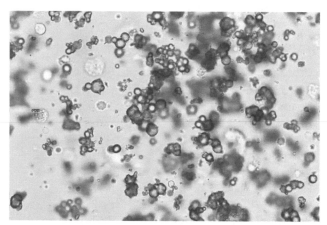

FIG. 29.2 Unstained urine sediment. Wet-drop preparation, ×40. (Courtesy Dr Judith Leidinger)

Four months later a urine sample was submitted for urinalysis and sediment examination. The results of the urine examination are presented in the Table and in **Fig. 29.2**.

URINALYSIS

Item	Result	Reference Interval
Colour	**Medium-Yellow**	Yellow
Transparency	**Turbid**	Clear
USG	1.038	1.020–1.045
Dipstick evaluation		
pH	7	6–7
Leucocytes	Negative	Negative
Nitrite	Negative	Negative
Protein (SSA method)	**++**	Trace
Glucose	Negative	Negative

Item	Result	Reference Interval
Ketone bodies	Negative	Negative
Urobilinogen	Negative	Negative to +
Bilirubin	Negative	Negative
Blood	**+++**	Negative
Protein: creatinine ratio	**1.49**	<0.5
Sediment analysis		
Quantity	**Increased**	
Erythrocytes	Maximum 1/hpf	<5/hpf
Crystals	**>10/lpf**	Variable/lpf

hpf = ×40 objective; lpf = ×10 objective.

QUESTIONS

1 What organisms are apparent in the lymph node aspirate smear?
2 What is your interpretation of the haematological findings?
3 What other biochemistry analyte would be good to look at in this case?
4 How would you describe the crystals present in the urine sediment?
5 What are the most important differentials?
6 Which medication can cause these crystals?
7 What is the mechanism of formation?

CASE 30

A 1.5-year-old male Golden Retriever presented for acute lethargy, anorexia and one episode of seizures. Some hours ago, he had been unattended in the garage. It is winter time and snowy outside.

ACID–BASE AND BLOOD GAS DATA

Analyte (units)	Result	Reference Interval
Arterial pH	**7.24**	7.36–7.44
$PaCO_2$ (mmHg)	**24**	36–44
PaO_2 (mmHg)	95	85–95
Plasma HCO_3^- (mmol/l)	**10**	18–26
Serum Na^+ (mmol/l)	145	145–155
Serum K^+ (mmol/l)	**6.5**	4–5
Serum Cl^- (mmol/l)	107	105–115
Anion gap	?	15–25

QUESTIONS

1 What is your assessment of the arterial pH?
2 What is your assessment of the underlying aetiology?
3 What is the anion gap (AG) in this case?
4 Why is the K^+ increased in this case?
5 What is a likely underlying aetiological mechanism for the condition in this dog?
6 What further test may strengthen your diagnosis?

CASE 31

A 4-year-old female Border Terrier being treated for superficial pyoderma with trimethoprim–sulphadiazine presented for abdominal pain, inappetence, vomiting and oliguria.

HAEMATOLOGY

Unremarkable. There is a mild lymphopaenia, likely to be stress related.

BIOCHEMISTRY

Analyte (units)	Result	Result (3 days later)	Reference Interval
Total protein (g/l)	65	67	55–75
Albumin (g/l)	35	38	25–40
Globulins (g/l)	30	29	23–35
Glucose (mmol/l)	**8.6**	6.3	3.3–6.5
ALP (U/l)	**434**	**256**	0–130
ALT (U/l)	**679**	**145**	0–85
Anion gap	**31**	**35**	12–25
Urea (mmol/l)	**21.4**	**47.4**	3.3–8.0
Creatinine (µmol/l)	**397**	**771**	45–150
Phosphate (mmol/l)	**2.97**	**3.65**	0.78–1.41

URINALYSIS

Item	Result	Reference Interval
USG	**1.010**	>1.030
Dipstick evaluation		
pH	6.5	
Protein	+	Negative to trace
Glucose	Negative	Negative
Ketone bodies	Negative	Negative
Bilirubin	Negative	Negative
Blood	Negative	Negative

Urine sediment analysis

No abnormalities observed apart from a few crystals (**Fig. 31.1**).

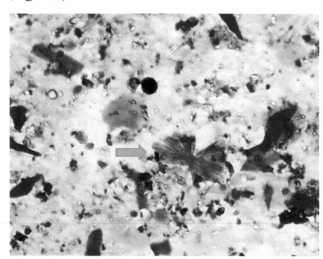

FIG. 31.1 Centrally waisted sheaves composed of needle-like crystals (orange arrow). Sedistained urine, wet drop preparation, ×40.

QUESTIONS

1 How would you describe the azotaemia, and what does this indicate?
2 How would you explain the high anion gap?
3 What is the crystal indicated by the arrow?
4 What is the main differential diagnosis for this case?

CASE 32

A 15-year-old male Yorkshire Terrier had PU/PD for several weeks, progressive weakness and lethargy.

HAEMATOLOGY

Unremarkable.

BIOCHEMISTRY

Analyte (units)	Result	Reference Interval
Total protein (g/l)	**84.1**	54–71
Albumin (g/l)	**34.9**	26–33
Globulins (g/l)	**49.2**	27–44
Glucose (mmol/l)	**38.21**	3.66–6.31
Total bilirubin (µmol/l)	0.1	0–3.4
Cholesterol (mmol/l)	**8.65**	3.5–7.0
Triglycerides (mmol/l)	**6.52**	0.29–3.88
ALP (U/l)	**742**	0–97
ALT (U/l)	**145**	0–55
GLDH (U/l)	**51**	0–12
Urea (mmol/l)	**3.49**	3.57–8.57
Creatinine (µmol/l)	55	35–106
Sodium (mmol/l)	146	141–152
Chloride (mmol/l)	100	100–120
Potassium (mmol/l)	3.9	3.6–5.35
Ionised calcium (mmol/l)	1.3	1.16–1.31
Phosphate (mmol/l)	**1.93**	0.7–1.6
Comment: The plasma was markedly lipaemic		

URINALYSIS

Item	Result	Reference Interval
USG	1.038	>1.030
Dipstick evaluation		
pH	6	Acidic
Bilirubin	Negative	Negative to trace
Blood	Negative	Negative
Glucose	**3+**	Negative
Ketone bodies	Negative	Negative
Protein	**1+**	Negative
Sediment analysis		
Erythrocytes	<5	0–5/hpf
Leucocytes	<5	0–5/hpf
Epithelial cells	None	Rare/lpf
Crystals	None	Variable/lpf
Casts	None	Variable/lpf
Bacteria	None	None

QUESTIONS

1 Describe and discuss the significant biochemistry and urinalysis findings.
2 What further tests would you recommend, and why?

CASE 33

The owner of a 10-year-old female mixed-breed dog is concerned regarding the cause for continued proteinuria in his dog. The urine protein:creatinine ratio is persistently increased, but there is no current increase in urea or creatinine and no increase in blood pressure with repeated measurements.

URINE PROTEIN ELECTROPHORESIS

Analyte	Result (%)	Result (g/l)
Total protein		1.88
Albumin	65.02	1.22
Alpha-1 globulins	10.95	0.21
Alpha-2 globulins	6.03	0.11
Beta globulins	13.67	0.26
Gamma globulins	4.33	0.08
Atypical bands	None	None

The urine protein:creatinine ratio is 1.6 (reference interval, <0.5).

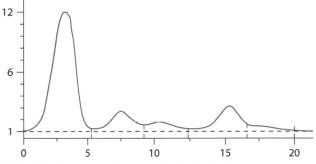

FIG. 33.1 Agarose gel urine protein electrophoresis. The albumin peak is to the left.

FIG. 33.2 Gel corresponding to the densitometry tracing in **Fig. 33.1**. Albumin is located at the bottom of the picture.

QUESTIONS

1 What is your interpretation of these findings?
2 What other categories of renal proteinuria can be determined by agarose gel urine protein electrophoresis?
3 What are the indications for agarose gel urine protein electrophoresis and the pitfalls in the use of agarose gel urine protein electrophoresis?

CASE 34

A 1-year-old female neutered DSH cat was involved in a road traffic accident and presented to the veterinary surgeon with hindlimb ataxia. Radiographic studies revealed a fractured femur, which was repaired on the following day. After recovery from anaesthesia the patient appeared depressed and blood samples were taken for analysis. Urine was not collected.

BIOCHEMISTRY

Analyte (units)	Result	Reference Interval
Total protein (g/l)	**86**	55–78
Albumin (g/l)	40	26–40
Globulins (g/l)	46	19–48
Urea (mmol/l)	**62.8**	3.5–8.0
Creatinine (µmol/l)	**1,148**	40–180
Calcium (mmol/l)	2.63	2.0–2.8
Phosphorus (mmol/l)	**5.3**	0.81–1.61
Sodium (mmol/l)	142	141–155
Potassium (mmol/l)	**7.4**	3.5–5.5

QUESTION

1 What is your assessment of the significant profile changes, and what are the possible causes?

CASE 35

A 3-year-old male neutered mixed-breed dog presented because of prolonged bleeding at the sites of fine needle aspirates and biopsies during work up for surgical removal of a cutaneous tumour. Coagulation tests are requested to characterise the possible haemostatic problem.

COAGULATION PROFILE

Analyte (units)	Result	Reference Interval
aPTT (seconds)	11	9–13
PT (seconds)	7	7–9
Platelet count (10^9/l)	**55**	200–500
Buccal mucosal bleeding time (BMBT) (seconds)	**368**	<210

QUESTION

1 What is your interpretation of these findings?

CASE 36

A 9-month-old Warmblood foal presented because it was very thin, had occasional episodes of diarrhoea and colic and had a poor hair coat. Its deworming programme was up to date.

EXAMINATION FINDINGS

There was slight oedema in the area of the throatlatch and ventrally.

HAEMATOLOGY

Measurand (units)	Result	Reference Interval
RBC count (10^9/l)	4.5	5–12
Haemoglobin (g/l)	75	80–150
Haematocrit (l/l)	0.22	0.35–0.45
MCV (fl)	50	40–60
MCH (pg)	16.8	12.5–17.5
MCHC (g/l)	322	320–360
Platelet count (10^9/l)	213	75–50
WBC count (10^9/l)	19.5	5.5–16.0
Neutrophils (10^9/l)	15.0	2.5–12.5
Band neutrophils (10^9/l)	0	0–0.3
Lymphocytes (10^9/l)	2	1.5–3.0
Eosinophils (10^9/l)	1.5	0–1.5
Monocytes (10^9/l)	1	0.0–0.5
Basophils (10^9/l)	0	Rare

BLOOD SMEAR EVALUATION

Platelet estimate adequate. No abnormalities of erythrocyte or leucocyte morphology.

BIOCHEMISTRY

Analyte (units)	Result	Reference Interval
Total protein (g/l)	42	55–72
Albumin (g/l)	15	22–40
Globulins (g/l)	27	28–51
ALP (U/l)	180	20–120
Total bilirubin (µmol/l)	30	0–25
Glucose (mmol/l)	7	4.11–8.83
Urea (mmol/l)	10	5.7–12.9
Creatinine (µmol/l)	178	71–200
Sodium (mmol/l)	130	144–160
Potassium (mmol/l)	6.2	3.5–5.8
Phosphorus (mmol/l)	3	1.00–2.42
Calcium (mmol/l)	1.7	1.95–2.83
Chloride (mmol/l)	90	109–122

QUESTIONS

1 What is your evaluation of the laboratory data?
2 What is your diagnosis/interpretation?
3 What pathophysiology is likely underlying the findings in this case?
4 What other tests would you recommend performing?

CASE 37

A 5-year-old female neutered English Springer Spaniel presented because of acute weakness and exercise intolerance.

EXAMINATION FINDINGS

The dog was lethargic with pale mucous membranes. Further abnormalities included dyspnoea, tachycardia and a bounding pulse. Radiographs of the thorax revealed a mild thoracic effusion, which was bloody when aspirated.

HAEMATOLOGY

Measurand (units)	Result	Reference Interval
RBC count (10^{12}/l)	3.04	5.5–8.5
Haemoglobin (g/l)	71	79–150

Measurand (units)	Result	Reference Interval
Haematocrit (l/l)	0.21	0.37–0.55
MCV (fl)	67.9	60–77
Platelet count (10^9/l)	232	150–500
WBC count (10^9/l)	17	6–17
Neutrophils (10^9/l)	14.1	3.0–11.5
Band neutrophils (10^9/l)	0	<0.5
Lymphocytes (10^9/l)	1.87	1.0–3.6
Monocytes (10^8/l)	1.02	0.04–1.35
Eosinophils (10^9/l)	0.09	<1.25
Basophils (10^9/l)	0	<0.04

BLOOD FILM EVALUATION

Normocytic-normochromic erythrocytes, mild anisocytosis of erythrocytes and mild mature neutrophilia. The platelets were adequate in number and the morphology was within normal limits.

Analyte (units)	Result	Reference Interval
Chloride (mmol/l)	**98**	102–110
Potassium (mmol/l)	**3.2**	3.35–4.37
Calcium (mmol/l)	**1.17**	1.23–1.43
Phosphate (mmol/l)	1.63	0.79–2.1

BIOCHEMISTRY

Analyte (units)	Result	Reference Interval
Total protein (g/l)	**51.7**	55–70
Albumin (g/l)	**25.5**	30–37
Globulins (g/l)	26.2	23–36
Glucose (mmol/l)	**11.17**	3.3–6.5
Bilirubin (µmol/l)	0.1	<3.6
Cholesterol (mmol/l)	5.67	3.3–8.6
Triglycerides (mmol/l)	**0.79**	<0.75
ALP (U/l)	93	<131
ALT (U/l)	22	<85
GLDH (U/l)	1	<10
Urea (mmol/l)	8.9	3.03–9.82
Creatinine (µmol/l)	68	53–123
Sodium (mmol/l)	**136**	147–152

COAGULATION PROFILE

Analyte (units)	Result	Reference Interval
PT (seconds)	**154.4**	7–10 (<15)
aPTT (seconds)	**38.4**	9.5–10.5
Fibrinogen (g/l)	**4.75**	2–4

QUESTIONS

1 Discuss the significant haematological and biochemistry findings.
2 Describe and discuss the coagulation profile. What is the most likely aetiology of the disease?
3 What are the prognosis, treatment and monitoring of this disease?

CASE 38

A 12-year-old male neutered cross-bred dog presented with exercise intolerance and poor hair coat. He had been receiving phenobarbitone (phenobarbital) for a number of years. A full thyroid panel and drug monitoring was performed.

ENDOCRINOLOGY

Analyte (units)	Result	Reference Interval
Phenobarbitone (µg/ml)	32.5	15–40
T4 (nmol/l)	**<6**	13–52
cTSH (ng/ml)	0.31	<0.41
TgAA (%)	**1,010**	<200% negative; >200% positive
FT4D (pmol/l)	**2**	7–40

T4 = thyroxine; cTSH = canine thyrotropin (thyroid stimulating hormone); TgAA = thyroglobulin autoantibodies; FT4D = free T4 measured by equilibrium dialysis

QUESTIONS

1 What is your diagnosis?
2 Comment on the profile abnormalities, the underlying pathophysiology and the degree of confidence each result contributes to the diagnosis.

CASE 39

An owner noted anorexia in her 3-year-old male cat. An assessment of acute-phase proteins (APPs) was performed to rule in/out possible inflammatory disease.

BIOCHEMISTRY

Analyte (units)	Result	Reference Interval
Serum amyloid A (mg/l)	**120**	0–10
Haptoglobin (g/l)	**23**	0–4
Albumin (g/l)	**19.9**	21.0–33.0

QUESTIONS

1 How do you interpret the clinical chemistry data?
2 What actions does haptoglobin perform in the body?

CASE 40

A 13-year-old male neutered DSH cat presented because of difficulty breathing and not wanting to eat. The cat seemed fine the night before. There is a previous history of bronchitis. Vaccination against calicivirus, herpesvirus, panleucopaenia and feline leukaemia virus and deworming are up to date.

EXAMINATION FINDINGS

T = 38.5°C (101.3°F); weight = 9.4 kg (20.75 lb); HR = 190 bpm; RR = 45 bpm; mucous membranes pale; respiratory wheeze auscultated.

HAEMATOLOGY

Measurand (units)	Result	Reference Interval
RBC count (10⁹/l)	**4.25**	5–10
Haemoglobin (g/l)	**63.5**	80–150
Haematocrit (l/l)	**0.17**	0.30–0.45
MCV (fl)	46	39–55
MCH (pg)	15	12.5–17.5
MCHC (g/l)	323	320–360

Measurand (units)	Result	Reference Interval
Aggregated reticulocytes (10⁹/l)	0	0–60
Platelets (10⁹/l)	200	190–400
WBC count (10⁹/l)	**20**	5.5–19.5
Neutrophils (10⁹/l)	**13.45**	2.5–12.5
Lymphocytes (10⁹/l)	4.847	1.5–7.0
Eosinophils (10⁹/l)	0.131	0–1.5
Monocytes (10⁹/l)	**1.572**	0.0–0.85
Basophils (10⁹/l)	0	Rare
NRBCs (per 100 WBCs)	**32**	Rare

BLOOD SMEAR EVALUATION

Many NRBCs, no polychromasia.

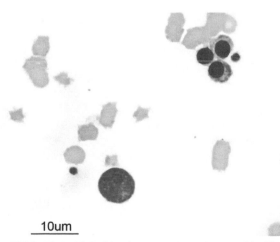
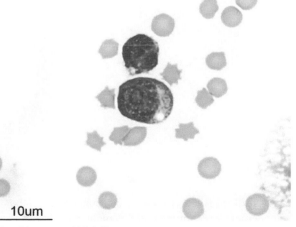

FIGS. 40.1, 40.2 Blood smears from this cat. Modified Wright–Giemsa, ×100 (oil).

INFECTIOUS DISEASES TESTS

Test	Result
FIV antibodies (ELISA)	Negative
FeLV antigen (ELISA)	Negative
FCoV antibodies (IFA)	Negative
Mycoplasma haemofelis (PCR)	Negative
Mycoplasma haemominutum (PCR)	Negative
Candidatus mycoplasma turicensis (PCR)	Negative

QUESTIONS

1 Does the anaemia appear regenerative?
2 What is the significance of the blood smear pictures?

CASE 41
A 4-year-old male neutered mixed-breed dog presented for anorexia, lethargy and diarrhoea.

HAEMATOLOGY

Measurand (units)	Result	Reference Interval
RBC count (10¹²/l)	**4.47**	5.5–8.5
Haemoglobin (g/l)	**73**	120–180
Haematocrit (l/l)	**0.25**	0.37–0.55
MCV (fl)	**56.2**	60–77
MCH (pg)	**16.3**	19.5–24.5
MCHC (g/l)	**289**	320–370
RDW (%)	**20.5**	13.2–17.8
Platelet count (10⁹/l)	462	175–500
WBC count (10⁹/l)	15.13	6–17
Neutrophils (10⁹/l)	9.9	3.0–11.5
Lymphocytes (10⁹/l)	2.08	1.0–4.8
Monocytes (10⁹/l)	0.6	0.2–1.5
Eosinophils (10⁹/l)	**2.5**	0.1–1.3

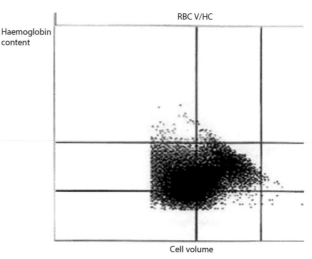

FIG. 41.2 Distribution of red blood cells according to cell volume and haemoglobin content. Normocytic-normochromic RBCs are present in the centre. A large number of hypochromic-microcytic cells are visible in the bottom left quadrant.

BLOOD SMEAR EVALUATION

RBCs: small number of polychromatophils, large number of hypochromic cells, moderate number of codocytes, moderate anisocytosis; WBCs: no significant abnormalities; platelets: no platelet clumps.

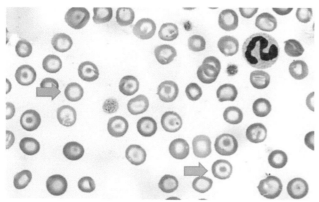

FIG. 41.1 Blood smear, high magnification. Large number of hypochromic cells (orange arrow), moderate number of codocytes (blue arrow).

BIOCHEMISTRY

Analyte (units)	Result	Reference Interval
Total protein (g/l)	73	55–75
Albumin (g/l)	38	25–40
Globulins (g/l)	35	23–35
Glucose (mmol/l)	5	3.3–6.5
ALP (U/l)	26	0–130
ALT (U/l)	25	0–85
Urea (mmol/l)	**18.5**	3.3–8.0
Creatinine (µmol/l)	128	45–150
Sodium (mmol/l)	148	135–155
Chloride (mmol/l)	115	105–120
Potassium (mmol/l)	**5.3**	3.35–4.37
Calcium (mmol/l)	2.6	2.30–2.80
Phosphate (mmol/l)	1.4	0.78–1.41

QUESTIONS

1 How would you interpret this anaemia?
2 What is the significance of the codocytes?
3 What is the significance of the eosinophilia?
4 How would you explain the high urea?
5 Give a possible explanation for this case. What further investigations would you suggest?

CASE 42

A 2-year-old Thoroughbred filly in training had a history of moderate weight loss and recurrent, mild colic of 3 months' duration. Appetite was poor but the faeces appeared normal.

HAEMATOLOGY

Measurand (units)	Result	Reference Interval
RBC count (10¹²/l)	**7.6**	8–12
Haemoglobin (g/l)	**75**	100–180
Spun PCV (%)	**27**	35–50
MCV (fl)	**35**	36–49
MCHC (g/l)	**280**	300–370
WBC count (10⁹/l)	**14.2**	5.5–12.5
Neutrophils (10⁹/l)	**10.0**	2.6–6.7
Band neutrophils (10⁹/l)	**0.5**	<0.10
Lymphocytes (10⁹/l)	1.6	1.5–5.5
Monocytes (10⁹/l)	**1.8**	<1
Eosinophils (10⁹/l)	0.2	<1
Basophils (10⁹/l)	0.1	<0.2

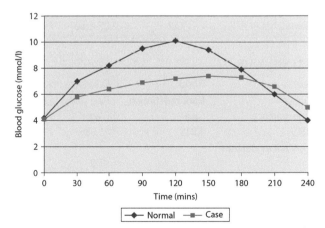

FIG. 42.1 Note the thin condition of the filly and the somewhat depressed demeanor.

BIOCHEMISTRY

Analyte (units)	Result	Reference Interval
Total protein (g/l)	**38**	47–67
Albumin (g/l)	**19**	25–37
Globulins (g/l)	19	19–37
GGT (U/l)	18	<20
ALP (U/l)	**290**	<130
GLDH (U/l)	**8**	<8
AST (U/l)	**405**	<200
CK (U/l)	**380**	<80

ADDITIONAL TESTING

Oral glucose absorption test

Time (minutes)	Blood glucose (mmol/l)	
	Patient	Results from a healthy horse for comparison
0	4.1	4.2
30	5.8	7.0
60	6.4	8.2
90	6.9	9.5
120	7.2	10.1
150	7.4	9.4
180	7.3	7.9
210	6.6	6.0
240	5.0	4.0

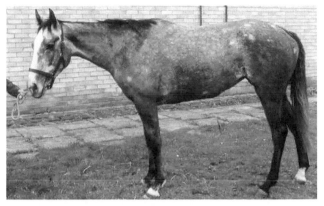

FIG. 42.2 Results of an oral glucose absorption test on the filly.

Faecal parasitology
Negative.

Peritoneal fluid analysis

Analyte (units)	Result	Reference Interval
Appearance	Clear, deep yellow	Clear
Total protein (g/l)	**22**	<15
Nucleated cell count (10⁹/l)	**12.5**	<3

Cytology of the peritoneal fluid

80% large mononuclear cells, 10% neutrophils, 10% lymphocytes.

Faecal occult blood

Weak positive.

1 Discuss the laboratory findings and their significance.
2 What is your interpretation of these findings, and what are your recommendations?

CASE 43

A 4-year-old male Border Collie-cross presented for acute onset of depression and gross haematuria.

HAEMATOLOGY

Measurand (units)	Result	Reference Interval
RBC count (10¹²/l)	**5.48**	5.5–8.5
Haemoglobin (g/l)	131	120–180
Haemocrit (l/l)	0.39	0.38–0.57
MCV (fl)	71.3	61–80
MCH (pg)	23.5	20–26
MCHC (g/l)	329	300–360
RDW (%)	14.2	10–16.0
Platelet count (10⁹/l)	361	150–450
WBC count (10⁹/l)	10.9	6–15
Neutrophils (10⁹/l)	7.41	2.50–12.50
Lymphocytes (10⁹/l)	2.83	0.50–4.80
Monocytes (10⁹/l)	0.44	<0.80
Eosinophils (10⁹/l)	0.22	0.05–0.80

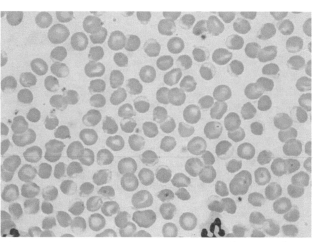

FIG. 43.1 Blood film. Modified Wright–Giemsa, ×50 (oil).

URINALYSIS

Item	Result	Reference Interval
Colour	**Dark red–brown**	Pale yellow to straw
Transparency	Clear	Clear
USG	**1.031**	>1.035
Dipstick evaluation		
ph	6.0	<7.0
Glucose	Negative	Negative
Protein	**3+**	Negative to trace
Bilirubin	**1+**	Negative to trance
Blood	**4+**	Negative
Sediment analysis		
Erythrocytes	<5	<5
Leucocytes	**1–2**	0–1
Epithelial cells	None	Variable
Crystals	None	Variable
Casts	None	None to few

1 What is your evaluation of the urinalysis findings?
2 What is your evaluation of the haematological findings and the photomicrograph of the peripheral blood film?
3 What conditions/differential diagnoses do you suspect, and what is the pathophysiological basis for this condition?

CASE 44
A 3-year-old female neutered DSH cat presented because of pollakiuria and slight stranguria.

URINALYSIS

Item	Result	Reference Interval
Colour	Light yellow	Yellow
Transparency	**Turbid**	Clear
USG	1.020	1.020–1.060
Dipstick evaluation		
pH	**8**	Acidic
Leucocyte esterase	**+++**	Negative
Nitrite	Negative	Negative
Protein	Negative	Traces
Glucose	Negative	Negative
Ketone bodies	Negative	Negative
Bilirubin	Negative	Negative
Blood	**++**	Negative

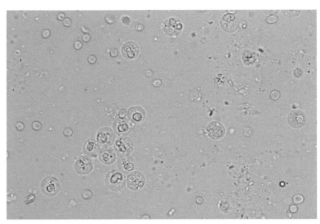

FIG. 44.1 Unstained urine sediment, ×40. (Courtesy Dr Judith Leidinger)

QUESTIONS

1 What cells can be seen in **Fig. 44.1**?
2 What do they indicate in urine?
3 Does the ratio of these cells indicate inflammation or bleeding?
4 Is the +++ positive leucocyte esterase test on the dipstick an indication of pyuria?
5 Is the nitrite test available on some dipsticks suitable for use in dogs and cats?

CASE 45
A 3-year-old female Holstein cow presented approximately 4 months following breeding with decreased milk production and partial anorexia of 3 weeks' duration.

EXAMINATION FINDINGS

A distended abdomen was observed, with 'ping' following percussion and auscultation of the left abdomen. Thirty-five litres of abomasal reflux were removed by orogastric tube.

HAEMATOLOGY

Measurand (units)	Result	Reference Interval
RBC count (10^{12}/l)	**8.7**	5.0–7.5
Haemoglobin (g/l)	**13.7**	85–132
Haematocrit (l/l)	**0.41**	0.24–0.36
MCV (fl)	49.0	37.8–56.0
MCH (pg)	16.1	14.2–20.1

Measurand (units)	Result	Reference Interval
MCHC (g/l)	330	317–404
Platelet count (10^9/l)	507	220–640
WBC count (10^9/l)	10	3.8–11.0
Neutrophils (10^9/l)	**5.5**	0.7–4.9
Lymphocytes (10^9/l)	4.2	1.0–5.8
Monocytes (10^9/l)	0.3	0.0–0.9
Eosinophils (10^9/l)	0	0.0–1.9
Basophils (10^9/l)	0	0.0–0.1
Fibrinogen (g/l) (heat precipitation method)	**0.8**	0.2–0.6

BLOOD SMEAR EVALUATION

RBC and WBC morphology were within expected limits. The platelet estimate was adequate.

BIOCHEMISTRY

Analyte (units)	Result	Reference Interval
Total protein (g/l)	**78**	65–76
Albumin (g/l)	**42**	23–39
Glucose (mmol/l)	3.9	2.6–3.9
Creatinine (µmol/l)	**184.2**	61–133
Sodium (mmol/l)	140	140–146
Potassium (mmol/l)	**2.7**	3.5–4.6
Chloride (mmol/l)	**82**	98–110
TCO$_2$ (mmol/l)	**40**	22–34

QUESTIONS

1 What is your assessment of these findings and the physiological bases for them?
2 What is your diagnosis?
3 What might you expect to find in the urine, and why?
4 What treatment is needed?

CASE 46

A 5-year-old female neutered German Shepherd Dog presented because of loss of appetite and frequent coughing.

EXAMINATION FINDINGS

Unremarkable except for a wet cough.

HAEMATOLOGY

Measurand (units)	Result	Reference Interval
RBC count (10^{12}/l)	6.81	5.5–8.5
Haemoglobin (g/l)	162	130–195
Haematocrit (l/l)	0.49	0.37–0.55
MCHC (g/l)	326	325–379
MCV (fl)	71.9	60–77
Platelet count (10^9/l)	288	150–500
WBC count (10^9/l)	**40.11**	6–17
Neutrophils (10^9/l)	**19.32**	3.0–11.5

Measurand (units)	Result	Reference Interval
Band neutrophils (10^9/l)	**0.75**	0.0–0.5
Lymphocytes (10^9/l)	**7.01**	1.0–3.6
Monocytes (10^9/l)	**3.53**	0.04–1.35
Eosinophils (10^9/l)	**9.3**	0.0–1.25
Basophils (10^9/l)	**0.2**	0.0–0.04

QUESTIONS

1 Describe and discuss the haematological abnormalities.
2 What preformed proteins are released from the eosinophilic-specific granules, and what actions do they perform?

CASE 47

Blood samples were collected from a 4-year-old female neutered DSH cat as part of an investigation into polydipsia.

BIOCHEMISTRY

Analyte (units)	Result	Reference Interval
Total protein (g/l)	66	55–78
Albumin (g/l)	37	26–40
Globulins (g/l)	29	19–48
ALP (U/l)	0	0–55
ALT (U/l)	55	30–60
Urea (mmol/l)	**8.2**	3.5–8.0
Creatinine (µmol/l)	113	40–180
Calcium (mmol/l)	**0**	2.0–2.8
Phosphorus (mmol/l)	1.2	0.81–1.61
Sodium (mmol/l)	155	141–155
Potassium (mmol/l)	**24.8**	3.5–5.5

QUESTION

1 There is no clear cause of the polydipsia, but what is your interpretation of the abnormalities present?

CASE 48

A 24-year-old Thoroughbred horse is reported to have weight loss, poor body condition and lethargy.

SERUM PROTEIN ELECTROPHORESIS

Serum protein electrophoresis shows an increased total protein of 96 g/l.

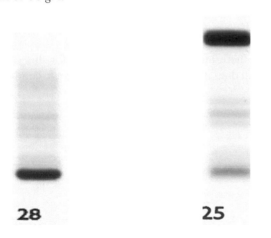

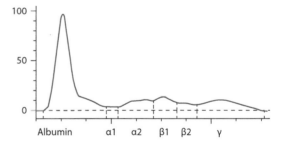

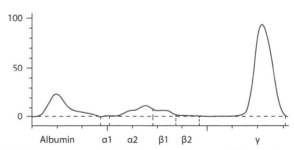

FIG. 48.1 Stained agarose gel (albumin is located at the bottom). Left gel (28) is from a horse that is within normal limits. Right gel (25) is from this patient.

FIG. 48.2 Densitometry tracing of agarose gel. Top tracing is from a horse that is within normal limits. Bottom tracing is from this patient.

QUESTIONS

1 What is your interpretation of this electrophoresis?
2 What is the most likely clinical diagnosis?

CASE 49

A 2-month-old male Irish Setter puppy displayed an omphalophlebitis shortly after birth. Osteomyelitis and enlarged peripheral lymph nodes were also noted.

HAEMATOLOGY

The erythron and thrombon are unremarkable.

Measurand (units)	Result	Reference Interval
WBC count (10^9/l)	90	6–17
Neutrophils (10^9/l)	85.4	3.0–11.5
Lymphocytes (10^9/l)	3.2	1.0–3.6
Monocytes (10^9/l)	0.6	0.04–1.35
Basophils (10^9/l)	0	0.0–0.4
Eosinophils (10^9/l)	1.2	0.0–1.25

QUESTIONS

1 What is the most likely diagnosis based on the haematological abnormalities, breed, age and clinical signs? What test could you perform to confirm your diagnosis?
2 Describe the underlying clinicopathological abnormality.
3 Summarise all the events and involved structures in the adhesion and transmigration of leucocytes from the vascular endothelium to a site of injury.

CASE 50

A 6-month-old female DSH cat is under general anaesthesia for ovariohysterectomy. Acid–base and blood gas data is obtained to evaluate the quality of the anaesthesia because no capnograph is present.

ACID–BASE AND BLOOD GAS DATA

Analyte (units)	Result	Reference Interval
Arterial pH	7.21	7.36–7.44
$PaCO_2$ (mmHg)	70	36–44
PaO_2 (mmHg)	35	85–95
Plasma HCO_3^- (mmol/l)	27	18–26
Serum Na^+ (mmol/l)	145	145–155
Serum K^+ (mmol/l)	6.5	4–5
Serum Cl^- (mmol/l)	104	105–115
Anion gap	?	15–25

QUESTIONS

1 What is the anion gap (AG) in this case?
2 What is your assessment of the arterial pH?
3 What is your assessment of the likely underlying aetiology for this arterial pH?
4 Is there appropriate compensation for this condition, and does it suggest an acute or a chronic condition?

CASE 51

A 2.5-year-old female Rough-coated Collie has grey faeces and an increased faecal volume. The owners have also noted weight loss and an increased appetite.

BIOCHEMISTRY

Analyte (units)	Result	Reference Interval
Total protein (g/l)	62.2	54–71
Albumin (g/l)	31.1	26–33
Globulins (g/l)	31.2	27–44
Glucose (mmol/l)	4.5	3.66–6.31
Cholesterol (mmol/l)	**3.1**	3.5–7.0
Triglycerides (mmol/l)	**0.20**	0.29–3.88
ALP (U/l)	95	0–97
ALT (U/l)	**71**	0–55
Urea (mmol/l)	8.11	3.57 8.57
Creatinine (µmol/l)	68	35–106
Sodium (mmol/l)	149	141–152
Chloride (mmol/l)	106	100–120
Potassium (mmol/l)	3.8	3.6–5.35
Ionised calcium (mmol/l)	1.28	1.16–1.31
Phosphate (mmol/l)	0.81	0.7–1.6
cTLI (µg/l)	**1.8**	5–35

QUESTIONS

1 How do you interpret the laboratory findings?
2 What further diagnostics are necessary in this patient, and why?

CASE 52

A 15-month-old Saler-cross heifer weighing 453 kg (1,000 lb) was part of a herd of similar heifers on irrigated pasture who were current on vaccinations and supplemented with vitamins and minerals. This heifer was found yesterday with bloody scours.

EXAMINATION FINDINGS

Haematochezia, diarrhoea, rectal oedema and staggering were observed. This progressed to lateral recumbency with opisthotonos. T = 40°C (104°F).

HAEMATOLOGY

Measurand (units)	Result	Reference Interval
RBC count (10¹²/l)	**4.82**	5.0–7.2
Haemoglobin (g/l)	**69**	87–124
Haematocrit (l/l)	**20.3**	0.25–0.33
MCV (fl)	42.1	38–51
MCH (pg)	14.3	14–19
MCHC (g/l)	340	340–380

Measurand (units)	Result	Reference Interval
Platelet count (10⁹/l)	**975**	252–724
WBC count (10⁹/l)	**5.34**	5.9–14.0
Neutrophils (10⁹l)	**1.02**	1.8–7.2
Band neutrophils (10⁹/l)	0	0.0–0.3
Lymphocytes (10⁹/l)	3.83	1.7–7.5
Monocytes (10⁹/l)	0.49	(0.0–0.9)
Eosinophils (10⁹/l)	0	0.0–1.3
Basophils (10⁹/l)	0	0.0–0.3
Fibrinogen (g/l) (heat precipitation method)	4	2–4
Total protein (g/l) (refractometer)	**49**	55–80
Fibrinogen:total protein ratio (%)	8	<10

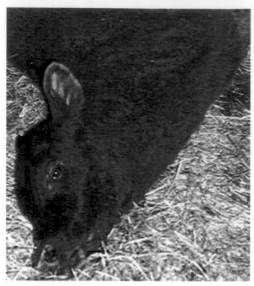

FIG. 52.1 Opisthotonous in the affected heifer.

BLOOD SMEAR EVALUATION

2+ polychromasia; 1+ anisocytosis.

BIOCHEMISTRY

Analyte (units)	Result	Reference Interval
Albumin (g/l)	**24**	31–41
Urea (mmol/l)	2.5	2.1–13.6
Creatinine (µmol/l)	106	62–115
Phosphorus (mmol/l)	**1.45**	1.49–2.36
Calcium (mmol/l)	2.63	2.23–2.73
Sodium (mmol/l)	139	135–144
Chloride (mmol/l)	**104**	92–102
Potassium (mmol/l)	4	3.5–5.0
TCO_2 (mmol/l)	29	24–32
Anion gap	**10**	15–22

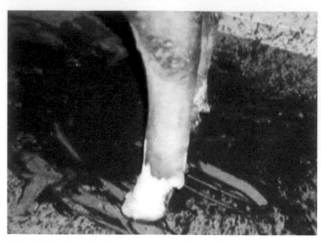

FIG. 52.2 Bloody diarrhoea in an affected herd mate.

QUESTIONS

1 What is your assessment of these findings?
2 What additional laboratory tests would you recommend?

CASE 53

A 4-year-old female Bernese Mountain Dog presented for intermittent diarrhoea of 4 months' duration, with no response to broad-spectrum antibiotics.

EXAMINATION FINDINGS

Unremarkable apart from a focal alopecia at the chin.

HAEMATOLOGY

Unremarkable.

BIOCHEMISTRY

Analyte (units)	Result	Reference Interval
Total protein (g/l)	**32.3**	55–70
Albumin (g/l)	**15.4**	30–37
Globulins (g/l)	**16.9**	23–36
Glucose (mmol/l)	6.18	3.3–6.5
Bilirubin (µmol/l)	1	<3.6
Cholesterol (mmol/l)	**2.32**	3.3–8.6
Triglycerides (mmol/l)	**0.95**	<0.75
ALP (U/l)	54	<131
ALT (U/l)	**165**	<85
GLDH (U/l)	**11**	<10
Urea (mmol/l)	3.72	3.03–9.82
Creatinine (µmol/l)	96	53–123
Sodium (mmol/l)	148	147–152
Chloride (mmol/l)	**114**	102–110
Potassium (mmol/l)	3.8	3.35–4.37
Ionised calcium (mmol/l)	**1.06**	1.23–1.43
Phosphate (mmol/l)	1.41	0.79–2.1

QUESTIONS

1 Describe and discuss the significant biochemistry findings.
2 What further tests are required to determine the aetiology of the significant abnormalities in this dog?

CASE 54

A blood smear from a 1-year-old Miniature Poodle is sent to a referral laboratory. No history is provided.

BLOOD SMEAR EVALUATION

The RBCs display a marked anisocytosis characterised by a dominance of macrocytic erythrocytes. In addition, metarubricytes are often noted and neutrophils appear hypersegmented. Few to moderate numbers of giant neutrophils can be seen.

QUESTIONS

1 What is the most likely diagnosis based on the present findings?
2 What further diagnostics would you perform to support your diagnosis?
3 How do you interpret the condition for the well-being of the patient?

CASE 55

A 9 year-old male Siberian Husky presented in emergency for acute onset of bilateral blepharospasm. One month ago the dog had an isolated episode of epistaxis.

EXAMINATION FINDINGS

Bilateral uveitis with secondary glaucoma and retinal detachment. Blood pressure was normal (105 mmHg).

HAEMATOLOGY

Unremarkable except for platelets of $16 \times 10^9/l$ (reference interval, 148–484).

SERUM PROTEIN ELECTROPHORESIS

Total protein = **112** g/l (reference interval, 55–70).

Analyte (units)	Result	Reference Interval
Albumin (%)	**21.7**	48.1–59.3
Alpha-1 globulin (%)	**0.8**	3.2–4.8
Alpha-2 globulin (%)	**10.4**	12.0–16.4
Beta-1 globulin (%)	**1.8**	2.7–4.1
Beta-2 globulin (%)	11.3	10.5–19.7
Gamma globulins (%)	**54.0**	6.6–12.2
Albumin:globulin ratio	0.3	

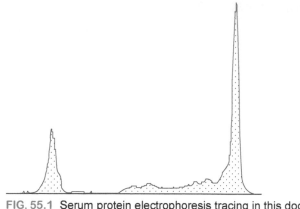

FIG. 55.1 Serum protein electrophoresis tracing in this dog.

SCREENING FOR INFECTIOUS DISEASES

Ehrlichia canis antibody >1:512; *Dirofilaria immitis* antigen: negative; *Leishmania* PCR (bone marrow): negative; *Ehrlichia canis* PCR: negative; *Babesia canis* PCR: negative; *Anaplasma phagocytophilum* PCR: negative.

QUESTIONS

1 What are the common clinicopathological findings in canine monocytic ehrlichiosis (*E. canis*)?
2 What does the serum protein electrophoresis tracing indicate?

CASE 56

A 6-year-old male neutered German Shorthair Pointer had been inappetent for 2 days, had vomited once each day and was lethargic.

BIOCHEMISTRY

Analyte (units)	Result	Reference Interval
Sodium (mmol/l)	**133.6**	135–155
Potassium (mmol/l)	**6.2**	3.6–5.6
Na:K ratio	**21.55**	28.8–40.0
Chloride (mmol/l)	102	100–116

ACTH STIMULATION TEST

Analyte (units)	Result	Reference Interval
Basal cortisol (nmol/l)	**12.1**	25–125
Cortisol 1 hour post ACTH (nmol/l)	**14.8**	125–520

QUESTIONS

1 What is your interpretation of these findings?
2 What is the pathophysiology associated with these findings?

CASE 57

A 5-year-old female Golden Retriever presented because of anorexia.

EXAMINATION FINDINGS

Hepatic disease was suspected based on clinical examination, biochemistry profile and ultrasound findings. A liver biopsy was planned to confirm this suspicion. There were no clinical signs of bleeding tendencies and no history of treatment with any medication within the past 12 months. Plasma-based coagulation screening and a platelet count were performed prior to biopsy.

COAGULATION PROFILE

Analyte (units)	Result	Reference Interval
aPTT (seconds)	**60**	10–13
PT (seconds)	7	7–9
Platelet count (10⁹/l)	Aggregates observed in blood film	200–500
Fibrinogen (g/l)	3.4	1–4

The reason for the markedly prolonged aPTT was pursued by performing an aPTT re-run immediately after mixing equal volumes of the patient's plasma sample and a pool of normal canine plasma. Result of re-run: aPTT mixing study = 64 seconds.

QUESTIONS

1 What is your interpretation of this finding?
2 Does the finding confirm that a coagulopathy is present in this dog?

CASE 58

A 12-year-old Shetland pony mare with a 1-week-old foal at foot was dull and inappetent, having been apparently normal the previous day.

EXAMINATION FINDINGS

The mare was moderately jaundiced and had a small area of midline ventral oedema. Serum taken for biochemistry appeared turbid after centrifugation.

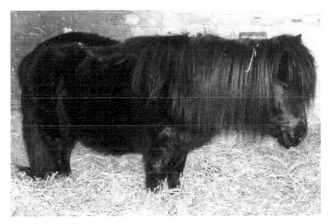

FIG. 58.1 Note the dull demeanour and slight ventral oedema in this mare.

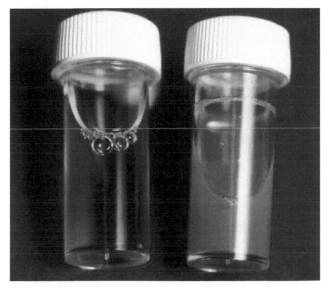

FIG. 58.2 Note the serum appearance following centrifugation. Normal horse on the left; this pony on the right.

HAEMATOLOGY

Unremarkable.

BIOCHEMISTRY

Analyte (units)	Result	Reference Interval
Total protein (g/l)	**75.4**	60–73
Albumin (g/l)	25.3	25–37
Globulins (g/l)	**50.1**	35–48
Triglycerides (mmol/l)	**10.2**	<1.0
Cholesterol (mmol/l)	**4.5**	2.3–3.6
Glucose (mmol/l)	**1.8**	2.8–5.5
GGT (U/l)	**220**	<20
GLDH (U/l)	**80**	<8
Bile acids (µmol/l)	**56**	<15
Total bilirubin (µmol/l)	**164**	9–48
Direct (conjugated) bilirubin (µmol/l)	**30**	<17
Urea (mmol/l)	**27.2**	2.5–8.3
Creatinine (µmol/l)	**262**	<177
Calcium (mmol/l)	3.2	2.6–3.3
Phosphorus (mmol/l)	**0.4**	0.5–1.6

QUESTIONS

1 Discuss the laboratory findings and their significance.
2 What is your interpretation?
3 What is the prognosis?

CASE 59

A 13-year-old male mongrel dog was lethargic and showing signs of severe respiratory distress. To avoid aggravation of the clinical signs, radiography and ultrasound were not performed.

CARDIAC BIOMARKER

NT-proBNP = 1,800 pmol/l.

QUESTIONS

1 Give a short overview of the pathophysiology of NT-proBNP. Where does it come from, why does it increase and what actions does it perform?

2 How do you interpret the NT-proBNP result in this patient? Discuss potential differential diagnoses.
3 What pre-analytical precautions do you need to consider?

CASE 60

A 9-year-old female Dachshund dog weighing 7.8 kg (17 lb) had been coughing and shown haematuria for 1 week, without response to broad-spectrum antibiotics and mucolytic treatment. Weight loss of 2.5 kg was noted within the last 4 months.

EXAMINATION FINDINGS

Dry, choking cough. Several haematomas were observed at the injection sites. Three firm mammary tumours were palpated at the mammary complex of the right side. There was a firm subcutaneous mass over the distal right costal arch.

Thoracic radiographs revealed an interstitial lung pattern and a clearly visible pleural fissure indicative of slight thoracic effusion. A moderate hepatosplenomegaly was detected on abdominal radiographs. A calcified mass was observed caudal to the costal arch consistent with a subcutaneous tumour.

HAEMATOLOGY

Measurand (units)	Result	Reference Interval
RBC count (10¹²/l)	**4.97**	5.5–8.5
Haemoglobin (g/l)	**69**	74–112
Haematocrit (l/l)	**0.33**	0.37–0.55
MCHC (g/l)	339	316–356
MCV (fl)	66.8	60–77
Platelet count (10⁹/l)	**44**	150–500
WBC count (10⁹/l)	**18.3**	6–17
Neutrophils (10⁹/l)	**14.57**	3.0–11.5
Band neutrophils (10⁹/l)	0	<0.5
Lymphocytes (10⁹/l)	1.54	1.0–3.6
Monocytes (10⁹/l)	**1.75**	0.04–1.35
Eosinophils (10⁹/l)	0.37	<1.25
Basophils (10⁹/l)	0.04	<0.04

BLOOD SMEAR EVALUATION

Slight anisocytosis and polychromasia of erythrocytes. Several target cells are present. There is slight mature neutrophilia and monocytosis. Approximately 10–30% of neutrophils display mild signs of toxicity (e.g. slightly basophilic foamy cytoplasm). Several reactive lymphocytes and rare lymphatic blasts are present. The number of platelets appears markedly decreased. The majority of platelets present are large or giant platelets.

BIOCHEMISTRY

Unremarkable.

COAGULATION PROFILE

Analyte (units)	Result	Reference Interval
PT (seconds)	**>120**	6.5–8.2
aPTT (seconds)	**>180**	10–14
Fibrinogen (g/l)	**<0.06**	2.0–4.0
D-dimers (ng/ml)	**1.9**	<0.4
Antithrombin (%)	**80**	109–128

QUESTIONS

1 Describe and discuss the significant haematological findings, as well as the coagulation profile.
2 What is the most likely aetiology of the abnormalities, and what prognosis is associated with the diagnosis?

CASE 61
A 13-year-old male neutered DSH cat was found hung in a partially opened window. He had been there for approximately 4 hours.

EXAMINATION FINDINGS

The cat is panting severely and has haemorrhages on the tongue. Moderate lethargy is noted.

HAEMATOLOGY

Measurand (units)	Result	Reference Interval
RBC count (10¹²/l)	6.38	5–10
Haemoglobin (g/l)	75	49–93
Haematocrit (l/l)	0.26	0.24–0.45
MCV (fl)	47.3	40–55
MCI I (pg)	10.5	7.7–11
MCHC (g/l)	326	325–379
Platelet count (10⁹/l)	323	180–550
WBC count (10⁹/l)	10.2	6–18
Neutrophils (10⁹/l)	9.22	2.5–12.5
Lymphocytes (10⁹/l)	**0.8**	1.5–7.0
Monocytes (10⁹/l)	0.10	0.04–0.85
Eosinophils (10⁹/l)	0.10	0.00–1.50
Basophils (10⁹/l)	0	0.00–0.04

BIOCHEMISTRY

Analyte (units)	Result	Reference Interval
Total protein (g/l)	60.6	54.7–78.0
Albumin (g/l)	23.3	21–33

Analyte (units)	Result	Reference Interval
Globulins (g/l)	37.3	26–51
Glucose (mmol/l)	**7.1**	3.89–6.11
ALP (U/l)	24	0–39.7
ALT (U/l)	**305**	0–70
CK (U/l)	**149,800**	0–205
Urea (mmol/l)	**21.22**	7.14–10.7
Creatinine (μmol/l)	**238**	0–168
Sodium (mmol/l)	155	147–156
Chloride (mmol/l)	**114**	115–130
Potassium (mmol/l)	3.60	3.6–4.8
Ionised calcium (mmol/l)	1.20	1.17–1.32
Phosphate (mmol/l)	1.9	0.8–1.9

QUESTIONS

1 What is the most likely explanation for the haematological and biochemical abnormalities? Describe the pathomechanism.
2 What further analyses would you recommend?
3 What isoenzymes of creatine kinase (CK) can occur?

CASE 62
A urinalysis was performed as part of a regular health check of a 14-year-old Standardbred gelding.

URINALYSIS

The dipstick test was unremarkable. USG by refractometry = 1.034; pH = 9.0.

Urine sediment analysis
See **Fig. 62.1**.

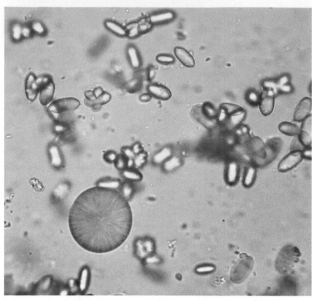

FIG. 62.1 Unstained urine sediment, ×40. (Courtesy Dr Judith Leidinger)

QUESTIONS

1 What are the boat-shaped to ovoid structures?
2 What is the origin of the spherical structure?
3 What happens when diluted (5–10%) acetic acid is added to the sediment?
4 What is the clinical importance of these structures?

CASE 63
A 15-year-old Thoroughbred-cross gelding is overweight, with fat deposits within the sheath, and he has a 'cresty' neck.

HAEMATOLOGY

Measurand (units)	Result	Reference Interval
RBC count (10⁹/l)	**4.6**	5–12
Haemoglobin (g/l)	**70**	80–150
Haematocrit (l/l)	**0.21**	0.35–0.45
MCV (fl)	52	40–60
MCH (pg)	15.8	12.5–17.5
MCHC (g/l)	342	320–360
Platelet count (10⁹/l)	330	75–350
WBC count (10⁹/l)	16	5.5–16.0
Neutrophils (10⁹/l)	**14**	2.5–12.5
Band neutrophils (10⁹/l)	0	0–0.3
Lymphocytes (10⁹/l)	**1**	1.5–3.0
Eosinophils (10⁹/l)	0.6	0–1.5
Monocytes (10⁹/l)	0.4	0.0–0.5
Basophils (10⁹/l)	0	Rare

DEXAMETHASONE SUPPRESSION TEST

Analyte (units)	Result	Reference Interval
Baseline cortisol (nmol/l)	30	30–50
Cortisol 24 hours post dexamethasone administration (nmol/l)	35	<30

QUESTIONS

1 Describe and interpret the present laboratory abnormalities.
2 What laboratory tests may be helpful for further testing?
3 Why is time of year an important consideration?
4 Why is an insulin assay an important part of the work up of this case?

CASE 64

A 2-year-old female mongrel dog is presented because she is anaemic. Her haematocrit is monitored to determine if an effective response is present. The reticulocyte count is increased.

Analyte (units)	Day 1	Day 3	Day 7
Haematocrit (l/l)	0.250	0.300	0.341

QUESTION

1 Are the changes in the haematocrit between (1) day 1 and day 3, (2) day 1 and day 7, and (3) day 3 and day 7 likely to represent a significant change based on what we know about biological variation and critical difference (reference change value [RCV]) in the dog?

CASE 65

A 2-year-old male American Pitbull presented with lethargy and slight abdominal distension. The dog lives in Germany, but has travelled extensively throughout the Mediterranean with its owner.

BIOCHEMISTRY

Analyte (units)	Result	Reference Interval
Total protein (g/l)	78	55.3–69.84
Albumin (g/l)	24.1	29.6–37.01
Globulin (g/l)	53.9	22.9–35.6
Glucose (mmol/l)	5.83	3.3–6.53
Total bilirubin (µmol/l)	3.71	0–3.6
Cholesterol (mmol/l)	2.68	3.3–6.53
Triglycerides (mmol/l)	0.32	0.08–0.75
ALP (U/l)	236	0–130
ALT (U/l)	567	0–85
GLDH (U/l)	16	0–9.9
CK (U/l)	96	<143
Fasting bile acids (µmol/l)	57	<20
Urea (mmol/l)	3.86	3.3–9.82
Creatinine (µmol/l)	81	53–122
Sodium (mmol/l)	143	141–146
Chloride (mmol/l)	106	104–112

Analyte (units)	Result	Reference Interval
Potassium (mmol/l)	3.76	3.35–4.37
Ionised calcium (mmol/l)	1.33	1.23–1.43
Phosphorus (mmol/l)	1.19	0.79–2.1
Ionised magnesium (mmol/l)	0.62	0.47–0.63
PT (seconds)	9.7	6.52–8.16
aPTT (seconds)	14.3	9.85–14.22

QUESTIONS

1 What does the biochemistry profile indicate?
2 Why is assessment of coagulation status important in animals with liver disease?
3 On abdominal ultrasound, a large cystic mass was detected in the cranial abdomen, which could have originated from the liver. What parasitic disease has to be considered?

CASE 66

A 2-week-old cross-breed calf was kept on a hill farm with 16 other cross-breed calves. One calf was observed to be bleeding from the nose, with oozing of blood from the ear-tag hole and multiple small foci over the head and neck.

EXAMINATION FINDINGS

This particular calf is lethargic and depressed. He had appeared healthy since birth and was gaining weight well prior to the acute development of bleeding.

HAEMATOLOGY

Measurand (units)	Result	Reference Interval (calves aged 2 weeks – 6 months)
RBC count (10^{12}/l)	4	6.5–11.9
Haemoglobin (g/l)	43	85–141
Haematocrit (l/l)	0.13	0.23–0.42
MCV (fl)	32.5	26.6–44.3
MCH (pg)	10.8	9.1–15.6
MCHC (g/l)	331	310–322
Platelet count (10^9/l)	10	220–950
WBC count (10^9/l)	1.2	5.6–13.7
Neutrophils (10^9/l)	0.3	0.6–6.1

Measurand (units)	Result	Reference Interval (calves aged 2 weeks – 6 months)
Lymphocytes (10^9/l)	0.5	2.2–8.7
Monocytes (10^9/l)	0.4	0.8–1.2
Eosinophils (10^9/l)	0	0.0–0.3
Basophils (10^9/l)	0	0.0–1.0
Fibrinogen (g/l)	3.0	2.7–8.2

BLOOD SMEAR EVALUATION

Confirmed the marked leucopaenia and thrombocytopaenia. No polychromasia was observed.

QUESTIONS

1 What is your assessment of these results?
2 What are your differential diagnoses?

CASE 67

A 10-year-old male cross-breed dog is reported to have vomited 4 days ago and then become anorexic. He had been receiving meloxicam for arthritis, was polydipsic but now hardly drank any water.

EXAMINATION FINDINGS

The dog was flat on presentation, was dehydrated, a degree of mental obtundation was observed and hepatomegaly was identified on ultrasound.

HAEMATOLOGY

Measurand (units)	Results	Reference Interval
RBC count (10^{12}/l)	4.6	5.0–8.5
Haemoglobin (g/l)	110	120–180
Haematocrit (l/l)	0.34	0.37–0.55
MCV (fl)	66.1	60–80
MCH (pg)	23.2	19–23

Measurand (units)	Results	Reference Interval
MCHC (g/l)	351	310–340
Reticulocytes (10^9/l)	20	60–80
Platelet count (10^9/l)	476	200–500
WBC count (10^9/l)	17	6–15
Neutrophils (10^9/l)	12.8	3.0–11.5
Band neutrophils (10^9/l)	0.3	0.0–0.3
Lymphocytes (10^9/l)	2	1.0–4.8
Monocytes (10^9/l)	1.7	0.0–1.3
Eosinophils (10^9/l)	0	0.1–1.25
Basophils (10^9/l)	0.2	Rare

BLOOD FILM EVALUATION

Platelet count appears adequate. Neutrophils show mild toxicity.

BIOCHEMISTRY

Analyte (units)	Result	Reference Interval
Total protein (g/l)	64.2	54–77
Albumin (g/l)	28	25–37
Globulins (g/l)	36.2	23–52
ALP (U/l)*	**1,440**	0–50
ALT (U/l)*	**818**	0–25
GGT (U/l)*	**43**	0–27
GLDH (U/l)*	**240**	0–10
Cholesterol (mmol/l)	**11**	3.8–7.0
Total bilirubin (μmol/l)	7	0–16
Bile acids, fasting (μmol/l)	**44.1**	0–10
CK (U/l)*	**425**	0–190
Glucose (mmol/l)	**75.9**	3.8–7.0
Amylase (U/l)*	**6.350**	100–900
Lipase (U/l)*	**>3,000**	0–250
Urea (mmol/l)	**46.7**	1.7–7.4
Creatinine (μmol/l)	**525**	0–106
Sodium (mmol/l)	**135**	139–154
Potassium (mmol/l)	5.1	3.6–5.6
Chloride (mmol/l)	**74**	105–122
Calcium (mmol/l)	2.93	2.3–3.0
Phosphate (mmol/l)	**4.07**	0.80–1.60
*Analysis performed at 37°C		

URINALYSIS

Item	Result	Reference Interval
USG	**1.015**	>1.035
Dipstick evaluation		
pH	7	
Protein	Negative	Negative
Glucose	**3+**	Negative
Ketone bodies	Negative	Negative
Urobilinogen	Negative	Negative
Bilirubin	+	Negative to trace
Blood	Negative	Negative
Sediment analysis		
Leucocytes (cells/mm³)	<10	
Erythrocytes (cells/mm³)	Negative	
Epithelial cells	+/-	
Bacteria	Negative	
Crystals	Negative	
Casts	Occasional hyaline cast	

QUESTIONS

1 Identify and list the abnormalities, and explain their associations.
2 Provide a conclusion for the findings described in question 1 and classify the type of diabetes mellitus.
3 What is the significance of the occasional hyaline cast?
4 This is an emergency situation, which should be communicated with the clinician. What is the most important information regarding the treatment of this condition that you need to convey to the clinician?

CASE 68

A 2-year-old male DSH cat had been showing signs of dysuria and stranguria, as well as vomiting and lethargy, since yesterday.

EXAMINATION FINDINGS

Palpation revealed a painful caudal abdomen with a markedly distended bladder. Abdominal ultrasound demonstrated bladder stones.

HAEMATOLOGY

Measurand (units)	Result	Reference Interval
RBC count (10¹²/l)	9.74	5–10
Haemoglobin (g/l)	78	49–93
Haematocrit (l/l)	0.26	0.24–0.45

Measurand (units)	Result	Reference Interval
MCV (fl)	**39.6**	40–55
MCHC (g/l)	218.5	184–220
Platelet count (10⁹/l)	300	296–354
WBC count (10⁹/l)	14.8	6.0–18.0
Neutrophils (10⁹/l)	**13.59**	2.5–12.5
Lymphocytes (10⁹/l)	**0.84**	1.5–7.0
Monocytes (10⁹/l)	0.31	0.04–0.85
Eosinophils (10⁹/l)	0.07	0.00–1.50
Basophils (10⁹/l)	0	0.00–0.04

BIOCHEMISTRY

Analyte (units)	Result	Reference Interval
Total protein (g/l)	70.2	54.7–78.0
Albumin (g/l)	32.9	21–33
Globulins (g/l)	37.3	26–51
Glucose (mmol/l)	**15.34**	3.89–6.11
ALP (U/l)	15	0–39.7
ALT (U/l)	56	0–70
Urea (mmol/l)	**65.4**	7.14–10.7
Creatinine (µmol/l)	**948**	0–168
Sodium (mmol/l)	**144**	147–156
Chloride (mmol/l)	**112**	115–130
Potassium (mmol/l)	**6.80**	3.6–4.8
Ionised calcium (mmol/l)	**0.77**	1.17–1.32
Phosphate (mmol/l)	**3.11**	0.8–1.9

URINALYSIS

Item	Result	Reference Interval
USG	**1.020**	>1.035
Dipstick evaluation		
pH	8.5	
Blood	**3+**	negative
Protein	**3+**	negative to trace
Glucose	**2+**	negative
Ketone bodies	**1+**	negative

QUESTIONS

1 Describe the laboratory abnormalities present. Discuss a possible diagnosis and differential diagnoses.
2 What further analyses would you recommend?

CASE 69

A 5-year-old male Poodle presents with lethargy and a markedly increased RR.

ACID–BASE AND BLOOD GAS DATA

Analyte (units)	Result	Reference Interval
Arterial pH	**7.58**	7.36–7.44
PaCO$_2$ (mmHg)	**20**	36–44
PaO$_2$ (mmHg)	**100**	85–95
Plasma HCO$_3^-$ (mmol/l)	18	18–26
Serum Na$^+$ (mmol/l)	145	145–155
Serum Cl$^-$ (mmol/l)	110	105–115
Anion gap	20.5	15–25

QUESTIONS

1 What is your assessment of the arterial pH?
2 What is your assessment of the likely underlying aetiology for this arterial pH?
3 Is there appropriate compensation for this condition, and does it suggest an acute or chronic condition?
4 What might be the underlying causes for this condition?

CASE 70

A 10-year-old male Australian Shepherd Dog presented for lethargy and exercise intolerance.

EXAMINATION FINDINGS

The dog was very calm and lay down immediately.

HAEMATOLOGY

Measurand (units)	Result	Reference Interval
RBC count (10^{12}/l)	**4.74**	5.5–8.5
Haemoglobin (g/l)	**109**	130–195
Haematocrit (l/l)	**0.32**	0.37–0.55
MCV (fl)	67	60–77

Measurand (units)	Result	Reference Interval
MCHC (g/l)	**340**	335–379
Platelet count (10^9/l)	**31**	150–500
WBC count (10^9/l)	**149.9**	6–17
Neutrophils (10^9/l)	4.28	3.0–11.5
Lymphocytes (10^9/l)	**121.7**	1.0–3.6
Monocytes (10^9/l)	**4.06**	0.04–1.35
Basophils (10^9/l)	**11.29**	0.0–0.4
Eosinophils (10^9/l)	0.09	0.0–1.25

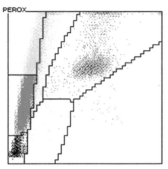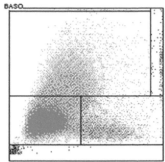

FIG. 70.1 ADVIA® peroxidase cytogram (left) and basophil cytogram (right) of this dog.

QUESTIONS

1 Describe how leucocytes are differentiated by the ADVIA® Haematology System and where various cell types can be seen on the physiological scattergrams.

2 What abnormalities are visible in this ADVIA® cytogram, and what is the most likely diagnosis based on the haematological results?

3 How do you interpret the basophilia reported by the ADVIA® Haematology System?

CASE 71

An 8-year-old female neutered Labrador Retriever presented because of progressive weight loss and lethargy.

HAEMATOLOGY

Leucocytosis of 70,000 cells/μl. The type of leucocytes predominating in the blood smear is shown (**Fig. 71.1**). The erythron and platelets are unremarkable; moderate neutropaenia.

QUESTIONS

1 Describe the cells on the blood smear and give a morphological diagnosis as well as possible differentials.

2 What immunocytochemical markers would you apply to help identify more specifically the cells visible on the blood smear?

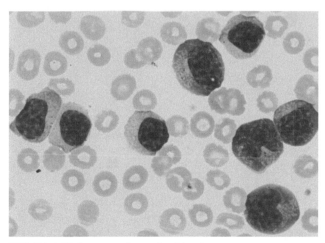

FIG. 71.1 Unknown cells on the blood smear. May–Grünwald–Giemsa, ×50.

CASE 72

You review the calcium data produced for the last week in your laboratory and note that there is a rise in the percentage of high calciums compared with what is normally seen. These animals did not have other laboratory abnormalities suggestive of underlying renal, adrenal, parathyroid or neoplastic disease.

QUESTIONS

1 What do you need to do in order to investigate a possible underlying cause for the increased number of high calcium results?
2 A review of recent quality control shows that the level 1 control ('normal') is within normal limits. The level 2 control ('abnormal' high) shows a shift in the data with the last four results exceeding +1 SD above the mean. What might this mean?

3 If you consistently have a high percentage of increased calcium results and the clinical conditions diagnosed do not correspond to conditions where high calcium is expected, no abnormal control material performance is identified and external quality assessment performance is acceptable, what else should you consider?

CASE 73

A stray cat of unknown age (looks adult) has been brought to the clinic (in Germany) for a health examination.

EXAMINATION FINDINGS

The cat is male, shows a dry hair coat and is poorly nourished. Otherwise, he appears healthy.

ELISA IN-HOUSE TEST

An ELISA in-house test was performed and the cat tested feline immunodeficiency virus (FIV) positive.

QUESTIONS

1 Which proteins do the most rapid tests detect?
2 How would you interpret the positive ELISA result?
3 What other tests for FIV do you know? Describe their advantages and disadvantages, if any.

CASE 74

A 1-year-old female neutered DSH cat was observed by her owner chewing on the leaves of a lily bouquet received as a gift.

BIOCHEMISTRY

Analyte	Result	Reference Interval
Total protein (g/l)	62.3	54.7–78.0
Albumin (g/l)	31.1	21–33
Globulins (g/l)	31.2	26–51
Glucose (mmol/l)	**13.2**	3.89–6.11
ALP (U/l)	21	0–39.7
ALT (U/l)	65	0–70
CK (U/l)	**806**	0–205

Analyte	Result	Reference Interval
Urea (mmol/l)	**20.4**	7.14–10.7
Creatinine (μmol/l)	**260**	0–168
Sodium (mmol/l)	149	147–156
Chloride (mmol/l)	124	115–130
Potassium (mmol/l)	4.2	3.6–4.8
Ionised calcium (mmol/l)	1.3	1.17–1.32
Phosphate (mmol/l)	**2.4**	0.8–1.9

URINALYSIS

Item	Result	Reference Interval
Appearance	Light yellow	Yellow
USG	**1.016**	>1.035
Dipstick evaluation		
pH	6.3	5.5–7.5
Blood	Negative	Negative
Protein	**3+**	Negative
Bilirubin	Negative	Negative
Glucose	**3+**	Negative
Ketone bodies	Negative	Negative
Sediment analysis		
Erythrocytes	2	<5/hpf
Leucocytes	None	<5/hpf
Epithelial cells	None	None to few
Crystals	None	None
Casts	None	None
Bacteria	None	None

QUESTIONS

1 Describe and interpret the laboratory abnormalities.
2 What kind of clinical signs might you expect from lily toxicity in this cat?
3 What histological findings might be present if this cat dies from lily toxicity?
4 What is the treatment and prognosis for lily toxicity?

CASE 75

An 8-year-old female neutered Golden Retriever presented for lethargy, anorexia, shifting leg lameness and back pain.

HAEMATOLOGY

Measurand (units)	Result	Reference Interval
RBC count (10¹²/l)	**4.10**	5.5–8.5
Haemoglobin (g/l)	**88**	120–180
Haematocrit (l/l)	**28.9**	0.37–0.55
MCV (fl)	70.5	60–77
MCHC (g/l)	**304**	320–370
Platelet count (10⁹/l)	**60**	175–500
WBC count (10⁹/l)	**5.2**	6–17
Neutrophils (10⁹/l)	**1.8**	3.0–11.5
Lymphocytes (10⁹/l)	1.3	1.0–4.8
Monocytes (10⁹/l)	1.4	0.2–1.5
Eosinophils (10⁹/l)	0.7	0.1–1.3

BLOOD FILM EVALUATION

RBCs: no polychromasia, moderate rouleaux; WBCs: few reactive lymphocytes; platelets: no platelet clumps.

BIOCHEMISTRY

Analyte (units)	Result	Reference Interval
Total protein (g/l)	**104**	55–75
Albumin (g/l)	**24**	25–40
Globulins (g/l)	**80**	23–35
Glucose (mmol/l)	5.3	3.3–6.5
ALP (U/l)	92	0–130
ALT (U/l)	57	0–85
Urea (mmol/l)	4	3.3–8.0
Creatinine (µmol/l)	88	45–150
Sodium (mmol/l)	142	135–155
Chloride (mmol/l)	105	105–120
Potassium (mmol/l)	**2.4**	3.35–4.37
Calcium (mmol/l)	**3.2**	2.30–2.80
Phosphate (mmol/l)	1.22	0.78–1.41

URINALYSIS

Item	Result	Reference Interval
USG	1.040	>1.030
Dipstick evaluation		
pH	6.5	
Protein	+++	Negative to trace
Glucose	Negative	Negative
Ketone bodies	Negative	Negative
Bilirubin	Negative	Negative
Blood	Negative	Negative

Urine sediment

Inactive sediment with no evidence of inflammation or infection.

QUESTIONS

1 How would you describe this anaemia, and what are possible causes?
2 How would you explain the presence of rouleaux?
3 How would you explain the high serum protein? What test would you suggest to investigate this?
4 How would you explain the proteinuria?
5 What are the differential diagnoses for this case? What test would you suggest to confirm your diagnosis?

CASE 76

An 8-year-old Clydesdale-Thoroughbred-cross mare presents because she is very nervous. She tends to kick when excited and there are no stocks at the farm that would allow rectal palpation. The owner suspects that she was bred by natural cover in the pasture by a neighbour's stallion approximately 2 months ago. The owner would like to know if she is pregnant.

QUESTIONS

1 What test would be suitable for diagnosis of equine pregnancy approximately 60 days post breeding?

2 What is a pitfall of this test?
3 What other laboratory test can be used for equine pregnancy during late gestation (>100 days)?

CASE 77

A 6-year-old female neutered Tervueren presented because of painful micturition.

EXAMINATION FINDINGS

The urinary bladder was painful on palpation.

URINALYSIS

Item	Result	Reference Interval
Colour	Light yellow	Yellow
Transparency	Turbid	Clear
USG	1.029	1.020–1.045
Dipstick evaluation		
pH	**8.0**	Acidic
Leucocyte esterase	+++	Negative
Nitrite	Negative	Negative
Protein	+	Negative to trace

Item	Result	Reference Interval
Protein (SSA)	+	Negative to trace
Glucose	Negative	Negative
Ketone bodies	Negative	Negative
Bilirubin	+	Negative to trace
Blood	+	Negative
Sediment analysis		
Amount	Increased	
Erythrocytes	**Moderate**	<5/hpf
Leucocytes	**Many**	<5/hpf
Squamous epithelial cells	Sparse	
Transitional epithelial cells	Sparse	
Crystals	Negative	

Urine culture

Significant amounts (>10^6 cfu/µl) of alpha-haemolysing streptococcal organisms.

The dog was treated for bacterial cystitis and a few days later a second urine specimen was submitted for sediment evaluation. Large crystals (**Fig. 77.1**) were found in moderate amounts.

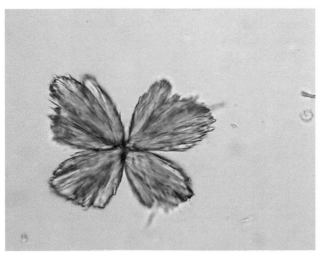

FIG. 77.1 Large crystals found in unstained urine sediment. Wet-drop preparation, ×40. (Courtesy Dr Judith Leidinger)

QUESTIONS

1 What crystal is shown in **Fig. 77.1**?
2 What test can be performed to verify the nature of these crystals?
3 Do they have any clinical significance?

CASE 78

A 1.3-year-old male neutered Maine Coon cat weighing 4.5 kg (10 lb) presents with a history of intermittent ptyalism and ataxia since the age of 4 months. Clinical signs appear to be associated with food intake. Recurrent vomiting and PU/PD have also been observed.

EXAMINATION FINDINGS

The cat appears underdeveloped for a male Maine Coon cat of this age and has a slightly dull hair coat. The most striking finding is the presence of copper-coloured irises (**Fig. 78.1**).

Abdominal radiographs reveal calcifications in the area of the renal pelvis of the left kidney.

HAEMATOLOGY

Unremarkable except for MCV of 34.3 fl (reference interval, 40–55).

BLOOD SMEAR EVALUATION

Several microcytic-normochromic erythrocytes. Leucocytes normal in number and morphology. Platelet count appears normal; several large aggregates are present.

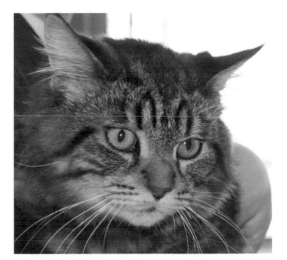

FIG. 78.1 Note the copper-coloured irises of this cat.

BIOCHEMISTRY

Analyte (units)	Result	Reference Interval
Total protein (g/l)	68.6	54.7–78.0
Albumin (g/l)	26.4	21–33
Globulins (g/l)	42.2	26–51
Glucose (mmol/l)	4.65	3.9–6.1
Bilirubin (µmol/l)	**2.9**	<3.4
Cholesterol (mmol/l)	**2.37**	2.46–3.37
Triglycerides (mmol/l)	0.34	<1.14
ALP (U/l)	**87**	<40
ALT (U/l)	**81**	<70
GLDH (U/l)	2	<11.3
Urea (mmol/l)	**4.51**	7.14–10.7
Creatinine (µmol/l)	108	<168
Sodium (mmol/l)	**158**	147–156
Chloride (mmol/l)	**114**	102–110
Potassium (mmol/l)	4.3	3.60–4.80
Ionised calcium (mmol/l)	**1.36**	1.17–1.32
Phosphate (mmol/l)	1.7	0.8–1.9

URINALYSIS (cystocentesis)

Item	Result	Reference Interval
USG	**1.014**	>1.035
Dipstick evaluation		
pH	7	
Bilirubin	0	Negative to trace
Blood	Trace	Negative
Glucose	0	Negative
Protein	0	Negative
Sediment analysis		
Erythrocytes	5	0–5/hpf
Leucocytes	5	0–5/hpf
Epithelial cells	0	0–5/hpf
Crystals	0	Variable
Casts	0	None
Bacteria	Some	None
hpf: ×40 magnification		

QUESTIONS

1 Describe and discuss the significant haematological and biochemistry findings as well as the urinalysis.
2 What further tests are required given the history and the haematological/biochemistry abnormalities?

CASE 79

A 3-year-old male neutered mixed-breed dog presented with a chronically infected wound on the leg.

HAEMATOLOGY

The erythron and thrombon are within their reference intervals.

Measurand (units)	Result	Reference Interval
WBC count (10⁹/l)	**34.1**	6–17
Neutrophils (10⁹/l)	**25.9**	3.0–11.5
Band neutrophils (10⁹/l)	**4.09**	<0.5
Lymphocytes (10⁹/l)	1.36	1.0–3.6
Monocytes (10⁹/l)	**1.71**	0.04–1.35
Eosinophils (10⁹/l)	0.68	0.0–1.25
Basophils (10⁹/l)	0	0.0–0.04

BLOOD SMEAR EVALUATION

Erythrocytes display a borderline anisocytosis. The RBCs are normocytic-normochromic, slight poikilocytosis with occasionally a codocyte present. Platelets are normal in number and morphology. No platelet clumps are seen. Neutrophils show a basophilic, foamy cytoplasm with prominent Döhle bodies visible. Rare large lymphocytes are present.

QUESTIONS

1 Describe and discuss the haematological abnormalities.
2 What aetiologies do you suspect for the development of toxic neutrophils?
3 What signs of toxicity can be seen in neutrophils, and what do they indicate?

CASE 80

A Cob mare known to be more than 18 years old presented because of thin body condition, ataxia and apparent blindness.

HAEMATOLOGY

Measurand (units)	Result	Reference Interval
RBC count (10¹²/l)	8.37	7.80–11.0
Haemoglobin (g/l)	162	130–170
Haematocrit (l/l)	0.45	0.34–0.46
MCV (fl)	**54**	38–49
MCH(pg)	**19.4**	14–19
MCHC (g/l)	358	310–390
Platelet count (10⁹/l)	111	100–350
WBC count (10⁹/l)	11.3	5–12
Neutrophils (10⁹/l)	**10.06**	2.5–7.5
Lymphocytes (10⁹/l)	1.02	1.5–4.0
Monocytes (10⁹/l)	0.23	<0.5
Eosinophils (10⁹/l)	0	0.0–0.5
Basophils (10⁹/l)	0	0.0–0.1
Fibrinogen (g/l) (heat precipitation method)	3	1–4

BIOCHEMISTRY

Analyte (units)	Result	Reference Interval
Total protein (g/l)	**85.4**	50–70
Albumin (g/l)	**24**	25–41
Globulins (g/l)	**61.4**	19–36
A:G ratio	**0.39**	0.6–2.0
ALP (U/l)	**1,305.7**	50–270
GGT (U/l)	**537.8**	10–45
AST (U/l)	**726.7**	100–370
CK (U/l)	**669.7**	20–225
LDH (U/l)	**1,162.9**	130–1,085
GLDH (U/l)	**24**	0–11
Cholesterol (mmol/l)	2.6	2–3
Total bilirubin (μmol/l)	36	9–50
Bile acids, fasting (μmol/l)	**61.1**	0.5–10.0
Urea (mmol/l)	**2.8**	3.3–7.4
Sodium (mmol/l)	132.1	132–146
Potassium (mmol/l)	3.4	3.3–5.4
Chloride (mmol/l)	98.2	89–108
Phosphorus (mmol/l)	**0.81**	0.9–1.8
Calcium (mmol/l)	2.76	2.5–3.6

SERUM PROTEIN ELECTROPHORESIS

Protein fraction (g/l)	Result	Reference Interval
Albumin	28.7	24–41
Alpha-1 globulin	0.92	0.5–3.0
Alpha-2 globulin	**11.87**	2–10
Beta-1 globulin	**11.76**	3–10
Beta-2 globulin	**9.1**	3–8
Gamma globulins	**23**	5–14

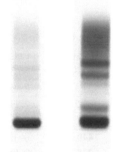

28   34

FIG. 80.1 Stained electrophoresis agar gel. Albumin band is at the bottom of the gel. Left gel (28) is from a horse that is within normal limits. Right gel (34) is from this patient.

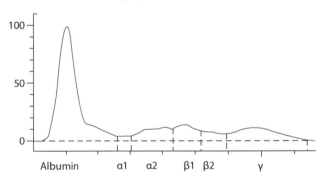

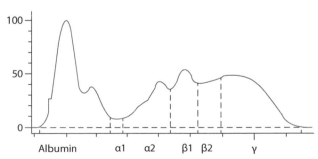

FIG. 80.2 Densitometry tracing of agar gel. Top tracing is from a horse that is within normal limits. Bottom tracing is from this patient.

QUESTIONS

1 What is your assessment of these laboratory findings?
2 What is the significance of the increased prominence of the 'shoulder' on the albumin peak and of the decreased definition between the beta-2 and gamma globulins apparent in the electrophoretic densitometry tracing?
3 What are likely differential diagnoses, and what further tests may be indicated?

CASE 81

A 4-year-old female spayed mongrel dog is being treated with potassium bromide and phenobarbitone as anti-epileptic therapy.

HAEMATOLOGY

Unremarkable.

BIOCHEMISTRY

Analyte (units)	Result	Reference Interval
Total protein (g/l)	62.3	55.3–69.84
Albumin (g/l)	31.1	29.6–37.01
Globulins (g/l)	31.2	22.9–35.6
Glucose (mmol/l)	6	3.3–6.53
ALP (U/l)	**440**	0–130
ALT (U/l)	**235**	0–85
Urea (mmol/l)	5.01	3.3–9.82
Creatinine (μmol/l)	66	53–122

Analyte (units)	Result	Reference Interval
Sodium (mmol/l)	142	141–146
Chloride (mmol/l)	**276**	104–112
Potassium (mmol/l)	4.2	3.35–4.37
Ionised calcium (mmol/l)	1.28	1.23–1.43
Phosphate (mmol/l)	1.8	0.79–2.10

QUESTIONS

1 What is the most likely explanation for the hyperchloraemia? Describe the mechanism for this finding.
2 What is the most likely explanation for the increased ALP and ALT enzyme activities?

CASE 82

A 3-year-old Holstein-cross dairy cow presented with a history of partial anorexia of 2 days' duration. The cow often stood with her head and neck extended. Milk production was decreased.

EXAMINATION FINDINGS

The cow was in a slightly thin body condition. T = 39.5°C (103.1°F); HR = 75 bpm (slightly increased). Respiration was shallow. Faeces were scant and slightly dry. There was no muffling of heart sounds on auscultation.

HAEMATOLOGY

Measurand (units)	Result	Reference Interval
RBC count (10^{12}/l)	6	5.0–7.2
Haemoglobin (g/l)	116	87–124
Haematocrit (l/l)	**0.35**	0.25–0.33
MCV (fl)	**57.8**	38–51
MCH (pg)	**19.3**	14–19
MCHC (g/l)	**334**	340–380

Measurand (units)	Result	Reference Interval
Platelet count (10^9/l)	367	252–724
WBC count (10^9/l)	**15**	5.9–14.0
Neutrophils (10^9L)	**11.1**	1.8–7.2
Band neutrophils (10^9/l)	**2.6**	0.0–0.3
Lymphocytes (10^9/l)	**0.4**	1.7–7.5
Monocytes (10^9/l)	0.9	0.0–0.9
Eosinophils (10^9/l)	0	0.0–1.3
Basophils (10^9/l)	0	0.0–0.3
Fibrinogen (g/l) (heat precipitation method)	**9.5**	2–4
Plasma protein (g/l) (refractometer)	**120**	55–80
Fibrinogen:total protein ratio (%)	**11.9**	<10

BIOCHEMISTRY

Analyte (units)	Result	Reference Interval
Albumin (g/l)	**41.5**	31–41
Glucose (mmol/l)	3	2.5–3.8
CK (U/l)	**233**	17–60
ALP (U/l)	**96**	3–86
GGT (U/l)	38	0–40
SDH (U/l)	12	0–15
Urea (mmol/l)	**23.8**	2.1– 13.6
Creatinine (µmol/l)	**150**	62–115
Phosphorus (mmol/l)	2.36	1.49 –2.36
Calcium (mmol/l)	2.62	2.23–2.73
Chloride (mmol/l)	**82**	92–102
Sodium (mmol/l)	**126**	135–144
Potassium (mmol/l)	**2.5**	3.5–5.0
TCO_2 (mmol/l)	**35**	24–32
Anion gap	**11.5**	12–22

SDH = sorbitol dehydrogenase; TCO_2 = total carbon dioxide.

PERITONEAL FLUID ANALYSIS

Cloudy, yellow, watery fluid obtained. Total protein by refractometry = 50 g/l. Cell counts and cytological evaluation are pending.

QUESTIONS

1 What is your assessment of these findings?
2 What is the most likely clinical diagnosis/differential diagnosis?

CASE 83

A 7-year-old female Irish Setter is presented because of sudden onset of anorexia, pyrexia and tachypnoea.

EXAMINATION FINDINGS

Abnormal findings are pale mucous membranes, tachycardia and panting, T = 39.4°C (102.9°F) and hepatosplenomegaly, which was noted at abdominal palpation.

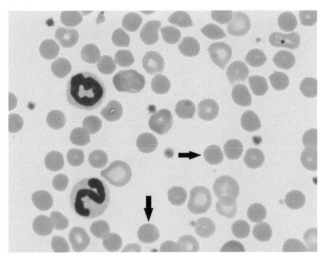

FIG. 83.1 Blood smear showing features typical of an immune-mediated haemolytic anaemia. There is moderate to marked anisocytosis of erythrocytes, polychromasia and a marked spherocytosis (arrows). A few platelets as well as two neutrophils are present. May–Grünwald–Giemsa, ×100 (oil).

QUESTIONS

1 List the main target autoantigens on the erythrocyte surface.
2 Which type of hypersensitivity is responsible for the development of immune-mediated haemolytic anaemia (IMHA)? Describe the pathogenesis.
3 What diseases may lead to secondary IMHA?

CASE 84

A 10-year-old Thoroughbred-cross mare presented with colic, pyrexia, anorexia and jaundice of 5 days' duration.

HAEMATOLOGY

Erythron variables were within the reference intervals and were unremarkable.

Measurand (units)	Result	Reference Interval
WBC count (10⁹/l)	**25.8**	6–12
Neutrophils (10⁹/l)	**16.6**	3–6.3
Band neutrophils (10⁹/l)	**3**	<0.17
Lymphocytes (10⁹/l)	1.8	1.3–4.3
Monocytes (10⁹/l)	**4**	<1
Eosinophils (10⁹/l)	0.4	<1

BIOCHEMISTRY

Analyte (units)	Result	Reference Interval
ALP (U/l)	**1,020**	<160
GGT (U/l)	**250**	<20
GLDH (U/l)	**95**	<8
Bile acids (μmol/l)	**62**	<15
Total bilirubin (μmol/l)	**215**	9–48
Direct (conjugated) bilirubin (μmol/l)	**80**	<17

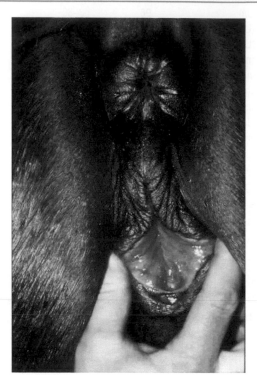

FIG. 84.1 Icteric vulvar mucous membrane.

QUESTIONS

1 Discuss the laboratory findings and their physiological significance.
2 What are your differential diagnoses based on these findings?
3 What tests should be carried out next in this mare?

CASE 85

A 9-year-old female German Shepherd Dog-cross had a history of acute fever up to 41.3°C (106.3°F) and anorexia. The dog was living in Germany but had been imported from Spain at the age of 18 months.

EXAMINATION FINDINGS

The dog was slightly lethargic with pale mucous membranes. Body temperature was 40.3°C (104.4°F). There was marked lameness of the left hindlimb. Thoracic and abdominal radiographs were unremarkable.

HAEMATOLOGY

Measurand (units)	Result	Reference Interval
RBC count (10¹²/l)	6.81	5.5–8.5
Haemoglobin (g/l)	100	80.6–122.1
Haematocrit (l/l)	0.45	0.39–0.56
MCV (fl)	66.3	60–77
Platelet count (10⁹/l)	**29**	150–500
WBC count (10⁹/l)	**4.8**	5.48–13.74
Neutrophils (10⁹/l)	3.89	2.78–8.73
Bands (10⁹/l)	0.24	<0.5
Lymphocytes (10⁹/l)	**0.38**	0.72–4.71
Monocytes (10⁹/l)	0.29	0.06–0.83
Eosinophils (10⁹/l)	0	<1.25
Basophils (10⁹/l)	0	<0.11

BLOOD SMEAR EVALUATION

The results of a blood smear evaluation are shown (**Figs. 85.1–85.3**).

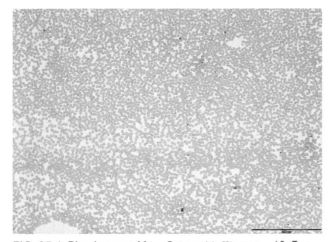

FIG. 85.1 Blood smear. May–Grünwald–Giemsa, ×10. Bar, 200 µm.

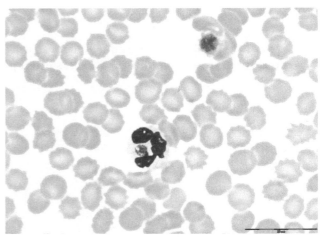

FIG. 85.2 Blood smear. May–Grünwald–Giemsa, ×100 (oil). Bar, 20 µm.

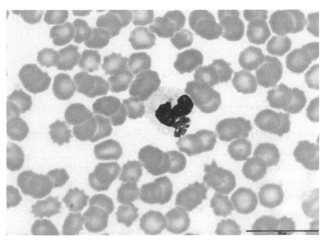

FIG. 85.3 Blood smear. May–Grünwald–Giemsa, ×100 (oil). Bar, 20 µm.

BIOCHEMISTRY

Analyte (units)	Result	Reference Interval
Total protein (g/l)	**74.3**	55.3–69.84
Albumin (g/l)	**28.2**	29.6–37.01
Globulins (g/l)	**46.1**	22.9–35.6

Other biochemistry parameters were unremarkable.

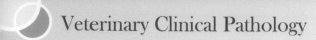

QUESTIONS

1 Have a look at the blood smear. What are the inclusions in the neutrophils?
2 Describe and discuss further abnormalities present on the smears.
3 Describe and discuss the haemogram.
4 Discuss the pattern of dysproteinaemia.
5 What recommendations do you have regarding treatment and prophylaxis?

CASE 86

A 10-month-old female Labrador Retriever was the smallest puppy of the litter. She appears blind from time to time. In addition, ataxia is often present.

HAEMATOLOGY

Measurand (units)	Result	Reference Interval
RBC count (10^{12}/l)	8	5.5–8.5
Haemoglobin (g/l)	143	130–195
Haematocrit (l/l)	0.48	0.37–0.55
MCV (fl)	**61**	62–73
MCH (pg)	**18.2**	21.7–42.2
MCHC (g/l)	**297**	335–379
Platelet count (10^9/l)	342	150–500
WBC count (10^9/l)	11	6–17
Neutrophils (10^9/l)	6.75	3.0–11.5
Lymphocytes (10^9/l)	3.1	1.0–3.6
Monocytes (10^9/l)	0.7	0.04–1.35
Basophils (10^9/l)	0.01	0.0–0.4
Eosinophils (10^9/l)	0.42	0.0–1.25

BIOCHEMISTRY

Analyte (units)	Result	Reference Interval
Total protein (g/l)	65.9	54–71
Albumin (g/l)	**25.5**	26–33
Globulins (g/l)	40.4	27–44
Glucose (mmol/l)	4.09	3.66–6.31
Total bilirubin (µmol/l)	0.62	0–3.4
Basal bile acids pre-prandial (µmol/l)	**61**	0–20
Bile acids post-prandial (µmol/l) (20 minutes post meal)	36	0–40
Bile acids post-prandial (µmol/l) 30 minutes post meal	30	0–40
Bile acids post-prandial (µmol/l) 40 minutes post meal	35	0–40
Cholesterol (mmol/l)	**2.68**	3.5–7.0
Triglycerides (mmol/l)	0.65	0.29–3.88
ALP (U/l)	**326**	0–97
ALT (U/l)	**103**	0–55
GLDH (U/l)	7	0–12
Urea (mmol/l)	**3.37**	3.57–8.57

Analyte (units)	Result	Reference Interval
Creatinine (µmol/l)	35	35–106
Sodium (mmol/l)	146	141–152
Chloride (mmol/l)	110	100–120
Potassium (10^9/l)	3.9	3.6–5.35
Ionised calcium (mmol/l)	**1.48**	1.16–1.31
Phosphate (mmol/l)	**2.65**	0.7–1.6

The bile acid challenge test was performed by giving two teaspoons of a high proteinaceous diet; 20, 30 and 40 minute post-prandial serum samples were obtained.

URINALYSIS

Item	Result	Reference Interval
USG	**1.024**	>1.030
Dipstick evaluation		
pH	8.5	
Bilirubin	**2+**	Negative to trace
Blood	Negative	Negative
Glucose	Negative	Negative
Ketone bodies	Negative	Negative
Protein	Negative	Negative to trace
Sediment analysis		
Erythrocytes	<5	0–5/hpf
Leucocytes	<5	0–5/hpf
Epithelial cells	None	
Crystals	None	Variable/lpf
Casts	None	
Bacteria	None	None

QUESTIONS

1 Describe and discuss the significant laboratory abnormalities, and indicate the most likely diagnosis.
2 What further tests would you recommend, and why?

CASE 87

A 1-year-old Whippet presented with lethargy after playing in the park. His owner mentioned that this occurred frequently after exercise, he sometimes appeared to have muscle cramps and that his urine was often port wine in colour after such episodes. On questioning it was apparent that his stool was sometimes dark yellow to orange in colour.

EXAMINATION FINDINGS

The dog had pale mucous membranes, tachycardia and a systolic heart murmur. Blood was submitted for a comprehensive profile, including haematology, biochemistry and urinalysis. NT-proBNP analysis was also requested to explore the possibility of cardiac disease given the clinical observations.

HAEMATOLOGY

Measurand (units)	Results	Reference Interval
RBC count (10^{12}/l)	**4.2**	5.0–8.5
Haemoglobin (g/l)	**113**	120–180
Haematocrit (l/l)	0.41	0.37–0.55
MCV (fl)	**97.6**	60–80
MCH (pg)	**26.9**	19–23
MCHC (g/l)	**276**	310–340
Platelet count (10^9/l)	-	200–500
WBC count (10^9/l)	10.7	6–15
Neutrophils (10^9/l)	5.7	3.0–11.5
Lymphocytes (10^9/l)	3.9	1.0–4.8
Monocytes (10^9/l)	0.9	0.0–1.3
Eosinophils (10^9/l)	0.3	0.1–1.25
NRBCs (cells/100 WBCs)	**126**	Up to 2–3 metarubricytes/ 100 WBCs
Reticulocytes (%)	**23.8**	
Reticulocytes (10^9/l)	**999.6**	0–60

BLOOD FILM EVALUATION

Polychromasia	**+++**
Metarubricytes and rubricytes	**Metarubricytes ++; rubricytes +**
Anisocytosis	**++**
Macrocytosis	**++**
Hypochromia	-
Spherocytes	-
Target cells	-
Howell–Jolly bodies	+
Platelets	Platelet count appears normal

BIOCHEMISTRY

Analyte (units)	Results	Reference Interval
Total protein (g/l)	66.8	54–77
ALP (U/l)*	47	0–50
ALT (U/l)*	21	0–25
Total bilirubin (µmol/l)	9.3	0–16

Analyte (units)	Results	Reference Interval
Bile acids (µmol/l)	5.8	0–10
CK (U/l)*	**557**	0–190
Glucose (mmol/l)	4.3	2.0–5.5
Amylase (U/l)*	800	100–900
Lipase (U/l)*	201	0–250
Urea (mmol/l)	6.6	1.7–7.4
Creatinine (µmol/l)	64	0–106
Sodium (mmol/l)	147	139–154
Potassium (mol/l)	**7.2**	3.6–5.6
Chloride (mmol/l)	109	105–122
Calcium (mmol/l)	2.43	2.3–3.0
Lead (µmol/l)	0.06	0.00–1.21
Phosphate (mmol/l)	1.03	0.89–1.60
NT-proBNP (pmol/l)	**1,238**	>1,000 (supports heart failure with clinical signs)
Coombs test	Negative @ 1:2	

* Analysis performed at 37°C.

URINALYSIS

Item	Results	Reference Interval
USG	1.035	>1.035
Dipstick evaluation		
pH	7	Acidic
Protein	**+++**	Negative to trace
Glucose	Negative	Negative
Ketone bodies	Negative	Negative
Urobilinogen	Negative	Negative
Bilirubin	**+**	Negative to trace
Haemoglobin	Negative	Negative
Biochemistry		
Protein (mg/dl)	6.937	
Creatinine (mmol/l)	20.58	
Protein:creatinine ratio	**2.95**	<0.5
Sediment analysis		
Erythrocytes (cells/mm³)	Negative	0–5/lpf
Leucocytes (cells/mm³)	<10	0–5/lpf
Epithelial cells	+/-	Rare/lpf
Crystals	Negative	Variable/lpf
Casts	Negative	Variable/lpf
Bacteria	Negative	None

QUESTIONS

1 Identify and list the abnormalities and explain their associations.
2 Is the automated low MCHC reported by the analyser genuine or not? Provide an explanation for your answer.
3 Two further samples over the following 3 months revealed similar findings. (1) Is the degree of regeneration appropriate for the degree of anaemia? (2) Is the number of nucleated RBCs appropriate for the degree of reticulocytosis?
4 Why is immune-mediated haemolytic anaemia (IMHA) not a consideration with this set of laboratory results?
5 Lead is within the reference interval, but which part of the haematological report may have prompted the veterinarian to request analysis of lead?
6 What is the most likely diagnosis with the excessive degree of erythrocyte regeneration, the mild degree of anaemia and evidence of clinical disease, particularly after exercise, along with this patient's breed?
7 What tests would be helpful in confirming a diagnosis?

CASE 88

An 8-year-old female neutered DSH cat presented for depression, anorexia and pale mucous membranes.

HAEMATOLOGY

Measurand (units)	Result	Reference Interval
RBC count (10¹²/l)	**1.77**	5.5–8.5
Haemoglobin (g/l)	**40**	120–180
Haematocrit (l/l)	**0.12**	0.37–0.55
MCV (fl)	68.2	60–77
MCH (pg)	22.4	19.5–24.5
MCHC (g/l)	329	320–370
RDW (%)	17.7	13.2–17.8
Reticulocytes (10⁹/l)	25.6	<50
Platelet count (10⁹/l)	**109**	175–500
WBC count (10⁹/l)	**3.8**	6–17
Neutrophils (10⁹/l)	**1.9**	3.0–11.5
Lymphocytes (10⁹/l)	**0.9**	1.0–4.8
Monocytes (10⁹/l)	0.5	0.2–1.5

BLOOD FILM EVALUATION

RBCs: no polychromasia; WBCs: no abnormalities seen; platelets: no platelet clumps seen.

BIOCHEMISTRY

Unremarkable.

QUESTIONS

1 How would you interpret this anaemia?
2 What further tests would you suggest? What is your diagnosis?

CASE 89

A 1-year-old female Miniature Schnauzer presented for vomiting.

EXAMINATION FINDINGS

A markedly painful cranial abdomen was noted.

ACID–BASE AND BLOOD GAS DATA

Analyte (units)	Result	Reference Interval
Arterial pH	**7.67**	7.36–7.44
PaCO₂ (mmHg)	40	36–44
PaO₂ (mmHg)	**100**	85–95
Plasma HCO₃⁻ (mmol/l)	**45**	18–26
Sodium (mmol/l)	145	145–155
Potassium (mmol/l)	**2.5**	4–5
Chloride (mmol/l)	**85**	105–115
Anion gap	17.5	15–25

QUESTIONS

1 What is your assessment of the arterial pH?
2 What is your assessment of the likely underlying aetiology for this arterial pH?
3 Is there appropriate compensation for this condition, and what does it suggest?
4 What might be the underlying causes for this condition?

CASE 90

A 5-year-old male gelded Exmoor pony had shown mild weight loss over the preceding 6 months but seemed otherwise well. At routine vaccination, a 15 cm diameter haematoma developed at the vaccination site on the neck.

HAEMATOLOGY

RBC and WBC variables are within the reference intervals.

Measurand (units)	Result	Reference Interval
Platelets (10⁹/l)	**180**	200–600

BIOCHEMISTRY

Analyte (units)	Result	Reference Interval
Total protein (g/l)	68.3	60–73
Albumin (g/l)	26	25–37
Globulins (g/l)	42.3	35–48
GGT (U/l)	**98**	<20
ALP (U/l)	**182**	<160
GLDH (U/l)	**15**	<8
Bile acids (μmol/l)	**15**	<15
Total bilirubin (μmol/l)	34	9–48
Urea (mmol/l)	7.2	2.5–8.3

HAEMOSTASIS

Analyte (units)	Result	Reference Interval
PT (seconds)	**25**	8–12.4
aPTT (seconds)	46	36–47

QUESTIONS

1 Discuss the laboratory findings and their significance.
2 What are your differential diagnoses?

CASE 91

An 8-year-old male Beagle presents with a limp in his right hindlimb a few hours after playing in the garden with another dog.

EXAMINATION FINDINGS

There are no external indications of trauma, but the knee joint is slightly swollen. Radiographs are unremarkable and both CBC and biochemistry parameters are normal. Aspiration of the joint produces fresh blood. There is no history of prior bleeding episodes, but the dog has never undergone any surgery or had any significant trauma.

COAGULATION PROFILE

Analyte (units)	Result	Reference Interval
aPTT (seconds)	10.5	<12.5
PT (seconds)	**45**	<9
Platelet count (10⁹/l)	346	200–500
D-dimer (g/l)	0.4	<0.5
Fibrinogen (g/l)	2	1–4

A TEG analysis shows a slightly prolonged R time, but otherwise normal tracing.

QUESTIONS

1 What is the likely defect?
2 What is the usual clinical severity of the defect in Beagles?
3 What advice would you give the owner regarding breeding?

CASE 92

A 3-year-old female neutered British shorthair cat is presented with anorexia, lethargy, weakness and PU/PD.

EXAMINATION FINDINGS

Examination revealed marked mental dullness, bradycardia (HR = 120 bpm), CRT >3 seconds, pale dry buccal mucous membranes and hypothermia (T = 32.7°C [90.9°F]). No arterial pulse could be felt.

HAEMATOLOGY

The results are unremarkable except for lymphocytes of $8.45 \times 10^9/l$ (reference interval, 1.5–7.0).

BIOCHEMISTRY

Analyte (units)	Result	Reference Interval
Total protein (g/l)	74.7	54.7–78.0
Albumin (g/l)	27.3	21–33
Globulin (g/l)	47.4	26–51
Glucose (mmol/l)	4.18	3.89–6.11
Total bilirubin (μmol/l)	2.69	0–3.4
Cholesterol (mmol/l)	**6.63**	2.46–3.37
Triglycerides (mmol/l)	1.03	0.57–1.14
ALP (U/l)	19	0–39.7
ALT (U/l)	57	0–70
GLDH (U/l)	1	0–11.3
CK (U/l)	**2,622**	<205
Fasting bile acids (μmol/l)	12	<20
Urea (mmol/l)	**23.53**	7.14–10.7
Creatinine (μmol/l)	**599**	0–168
Sodium (mmol/l)	**115**	141–150
Chloride (mmol/l)	**91**	110–125
Potassium (mmol/l)	**7.17**	3.6–4.8
Ionised calcium (mmol/l)	**1.47**	1.19–1.41
Phosphorus (mmol/l)	**3.76**	0.8–1.9
Ionised magnesium (mmol/l)	**0.67**	0.43–0.65

BLOOD GAS ANALYSIS (venous)

Analyte (units)	Result	Reference Interval
pH	**7.14**	7.31–7.40
PCO_2 (mmHg)	**31**	33.5–50.7
Sodium (mmol/l)	**121.1**	141–150
Potassium (mmol/l)	**7.99**	3.6–4.8
Ionised calcium (mmol/l)	**1.45**	1.12–1.32
Glucose (mmol/l)	4	3.8–6.1
Lactate (mmol/l)	1.6	0.4–2.2
Bicarbonate (mmol/l)	**10.4**	18.2–26.0
Base excess (mmol/l)	**−17.4**	−5.4–1.2

HORMONE TESTING

Analyte (units)	Result	Reference Interval
Aldosterone (ng/dl)	**<2.0**	5.4–15.5
Cortisol (μg/dl)	<0.3	<4

QUESTIONS

1 What is the most likely diagnosis?
2 What are the differential diagnoses for marked hyperkalaemia?
3 Why does metabolic acidosis develop in the condition diagnosed in this cat?

CASE 93
A 9-month-old Miniature Schnauzer had been recently bought and was presented by the owners for a health check.

URINALYSIS

Item	Result	Reference Interval
Colour	Dark yellow	Yellow
Transparency	**Turbid**	Clear
USG	1.048	1.020–1.045
Dipstick evaluation		
pH	6.0	Acidic
Leucocyte esterase	Negative	Negative
Nitrite	Negative	Negative
Protein	+	Trace
Protein (sulphasalicylic acid)	+	Trace
Glucose	Negative	Negative
Ketone bodies	Negative	Negative
Bilirubin	+	Negative to trace
Blood	+	Negative
Sediment analysis		
Amount	Increased	
Squamous epithelial cells	Sparse	
Transitional epithelial cells	Sparse	
Erythrocytes	Few	<5/ hpf
Leucocytes	Sparse	<5/ hpf
Crystals	Numerous	

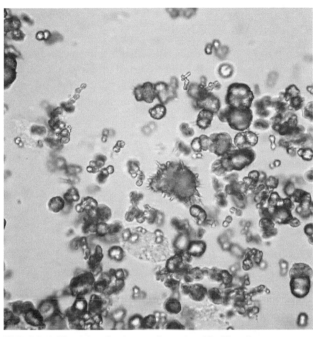

FIG. 93.1 Unstained urine sediment. ×40. (Courtesy Dr Judith Leidinger)

QUESTIONS

1 What is the nature of the crystals shown in **Fig. 93.1**?
2 What other crystals show a similar morphology?
3 What do they indicate?

CASE 94
A 14-year-old male mongrel dog presents for his annual health check. The owner reports that the dog is mildly lethargic and sleeps a lot, potentially due to his old age.

HAEMATOLOGY

Analyte (units)	Result	Reference Interval
RBC count (10¹²/l)	**4.2**	5.5–8.5
Haemoglobin (g/l)	**93**	130–195
Haematocrit (l/l)	**0.29**	0.37–0.55
MCHC (g/l)	322	320–379
MCV (fl)	69.5	62–73
Reticulocytes (cells/µl)	43,000	0–60,000
Platelet count (10⁹/l)	288	150–500
WBCs	Within normal limits	

QUESTIONS

1 Describe the abnormalities detected.
2 List possible causes for the finding and briefly describe the pathological mechanisms.

CASE 95

A 4-year-old male gelded pony developed severe, watery diarrhoea and recurrence of abdominal pain 2 days after recovery from a pelvic flexure impaction.

EXAMINATION FINDINGS

The pony was very dull and unwilling to stand. The oral mucous membranes were congested and had a 'toxic line' and petechial haemorrhages. Rectal temperature was 39.2°C (102.6°F) and there was oedema of the lower limbs.

HAEMATOLOGY

Measurand (units)	Result	Reference Interval
RBC count (10^{12}/l)	11.6	5.5–9.5
Haemoglobin (g/l)	170	80–140
Spun PCV (%)	55	24–45
MCV (fl)	47	40–56
MCHC (g/l)	301	300–370
Platelet count (10^9/l)	70	200–600
WBC count (10^9/l)	2.6	6–12
Neutrophils (10^9/l)	0.8	3.0–6.3
Band neutrophils (10^9/l)	0	<0.17
Lymphocytes (10^9/l)	1.3	1.3–4.3
Monocytes (10^9/l)	0.5	<1
Eosinophils (10^9/l)	0	<1
Basophils (10^9/l)	0	<0.3

BIOCHEMISTRY

Analyte (units)	Result	Reference Interval
Total protein (g/l)	86	60–73
Albumin (g/l)	38	25–37
Globulins (g/l)	48	35–48
Triglycerides (mmol/l)	3.5	<1.0
Glucose (mmol/l)	10.3	2.8–5.5
Urea (mmol/l)	18.2	2.5–8.3
Creatinine (µmol/l)	201	<177
Sodium (mmol/l)	128	134–150
Potassium (mmol/l)	6.3	2.7–5.9
Chloride (mmol/l)	88	96–102

HAEMOSTASIS

Analyte (units)	Result	Reference Interval
PT (seconds)	16	8.0–12.4

QUESTIONS

1 Discuss the laboratory findings and their significance.
2 What is your interpretation and any recommendations?

CASE 96

A 6-year-old male neutered DSH cat, which was slightly overweight, presented with anorexia, weight loss and depression over 1 week, with intermittent vomiting.

EXAMINATION FINDINGS

On examination the cat was depressed and had icteric mucous membranes.

HAEMATOLOGY

Measurand (units)	Result	Reference Interval
RBC count (10^{12}/l)	4.8	5–10
Haemoglobin (g/l)	75	80–150
Haematocrit (l/l)	0.24	0.24–0.45
MCV (fl)	41	39–55
MCHC (g/l)	313	300–360
Reticulocyte count (10^9/l)	45	0–60
Platelet count (10^9/l)	180	150–700

Measurand (units)	Result	Reference Interval
WBC count (10^9/l)	15.8	5.5–19.5
Neutrophils (10^9/l)	14.1	2.4–12.5
Band neutrophils (10^9/l)	0	0.0–0.3
Lymphocytes (10^9/l)	0.7	1.5–7.9
Monocytes (10^9/l)	0.9	0.0–0.9
Eosinophils (10^9/l)	0.1	0.0–1.5

BLOOD SMEAR EVALUATION

Erythrocytes showed 2+ acanthocytes, and occasional fragmented RBCs. The WBC morphology was normal. New methylene blue stain revealed 40% Heinz bodies (<5% are considered normal).

BIOCHEMISTRY

Analyte (units)	Result	Reference Interval
Total protein (g/l)	59	54–78
Albumin (g/l)	31	23–38
Globulins (g/l)	28	25–51
Total bilirubin (µmol/l)	**88**	0–5.1
Glucose (mmol/l)	**3.0**	3.7–6.8
ALT (U/l)	**332**	20–80
AST (U/l)	**410**	25–75
ALP (U/l)	**2,185**	11–210
GGT (U/l)	3	0–4
CK (U/l)	**523**	0–220
Urea (mmol/l)	**14.0**	6.1–11.4
Creatinine (µmol/l)	150	88–177
Calcium (mmol/l)	2.1	1.8–2.5
Phosphorus (mmol/l)	**1.1**	1.3–2.8
Sodium (mmol/l)	149	146–160
Potassium (mmol/l)	**3.2**	3.7–5.4
Chloride (mmol/l)	**109**	112–129
TCO₂ (mmol/l)	19	14–23

URINALYSIS (cystocentesis)

Item	Result	Reference Interval
Colour	Light yellow	Yellow
Transparency	Clear	Clear
USG	**1.020**	>1.030
Dipstick evaluation		
pH	7.0	
Bilirubin	**2+**	Negative to trace
Blood	**1+**	Negative
Glucose	Negative	Negative
Ketone bodies	Negative	Negative
Protein	1+	Negative to trace
Sediment analysis		
Erythrocytes	2	0–5/hpf
Leucocytes	0	0–5/hpf
Epithelial cells	2	None
Crystals	None	Variable/lpf
Casts	None	None
Bacteria	None	None/lpf
Others	1+ fat	

QUESTIONS

1 Interpret any abnormal laboratory results and discuss any pathophysiological mechanisms that could be causing changes in the laboratory values.

2 What further tests, laboratory or otherwise, are indicated in this case?

CASE 97
An 18-year-old pony mare presented during the summer with PU/PD of 3 months' duration.

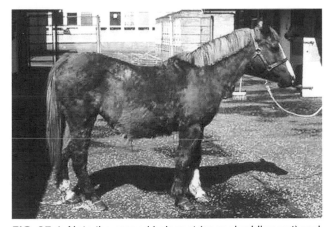

FIG. 97.1 Note the ragged hair coat (poor shedding out) and pot-bellied appearance.

HAEMATOLOGY

RBC variables are within reference intervals.

Measurand (units)	Result	Reference Interval
WBC count (10⁹/l)	**13.3**	6–12
Neutrophils (10⁹/l)	**10.9**	3.0–6.3
Band neutrophils (10⁹/l)	0	0.00–0.17
Lymphocytes (10⁹/l)	1.6	1.3–4.3
Monocytes (10⁹/l)	0.8	0.0–1.0
Eosinophils (10⁹/l)	0	0.0–1.0
Basophils (10⁹/l)	0	0.0–0.3

BIOCHEMISTRY

Analyte (units)	Result	Reference Interval
AST (U/l)	249	<290
GGT (U/l)	**45**	<20
GLDH (U/l)	**16**	<8
Bile acids (µmol/l)	14	<15
Urea (mmol/l)	7.2	2.5–8.3
Creatinine (µmol/l)	165	<177

ADDITIONAL TESTS

Requested after above results obtained.

Analyte (units)	Result	Reference Interval
Glucose (mmol/l)	**10.3**	2.8–5.5
Basal cortisol (nmol/l)	165	120–280
Cortisol following overnight dexamethasone suppression test – 40 µg/kg, IM (nmol/l)	**65**	<28

QUESTIONS

1 Discuss the laboratory findings and their significance.
2 What is your interpretation, and what is the underlying cause for this condition?

CASE 98

A 3-year-old female mongrel dog was spayed yesterday and lost some blood. Haematology was performed to evaluate the amount of inflammation and blood loss.

HAEMATOLOGY

Measurand (units)	Result	Reference Interval
RBC count (10¹²/l)	**4.08**	5.5–8.5
Haemoglobin (g/l)	**54**	74–112
Haematocrit (l/l)	**0.25**	0.37–0.55
MCHC (g/l)	199	196–221
MCV (fl)	73.9	60–77
Platelet count (10⁹/l)	457	150–500
WBC count (10⁹/l)	10.11	6.0–17.0
Neutrophils (10⁹/l)	8.10	3.0–11.5
Lymphocytes (10⁹/l)	1.01	1.0–3.6
Monocytes (10⁹/l)	0.53	0.04–1.35
Eosinophils (10⁹/l)	0.45	<1.25
Basophils (10⁹/l)	0.02	<0.04

QUESTIONS

1 This haematology case is referred to you for review because your technician says that the Rule of 3 has been violated. What is the Rule of 3?
2 What should be done if the Rule of 3 is violated?

CASE 99

A 6-year-old female Border Collie has been lethargic since yesterday. Today she is reluctant to get up.

HAEMATOLOGY

Measurand (units)	Result	Reference Interval
RBC count (10¹²/l)	**1.08**	5.5–8.5
Haemoglobin (g/l)	**46**	74–112
Haematocrit (l/l)	**0.14**	0.37–0.55
MCHC (g/l)	**328**	335–379
MCV (fl)	**80.1**	60–77
Reticulocyte count (cells/µl)	**210,000**	0–60,000
Platelet count (10⁹/l)	**66**	150–500

Measurand (units)	Result	Reference Interval
WBC count (10⁹/l)	**35**	6–17
Neutrophils (10⁹/l)	**27**	3.0–11.5
Band neutrophils (10⁹/l)	**2.5**	<0.5
Lymphocytes (10⁹/l)	2.97	1.0–3.6
Monocytes (10⁹/l)	**2.5**	0.04–1.35
Eosinophils (10⁹/l)	0.01	<1.25
Basophils (10⁹/l)	0.04	<0.04

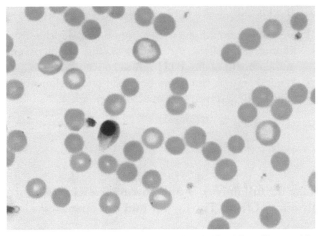

FIG. 99.1 Blood smear of the Border Collie. May–Grünwald–Giemsa, ×100 (oil).

QUESTIONS

1 Describe and discuss the significant haematological findings based on the results provided and present in the blood smear.
2 What further tests would you recommend, and why?

CASE 100

A 7-year-old male Tervueren had a 2-year history of occasionally rubbing his face and itching without evident cause. There was a 1-month history of seizures after exercise, associated with a weak pulse. Two days prior to referral he exhibited exercise intolerance, PU/PD and acute vomiting.

EXAMINATION FINDINGS

Unremarkable apart from a weak pulse. An ECG was also unremarkable.

HAEMATOLOGY

Unremarkable.

Analyte (units)	Result	Reference Interval
Potassium (mmol/l)	4.21	3.35–4.37
Ionised calcium (mmol/l)	**0.73**	1.32–1.51
Magnesium (mmol/l)	**0.45**	0.47–0.63
Phosphate (mmol/l)	**2.02**	0.70–1.60

BIOCHEMISTRY

Analyte (units)	Result	Reference Interval
Total protein (g/l)	66.8	55–70
Albumin (g/l)	**37.2**	30–37
Globulins (g/l)	29.6	23–36
Glucose (mmol/l)	5.45	3.3–6.5
Bilirubin (µmol/l)	3.02	<3.6
Cholesterol (mmol/l)	6.8	3.3–8.6
Triglycerides (mmol/l)	0.71	<0.75
ALP (U/l)	**200**	<131
ALT (U/l)	**203**	<85
GLDH (U/l)	**40**	<10
Amylase (U/l)	**2,651**	<1,157
Lipase (U/l)	**746**	<300
Osmolality (mOsm/kg)	306	289–313
Urea (mmol/l)	4.62	3.03–9.82
Creatinine (µmol/l)	57	53–123
Sodium (mmol/l)	148	147–152
Chloride (mmol/l)	106	102–110

URINALYSIS (cystocentesis)

Item	Result	Reference Interval
USG	**1.023**	>1.030
Dipstick evaluation		
pH	7.6	
Bilirubin	Negative	Negative
Blood	**+**	Negative
Glucose	Negative	Negative
Protein	**++**	Negative
UPCR	**0.7**	<0.2 (<1.0)
Sediment analysis		
Erythrocytes	<5	0–5/hpf
Leucocytes	**>5**	0–5/hpf
Epithelial cells	Negative	0–5/hpf
Crystals	Negative	Variable
Casts	Negative	None
Bacteria	Negative	Negative

hpf: ×40 magnification.

ADDITIONAL TEST

Serum parathormone (PTH) concentration determined at the time of presentation was 25 pg/ml (reference interval, 8–45 pg/ml).

QUESTIONS

1 Describe and discuss the significant biochemistry findings as well as the results of the urinalysis and measurement of the PTH serum concentration.
2 What diagnosis can be made based on the clinical and laboratory findings, and what is the prognosis?

CASE 101

A 12-year-old Quarter horse gelding presented because of dull hair coat and chronic weight loss over the last 3 months, despite increasing the amount of feed. The owner had not observed increased urination or abnormalities in the stool.

BIOCHEMISTRY AND URINALYSIS

The initial findings included azotaemia, hypercalcaemia and isosthenuric USG (1.014). The veterinarian was suspicious of chronic renal failure as a likely cause for the clinical signs and initial laboratory findings.

QUESTIONS

1 Compare and contrast AKI and chronic renal failure in the horse with regard to common clinical presentation, common clinicopathological findings and prognostic indicators.
2 What is the underlying mechanism for the development of hypercalcaemia in chronic renal disease in the horse?

CASE 102

A 3-year-old Arabian gelding presented for severe weight loss (Fig. 102.1), a poor appetite, dysphagia and mild colic (especially soon after eating) for the past 2 weeks. No therapy was administered other than an NSAID as required for the mild colic. Over the past 2 days, the horse developed urinary tenesmus.

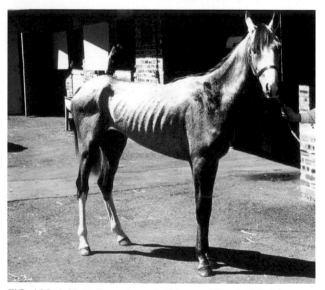

FIG. 102.1 Note the extremely thin condition in this horse.

HAEMATOLOGY

Measurand (units)	Result	Reference Interval
RBC count (10^{12}/l)	**10.74**	5.5–9.5
Haemoglobin (g/l)	**170**	80–140
Haematocrit (l/l)	**0.48**	0.24–0.45
MCV (fl)	45	40–56
MCHC (g/l)	354	340–380
Leucogram and platelets	No abnormality detected	

PERIPHERAL BLOOD SMEAR EVALUATION

No abnormalities were noted.

BIOCHEMISTRY

Analyte (units)	Result	Reference Interval
Total protein (g/l)	63.2	47–67
Albumin (g/l)	35.8	25–37
Globulins (g/l)	27.4	19–37
ALP (U/l)	**354**	<130
GGT (U/l)	17	<20
AST (U/l)	442	258–554
CK (U/l)	**364**	<80
GLDH (U/l)	5	<8
Bile acids (µmol/l)	12.5	1–15
Total bilirubin (µmol/l)	**102.2**	17–40
Urea (mmol/l)	**17.5**	2.5–8.3
Creatinine (µmol/l)	97	40–150

Analyte (units)	Result	Reference Interval
Calcium (mmol/l)	3.11	2.6–3.3
Glucose (mmol/l)	5.1	2.8–5.5
Magnesium (mmol/l)	0.74	0.6–1.0
Potassium (mmol/l)	3.9	2.7–5.9
Sodium (mmol/l)	140	134–150
Chloride (mmol/l)	**87**	98–118

QUESTIONS

1 What is your analysis of these results?
2 What is your primary diagnosis?

CASE 103

A 5-year-old female neutered indoor/outdoor DSH cat is reported to be 'not herself' over the last 2 days. There is suspected access to rodenticide recently put out in the apartment building in which this cat lives. No blood is observed in the urine or faeces.

EXAMINATION FINDINGS

The cat is quiet, but bright, alert and responsive.

HAEMATOLOGY

Within normal limits.

COAGULATION PROFILE

Analyte (units)	Result	Reference Interval
PT (seconds)	10	6–11
aPTT (seconds)	**64**	10–25

QUESTIONS

1 Why do these results rule out rodenticide toxicity?
2 What are your differential diagnoses, and why?

CASE 104

A 4-month-old male Maine Coon cat presented with a history of dyspnoea and lethargy of 2 weeks' duration. The referring veterinarian had administered diuretics.

EXAMINATION FINDINGS

The cat appeared underdeveloped for a male Maine Coon cat of this age and dull heart and respiratory sounds were detected on the right side of the thorax. Tachypnoea and severe mixed dyspnoea were also present. Radiography revealed a severe thoracic effusion.

HAEMATOLOGY

Measurand (units)	Result	Reference Interval
RBC count (10^{12}/l)	8.41	5–10
Haemoglobin (g/l)	81	49–93
Haematocrit (l/l)	0.35	0.24–0.45
MCV (fl)	41.4	40–55
Platelet count (10^9/l)	290	180–550
WBC count (10^9/l)	15.7	6.0–18.0
Neutrophils (10^9/l)	12.08	2.5–12.5
Lymphocytes (10^9/l)	**1.37**	1.5–7.0
Monocytes (10^9/l)	**1.24**	0.04–0.85
Eosinophils (10^9/l)	0.8	0.0–1.50
Basophils (10^9/l)	0.04	0.0–0.04
Large unstained cells [LUCs] (10^9/l)	0.12	0.0–0.58

LUCs: this variable is specific for the ADVIA 120/2120® Haematology System and includes plasma cells, reactive lymphocytes and lymphoblasts.

BIOCHEMISTRY

Analyte (units)	Result	Reference Interval
Total protein (g/l)	**78.3**	54.7–78.0
Albumin (g/l)	24.3	21–33
Globulins (g/l)	**53.7**	26–51
Glucose (mmol/l)	4.47	3.9–6.1
Bilirubin (μmol/l)	1.49	<3.4
Cholesterol (mmol/l)	2.77	2.46–3.37
Triglycerides (mmol/l)	0.34	<1.14
ALP (U/l)	33	<40
ALT (U/l)	**172**	<70
GLDH (U/l)	**102**	<11.3
Urea (mmol/l)	**11.93**	7.14–10.7
Creatinine (μmol/l)	46	<168
Sodium (mmol/l)	**157**	147–156
Chloride (mmol/l)	**113**	102–110
Potassium (mmol/l)	3.8	3.60–4.80
Phosphate (mmol/l)	1.85	0.8–1.9

THORACIC EFFUSION EXAMINATION

The fluid was yellow, highly viscous, slightly turbid and contained several fibrin clots. The following results were obtained:

Variable (units)	Result	Transudate	Modified Transudate	Exudate
Nucleated cell count (10^9/l)	0.5	<1	<5	>5
SG gravity (refractometer)	1.041	<1.017	>1.017	>1.025
Total protein (g/l)	68	<25	>25	>30

Editors' note: The criteria for classification as modified transudate and exudate may vary, depending on the source. Some sources use >7.5 or $>10.0 \times 10^9$/l as cut-offs for nucleated cell counts required for classification as an exudate. Some sources use >35 g/l total protein as a cut-off for classification as an exudate.

CYTOLOGY

Direct smears of the effusion were of low cellularity. On a granular eosinophilic highly proteinaceous background, a few non-degenerate neutrophils were present.

QUESTIONS

1 Describe and discuss the significant haematological and biochemistry findings, as well as the results of the fluid analysis.
2 What diagnosis can be made based on the clinical and laboratory findings, and what is the prognosis?

CASE 105

One animal out of a group of eight yearling to 3-year-old unbroken horses at pasture was found dead following a heavy rainstorm in the autumn with near freezing temperatures. Two animals were recumbent and two animals appeared stiff or weak and reluctant to move. One animal was observed urinating with red–brown discolouration of the urine. These horses did not have supplementary feeding. The horse with observed red–brown urine discolouration was brought to the veterinary clinic for further evaluation.

HAEMATOLOGY

Within normal limits.

BIOCHEMISTRY

Analyte (units)	Result	Reference Interval
Total protein (g/l)	66	47–67
Albumin (g/l)	37	25–37
Globulins (g/l)	29	19–37
ALP (U/l)	120	<130
GGT (U/l)	17	<20
AST (U/l)	**3,400**	258–554
CK (U/l)	**120,000**	<80
GLDH (U/l)	**15**	<8
Bile acids (µmol/l)	12.5	1–15

Analyte (units)	Result	Reference Interval
Glucose (mmol/l)	**8.5**	2.8–5.5
Urea (mmol/l)	7	2.5–8.3
Creatinine (µmol/l)	97	40–150
Calcium (mmol/l)	**2.45**	2.6–3.3
Magnesium (mmol/l)	0.65	0.6–1.0
Potassium (mmol/l)	3.9	2.7–5.9
Sodium (mmol/l)	140	134–150
Chloride (mmol/l)	102	98–118

QUESTIONS

1 What is your analysis of these results?
2 What are your differential diagnoses?

CASE 106

A 7-year-old mongrel dog presented as an emergency case after a car accident.

EXAMINATION FINDINGS

The dog was in lateral recumbency, had an increased HR and showed red mucous membranes with prolonged CRT.

ACID–BASE AND BLOOD GAS DATA

Analyte (units)	Result	Reference Interval
Arterial pH	**7.02**	7.36–7.44
PaCO$_2$ (mmHg)	40	36–44
PaO$_2$ (mmHg)	**35**	85–95
Plasma HCO$_3^-$ (mmol/l)	**10**	18–26
Serum Na$^+$ (mmol/l)	145	145–155
Serum K$^+$ (mmol/l)	**6.5**	4–5
Serum Cl$^-$ (mmol/l)	107	105–115
Anion gap	**34.5**	15–25

QUESTIONS

1 What is your assessment of the arterial pH?
2 What is your assessment of the likely underlying aetiology for this arterial pH?
3 Is there appropriate compensation for this condition, and what does it suggest?
4 What might be the underlying causes in this patient?

CASE 107

An 8-year-old female Border Collie presented for PU/PD and severe lethargy.

HAEMATOLOGY

Unremarkable.

BIOCHEMISTRY

Analyte (units)	Result	Reference Interval
Total protein (g/l)	62.2	54–71
Albumin (g/l)	31.1	26–33
Globulins (g/l)	31.2	27–44
Glucose (mmol/l)	**37.03**	3.66–6.31
Cholesterol (mmol/l)	**9.41**	3.5–7.0
Triglycerides (mmol/l)	0.59	0.29–3.88
ALP (U/l)	95	0–97
ALT (U/l)	**66**	0–55
GLDH (U/l)	**17**	0–12
Urea (mmol/l)	8.11	3.57–8.57
Creatinine (µmol/l)	68	35–106
Sodium (mmol/l)	**139**	141–152
Chloride (mmol/l)	106	100–120
Potassium (mmol/l)	**3.1**	3.6–5.35
Ionised calcium (mmol/l)	1.28	1.16–1.31
Phosphate (mmol/l)	0.81	0.7–1.6

BLOOD GAS ANALYSIS (venous)

Analyte (units)	Result	Reference Interval
pH	**7.1**	7.36 ± 0.02
PCO$_2$	**29.6**	43 ± 3
PO$_2$	58.7	58 ± 9
HCO$_3^-$	**9.0**	23 ± 1

URINALYSIS

Item	Result	Reference Interval
USG	1.042	>1.030
Dipstick evaluation		
pH	7.0	
Bilirubin	Negative	Negative to trace
Blood	Negative	Negative
Glucose	**2+**	Negative
Ketone bodies	**Positive**	Negative
Protein	Negative	Negative
Sediment analysis		
Erythrocytes	<5	0–5/hpf
Leucocytes	<5	0–5/hpf
Epithelial cells	None	
Crystals	None	Variable/hpf
Casts	None	
Bacteria	None	None

QUESTIONS

1 Describe and discuss the significant laboratory abnormalities, and discuss possible diagnoses.
2 How is the anion gap (AG) calculated, and how do you interpret the AG in this case? What differential diagnoses do you have for the increased AG detected in this dog?

CASE 108

A 4-year-old male neutered Fox Terrier weighing approximately 12 kg (26.4 lb) ate three sticks of sugar-free gum containing xylitol about 15 minutes ago.

BIOCHEMISTRY

Analyte (units)	Result	Reference Interval
Total protein (g/l)	62.2	54–71
Albumin (g/l)	31.1	26–33
Globulins (g/l)	31.2	27–44
Glucose (mmol/l)	**2.9**	3.66–6.31
Cholesterol (mmol/l)	6.4	3.5–7.0
Total bilirubin (µmol/l)	**5.6**	0–3.4
ALP (U/l)	**122**	0–97
ALT (U/l)	**157**	0–55
Urea (mmol/l)	8.11	3.57–8.57
Creatinine (µmol/l)	68	35–106

Analyte (units)	Result	Reference Interval
Sodium (mmol/l)	149	141–152
Chloride (mmol/l)	106	100–120
Potassium (mmol/l)	**3.1**	3.6–5.35
Ionised calcium (mmol/l)	1.28	1.16–1.31
Phosphate (mmol/l)	**2.1**	0.7–1.6

QUESTIONS

1 Describe the laboratory abnormalities present as well as the bases for these. What clinical signs do you expect in association with this history?
2 Would you expect this amount of ingestion to be toxic?

CASE 109
A 17-week-old male neutered Tiffanie cat presented for ill thrift. Feline coronavirus was known to be present within the breeding colony.

EXAMINATION FINDINGS

Pyrexia, pleural effusion, poor body condition.

PCR TESTING

A PCR test for feline coronavirus on the pleural effusion was positive.

PLEURAL FLUID PROTEIN ELECTROPHORESIS

Total pleural fluid protein (bromocresol green method) = 79 g/l.

FIG. 109.1 Stained agarose gel.

Protein fraction (g/l)	Result	
	(%)	(g/l)
Albumin	29.16	23.07
Alpha-1 globulin	2.66	2.10
Alpha-2 globulin	13.58	10.74
Beta globulins	12.28	9.72
Gamma globulins	42.32	33.48

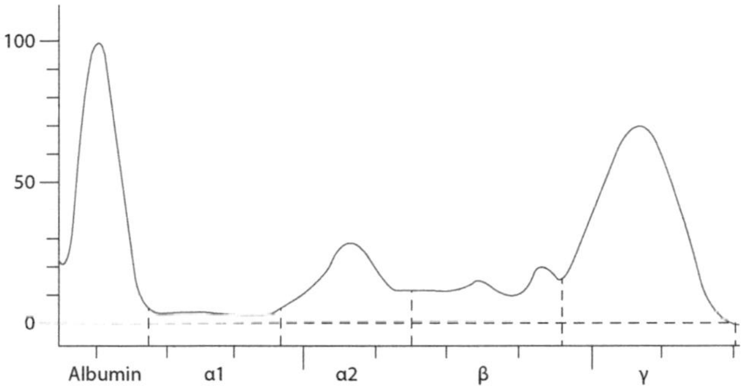

FIG. 109.2 Densitometry tracing of agarose gel.

QUESTIONS

1 What is your assessment of the fluid protein electrophoresis results?
2 What is the most likely clinical diagnosis?

CASE 110
A young female cat, thought to be neutererd (age unknown since recently rehomed) has recently started exhibiting clinical signs suggestive of oestrus (vocalisation, restlessness).

FELINE hCG STIMULATION TEST

Analyte (units)	Result	Reference Interval
Basal progesterone (nmol/l) taken 1–3 days after onset of oestral behaviour	2.2	<3.0
Progesterone (nmol/l) 7 days after hCG administration	22.0	>5.0 indicative of ovarian tissue

QUESTIONS

1 What is your interpretation of these test results?
2 How does the hCG protocol and testing differ in the dog and the cat?
3 What result would you expect in this cat if you performed a vaginal cytology?

CASE 111

A 1-year-old female DSH cat was spayed 1 week ago. During surgery, slight blood loss occurred. Haematology parameters are now assessed to determine recovery from anaemia. The haematology analyser used in this cat employed an impedance method.

HAEMATOLOGY

Measurand (units)	Result	Reference Interval
RBC count (10¹²/l)	6.9	5–10
Haemoglobin (g/l)	82	49–93
Haematocrit (l/l)	0.26	0.24–0.45
MCV (fl)	**36.2**	40–55
MCH (pg)	11	7.7–11.0
MCHC (g/l)	292	184–300
Platelet count (10⁹/l)	**109**	180–550
WBC count (10⁹/l)	7.1	6–18

BIOCHEMISTRY

No abnormalities are present.

QUESTIONS

1 What is the most likely explanation for the microcytic RBCs (decreased MCV)?
2 What further diagnostics can you perform to detect the cause of the microcytic RBCs?

CASE 112

An 8-year-old female neutered Cavalier King Charles Spaniel (CKCS) presented for tachypnoea that had been ongoing for 2 months. There was a history of recurrent infections (hypersalivation with mouth ulcers, urinary tract infection and kennel cough).

HAEMATOLOGY

Measurand (units)	Result	Reference Interval
RBC count (10¹²/l)	**3.28**	5.5–8.5
Haemoglobin (g/l)	**90**	120–180
Haematocrit (l/l)	**0.27**	0.37–0.55
MCV (fl)	73.2	60–77
MCH (pg)	23.3	19.5–24.5
MCHC (g/l)	320	320–370
RDW (%)	15.4	13.2–17-8
Platelet count (l0⁹/l)	**45**	175–500
WBC count (l0⁹/l)	**19.9**	6–17
Neutrophils (l0⁹/l)	11.2	3.0–11.5

Measurand (units)	Result	Reference Interval
Lymphocytes (l0⁹/l)	**7.2**	1.0–4.8
Monocytes (l0⁹/l)	0.8	0.2–1.5
Eosinophils (l0⁹/l)	0.7	0.1–1.3

BLOOD FILM EVALUATION

RBCs: no polychromasia, slight anisocytosis; WBCs: few reactive lymphocytes; platelets: no platelet clumps, mainly large platelets seen.

BIOCHEMISTRY

Unremarkable.

CYTOLOGY (bronchoalveolar lavage [BAL])

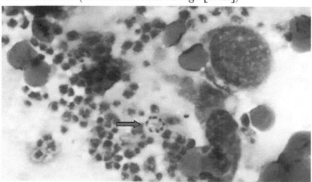
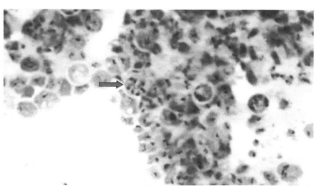

FIGS. 112.1, 112.2 Note the chronic and active inflammation with multiple organisms (orange arrows). Wright–Giemsa, ×100 (oil).

QUESTIONS

1 How would you classify this anaemia? Give a possible explanation for this classification.
2 Give a possible explanation for the lymphocytosis.
3 Give a possible explanation for the thrombocytopaenia.
4 What is the microorganism in the BAL?
5 What further investigations would you recommend?
6 What is your overall interpretation?

CASE 113

A 2-year-old female alpaca was one of several in a herd showing signs of progressive weight loss, decreased appetite and lethargy. The farmer initially thought it may just have been due to reduced nutritional value of the winter pasture, but he became more concerned as the animal's condition deteriorated.

EXAMINATION FINDINGS

The alpaca had an increased RR and HR. Her mucous membranes were moist, but pale. Samples were taken for an FBC, partial biochemistry and faecal analysis.

HAEMATOLOGY

Measurand (units)	Result	Reference Interval
RBC count (10^{12}/l)	**2.46**	11.20–14.4
Haemoglobin (g/l)	**25**	114–188
Haematocrit (l/l)	**0.07**	0.30–0.42
MCV (fl)	29	26–31
MCHC (g/l)	357	350–417
Reticulocytes (%)	**20**	<1.4
Reticulocytes (10^9/l)	**492**	12–79
NRBCs (cells/100 WBC)	**140**	Up to 2–3 (metarubricytes/100 WBCs)
Platelet count (10^9/l)	565	91–858
WBC count (10^9/l)	**2.0**	6.0–20.9
Neutrophils (10^9/l)	**1.5**	2.0–13.3
Lymphocytes (10^9/l)	**0.2**	2.0–6.8
Monocytes (10^9/l)	0.2	<0.8
Eosinophils (10^9/l)	0.1	<2.7
Basophils (10^9/l)	0	Rare

BLOOD FILM EVALUATION

The total WBC count has been corrected for the presence of NRBCs. The platelet count seemed adequate on the smear. No haemoparasites were detected.

BIOCHEMISTRY

Analyte (units)	Result	Reference Interval
Total protein (g/l)	52	48–65
Albumin (g/l)	28	9–45
Globulins (g/l)	24	1–30
GLDH (U/l)	**36**	0–9
GGT (U/l)	21	0–28
AST (U/l)	220	6–307
CK (U/l)	138	8–483
Total bilirubin (μmol/l)	**3.8**	0–3.4
Urea (mmol/l)	10.4	2.5–11.4
Creatinine (μmol/l)	120	82–171
Sodium (mmol/l)	145	143–154
Potassium (mmol/l)	7	3.5–8.6
Calcium (mmol/l)	1.86	1.5–2.9
Phosphate (mmol/l)	**0.2**	1.3–3.3
Magnesium (mmol/l)	**0.8**	0.9–1.1
Beta-hydroxy-butyrate (mmol/l)	0	0–0.2
Iron (μmol/l)	**40**	10–29
Glutathione peroxidase (U/g Hgb)	28	5–200
Copper (μmol/l)	8.5	6–15
Vitamin B_{12} (pmol/l)	166	150–2,000
Fibrinogen (g/l)	3.5	1–5

SUPPLEMENTARY TESTS

Faecal floatation: negative for parasites.
Haematest: negative for occult blood.
Urinalysis: no abnormalities detected.

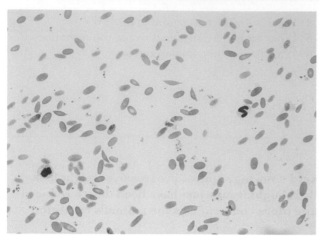 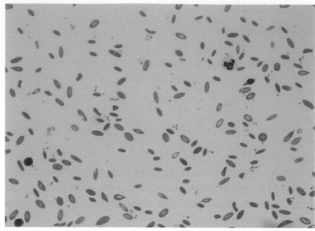

FIGS. 113.1, 113.2 Blood smear from an alpaca. Modified Wright–Giemsa, ×60.

QUESTIONS

1 Describe the abnormalities observed in these photomicrographs of the blood film.
2 List the abnormalities detected in the laboratory profile and their potential associations.
3 List differentials for regenerative anaemia in an alpaca.

4 Explain the pathophysiological mechanism by which hypophosphataemia causes haemolysis.
5 What other laboratory test would you like to perform to determine a potential cause of hypophosphataemia in this type of animal in the winter?

CASE 114

A 12-year-old Thoroughbred-Cleveland Bay mare is presented for investigation and treatment of lethargy and inappetence following an episode of azoturia (exertional rhabdomyolysis) 3 days previously. She was exercised 4 days earlier with some steep incline work undertaken. During this ride the owner noticed that the mare started sweating up excessively and became stiff in the hind quarters. The condition did not improve after turn out to pasture. On subsequent examination by the referring veterinarian, the mare was treated for exertional rhabdomyolysis (confirmed on biochemistry) with flunixin meglumine IV and box (stall) rest. After an initial response to treatment, the mare became inappetent, was unwilling to drink and was lethargic, prompting referral. The owner reported that the mare had suffered at least one previous episode of tying-up.

EXAMINATION FINDINGS

On presentation, the mare was quiet but alert and responsive. She was in good body condition (BCS 3/5), weighing 522 kg (1,150 lb). A mild tachycardia (48 bpm) was present but all other vital parameters were within normal limits. The oral mucous membranes were pale pink and tacky, with a CRT of 2 seconds. Gastrointestinal borborygmi were normal throughout the abdomen. The hind quarter musculature, in particular the gluteal mass and the caudal thigh muscles (semimembranosus and semitendinosus), were tense and painful on palpation.

IV and enteric fluid therapy were instituted following collection of initial specimens for laboratory evaluation.

HAEMATOLOGY

Unremarkable except for neutrophilia of $12.2 \times 10^9/l$ (reference interval, 2.7–6.8).

BIOCHEMISTRY

Analyte (units)	Result				Reference Interval
	Day 1	Day 2	Day 5	Day 7	
Total protein (g/l)	75.5				47–67
Albumin (g/l)	28.5				25–37
Globulins (g/l)	47				19–37
AST (U/l)	24,286	7,637			<240
CK (U/l)	16,435	1,669		4,289	<150
Total bilirubin (µmol/l)	102.2				17–40
Urea (mmol/l)	28.1	21.2	5.0		<6.8
Creatinine (µmol/l)	787	515			62–140
Calcium (mmol/l)	3.7				2.6–3.3
Glucose (mmol/l)	5.1				2.8–5.5
Potassium (mmol/l)	5.8				2.7–5.9
Sodium (mmol/l)	125				134–150
Chloride (mmol/l)	88				98–118

URINALYSIS

Item	Result	Reference Interval
USG	1.008	>1.025
Fractional excretion of electrolytes		
Sodium (%)	10.8	<1.0
Chloride (%)	8.8	0.1–1.6
Potassium (%)	292	15–65

Urine sediment analysis
Occasional RBCs, WBCs and granular casts.

QUESTIONS

1 What is your assessment of these results?
2 What is the most likely cause of the continued inappetence and lethargy in this mare?
3 What is the pathophysiological basis for myoglobinuric nephrosis?

CASE 115

A 12-year-old male neutered DSH cat presented with clinical signs of anaemia. He was fully vaccinated; the last vaccination was about 1 year previously.

HAEMATOLOGY

FBC revealed a moderate normocytic-normochromic regenerative anaemia (PCV = 20%).

BIOCHEMISTRY

The plasma was markedly haemolytic. A chemistry panel showed hyperproteinaemia and azotaemia (both urea and creatinine increased by about three times the upper reference limit).

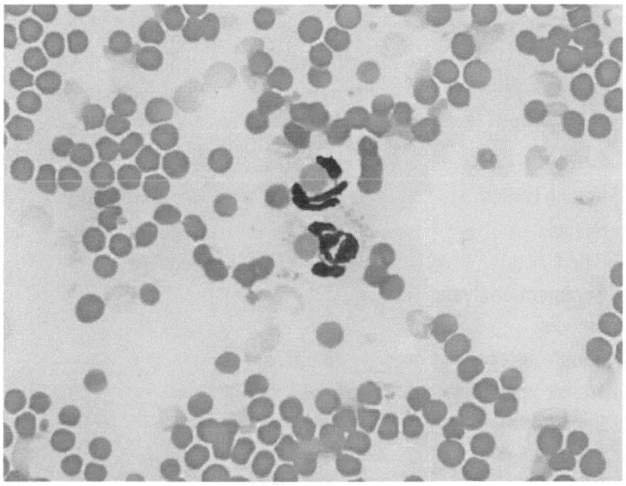

BLOOD FILM EVALUATION

See **Fig. 115.1**.

QUESTIONS

1 How would you describe the RBC morphology?
2 What is a strong indication for an immune-mediated anaemia in this case?
3 What additional test could be useful?

FIG. 115.1 Peripheral blood smear. May–Grünwald–Giemsa, ×100 (oil).

CASE 116

A 3-year-old female neutered cat presented for vomiting and polydipsia. She was suspected of having ingested antifreeze approximately 6 hours ago because the owner was changing antifreeze in the garage this morning.

BIOCHEMISTRY

Analyte (units)	Result	Reference Interval
Total protein (g/l)	60.6	54.7–78.0
Albumin (g/l)	26.3	21–33
Globulins (g/l)	34.3	26–51
Glucose (mmol/l)	**20**	3.89–6.11
ALP (U/l)	37	0–39.7
ALT (U/l)	23	0–70
CK (U/l)	198	0–205
Urea (mmol/l)	10.7	7.14–10.7
Creatinine (µmol/l)	164	0–168
Sodium (mmol/l)	155	147–156
Chloride (mmol/l)	127	115–130
Potassium (mmol/l)	4.7	3.6–4.8
Ionised calcium (mmol/l)	**0.87**	1.17–1.32
Phosphate (mmol/l)	**3.1**	0.8–1.9

QUESTIONS

1 Describe and discuss the laboratory abnormalities present. What are the bases for the changes that are present? How will the laboratory abnormalities change over the next few days if this is EG toxicity and it is left untreated?
2 What findings would you expect in a blood gas analysis over the same time frame?
3 What findings would you expect in an urinalysis over the same time frame?
4 What is the prognosis for EG toxicity?

CASE 117

A 2-year-old female neutered Beagle presents with a history of incoordination, ataxia, somnolence and seizures. She had vomited twice and showed marked polyuria. The owner reported that the dog had access to the garage and might have ingested some spilled liquid a few hours ago.

HAEMATOLOGY

FBC showed a polycythaemia (PCV = 62%).

BIOCHEMISTRY

Azotaemia (urea = 27.8 mmol/l; creatinine = 371 µmol/l); hyperkalaemia (6.0 mmol/l); hypocalcaemia (1.9 mmol/l).

URINALYSIS

Item	Result	Reference Interval
Colour	Pale yellow	
Transparency	Turbid	Clear
USG	**1.017**	1.020–1.045

Item	Result	Reference Interval
Dipstick evaluation		
pH	5.0	Acidic
Leucocyte esterase	+	Negative
Nitrite	Negative	Negative
Protein	++	Negative to trace
Protein (SSA)	++	Traces
Glucose	Negative	Negative
Ketone bodies	Negative	Negative
Bilirubin	Positive +	Negative to trace
Blood	+	Negative
Sediment analysis		
Amount	Increased	
Squamous epithelial cells	Negative	
Transitional epithelial cells	**Few**	
Erythrocytes	**Few**	Rare
Leucocytes	**Few**	Rare
Crystals	**Many (156)**	

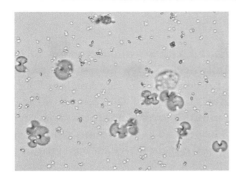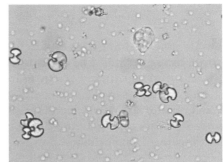

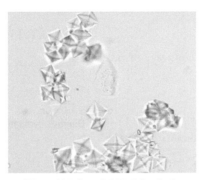

FIGS. 117.1–117.3 Unstained urine sediment. **Figs. 117.1** and **117.2** (top) show exactly the same aspect of urinary sediment but with different tiers in focus. **Fig. 117.3** (bottom) shows the same sediment in a different area of the preparation. Wet-drop preparations, ×40. (Courtesy Dr Judith Leidinger)

QUESTIONS

1 What are the crystals in focus in **Figs. 117.1** and **117.2**?
2 What are the crystals in focus in **Fig. 117.3**?

3 What is clinically the most important cause of the concurrent occurrence of the two crystals?

CASE 118
A 14-year-old female neutered DSH presented with weakness and cervical ventroflexion and weight loss.

EXAMINATION FINDINGS

A mid-intra-abdominal mass was palpated. Ultrasound determined that this was due to a unilateral adrenal mass.

BIOCHEMISTRY

Analyte (units)	Result	Reference Interval
Total protein (g/l)	60.6	54.7–78.0
Albumin (g/l)	23.3	21–33
Globulins (g/l)	37.3	26–51
Glucose (mmol/l)	5.3	3.89–6.11
ALP (U/l)	24	0–39.7
ALT (U/l)	55	0–70
CK (U/l)	**670**	0–205
Urea (mmol/l)	**13.3**	7.14–10.7

Analyte (units)	Result	Reference Interval
Creatinine (µmol/l)	**199**	0–168
Sodium (mmol/l)	**159**	147–156
Chloride (mmol/l)	210	115–130
Potassium (mmol/l)	**2.6**	3.6–4.8
Ionised calcium (mmol/l)	1.2	1.17–1.32
Phosphate (mmol/l)	**2.2**	0.8–1.9

QUESTIONS

1 Describe the present laboratory abnormalities. What is the most likely diagnosis?
2 What further laboratory findings are expected in this disease? What are their pathophysiological bases?
3 What other disease(s) or condition(s) is (are) commonly associated with this condition in cats?

CASE 119

A 7-year-old female neutered Springer Spaniel presented with a 3-month history of intermittent vomiting, multiple times per day. The vomiting usually occurs a few hours after eating and contains bile, mucus and ingesta in varying states of digestion. The dog has lost 5 kg (11 lb) body weight and has had a progressive decrease in appetite. She is fully vaccinated and is dewormed regularly with an appropriate dewormer, including monthly treatment for heartworm, and is fed a well balanced commercial pelleted dog food. There is no access to any other food sources. A previous trial therapy of an exclusion diet was carried out for 3 weeks, but with no clinical response.

EXAMINATION FINDINGS

The dog appeared thin, abdominal palpation was normal and she was well hydrated.

HAEMATOLOGY

Unremarkable. Plasma protein by refractometry = 49 g/l (reference interval, 60–80).

BIOCHEMISTRY

Analyte (units)	Result	Reference Interval
Total protein (g/l)	**44**	54–74
Albumin (g/l)	**21**	27–45
Globulins (g/l)	23	19–34
Total bilirubin (μmol/l)	**7**	0–6.8
Cholesterol (mmol/l)	**3.2**	3.4–9.6
ALT (U/l)	**135**	10–120
AST (U/l)	38	16–140
ALP (U/l)	**305**	35–280
Glucose (mmol/l)	5.2	3.5–6.0
Amylase (U/l)	1,200	50–1,250
Lipase (U/l)	93	30–560
Urea (mmol/l)	3.6	2.5–10.0
Creatinine (μmol/l)	98	80–150
Calcium (mmol/l)	2.4	2.25–2.80
Phosphorus (mmol/l)	0.93	0.89–1.95
Sodium (mmol/l)	152	145–158
Potassium (mmol/l)	4.8	4.1–5.5
Chloride (mmol/l)	106	106–127

URINALYSIS (cystocentesis)

Item	Result	Reference Interval
Colour	Pale yellow	Yellow
Transparency	Clear	Clear
USG	1.011	>1.030
Dipstick evaluation		
pH	6.9	
Protein	Negative	Negative to trace
Glucose	Negative	Negative
Bilirubin	**2+**	Negative to trace
Blood	Negative	Negative
Sediment analysis		
Leucocytes	2/hpf	>10/hpf
Erythrocytes	3/hpf	>10/hpf
Epithelial cells	Negative	
Crystals	Negative	
Casts	Occasional triple phosphate (struvite)	
Bacteria	Negative	Negative

FAECAL PARASITES

Negative.

QUESTIONS

1 Based on this history, how would you differentiate vomiting from regurgitation?
2 Give a list of possible differentials for the dog's chronic vomiting.
3 Evaluate the laboratory data and give explanations for the abnormalities seen.
4 Discuss a diagnostic plan.

CASE 120

An adult entire male stray cat (age unknown) presented because it was skinny, had a rough hair coat and had mild lymphadenopathy of the peripheral lymph nodes.

HAEMATOLOGY

Slight to moderate non-regenerative anaemia. Erythrocytes displayed these findings (**Fig. 120.1**).

QUESTIONS

1 Describe the findings visible on the blood smear. What is the most likely diagnosis in this patient?
2 State the underlying pathophysiological mechanism for the development of the non-regenerative anaemia.
3 What diagnostic test can you perform to confirm the suspicion raised by the finding on the blood smear?

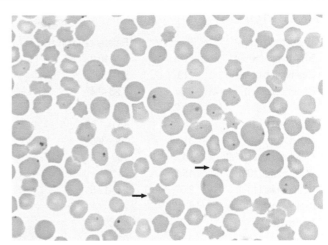

FIG. 120.1 Erythrocytes (arrows) of a male stray cat. May–Grünwald–Giemsa, ×100 (oil).

CASE 121

A 3-year-old female Hereford-Highland-cross cow with a calf at its side had withdrawn from the rest of a herd of 12 cows with calves at foot. They were turned out to fresh grass approximately 1 month ago, after being housed for the winter and fed hay and silage. One cow was found dead in the last week, but a possible cause was not investigated. There were scuff marks in the ground surrounding the dead cow, suggesting struggling or convulsions prior to death.

EXAMINATION FINDINGS

The cow was uncoordinated and staggered or fell sometimes, bellowed when approached and was aggressive to anyone approaching her. Nystagmus was present. Rapid HR (120 bpm) and RR (45 bpm). The heart sounds were quite loud.

HAEMATOLOGY

Haematology findings were within normal limits.

BLOOD SMEAR EVALUATION

RBC and WBC morphology within expected limits. The platelet estimate was adequate.

BIOCHEMISTRY

Analyte (units)	Result	Reference Interval
Total protein (g/l)	72	65–76
Albumin (g/l)	23.5	23–39
Creatinine (μmol/l)	72	61–133
Glucose (mmol/l)	3.9	2.6–3.9
Sodium (mmol/l)	**139**	140–146
Potassium (mmol/l)	**7.5**	3.5–4.6
Chloride (mmol/l)	105	98–110
Magnesium (mmol/l)	**0.32**	0.75–1.30
Calcium (mmol/l)	**1.9**	2.45–3.18

QUESTIONS

1 What is your assessment of these findings?
2 What is the most likely clinical diagnosis?
3 What are the physiological bases for these findings?

CASE 122

A 4-year-old female neutered British blue cat presented because of very thin body condition, inappetence, possible left kidney enlargement and possible polydipsia.

HAEMATOLOGY

Measurand (units)	Result	Reference Interval
RBC count (10^{12}/l)	7.75	5.5–10.0
Haemoglobin (g/l)	119	90–150
Haematocrit (l/l)	0.31	0.26–0.47
MCV (fl)	41.2	35.1–53.9
MCH (pg)	15.4	13.0–17.5
MCHC (g/l)	**373**	280–360
Platelet count (10^9/l)	**94**	150–550
WBC count (10^9/l)	**15.8**	6–15
Neutrophils (10^9/l)	8.37	2.5–12.5
Lymphocytes (10^9/l)	6	2–7
Monocytes (10^9/l)	1.26	<0.60
Eosinophils (10^9/l)	0.16	0.00–0.70

BLOOD FILM EVALUATION

Some platelet clumping; true count probably higher than indicated. Few large form platelets. Platelet estimate adequate.

BIOCHEMISTRY

Analyte (units)	Result	Reference Interval
Total protein (g/l)	**109.3**	60–80
Albumin (g/l)	27.3	25–45
Globulins (g/l)	**82**	25–45
A:G ratio	**0.33**	0.6–1.5
ALT (U/l)	**200**	5–60
ALP (U/l)	31	<60
GGT (U/l)	1.4	1–9
Total bilirubin (µmol/l)	**59.7**	0.1–5.1
Bile acids (µmol/l)	**196.9**	1–5
Cholesterol (mmol/l)	5.5	2.2–4.0
Triglycerides (mmol/l)	0.76	0.3–1.2
Amylase (U/l)	**1,462**	100–1,200
Lipase (U/l)	29.6	0.1–89.0
CK (U/l)	**1,152**	20–225
Urea (mmol/l)	7	2.5–9.9
Creatinine (µmol/l)	98.2	20.0–177
Sodium (mmol/l)	147.2	145–157
Potassium (mmol/l)	3.50	3.5–5.5
Na:K ratio	**42.06**	28–40
Chloride (mmol/l)	109.9	100–124
Phosphorus (mmol/l)	1.36	0.9–2.2
Calcium (mmol/l)	2.19	2.05–2.95

SERUM PROTEIN ELECTROPHORESIS

Fraction (g/l)	Result	Reference Interval
Albumin	**24.05**	25–45
Alpha-1 globulin	4.08	2–5
Alpha-2 globulin	**16.01**	2–5
Beta globulin	**16.2**	6–11
Gamma globulins	**48.95**	12–32

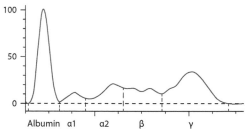

FIG. 122.1 Stained agarose gel electrophoresis. Albumin band is at the bottom of the gel. Left gel (26) is from a cat with a normal electrophoretic pattern. Right gel (23) is from this patient.

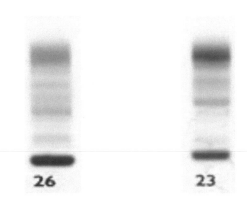
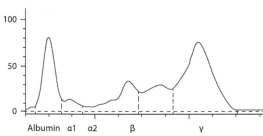

FIG. 122.2 Densitometry tracing of agarose gel. Top tracing is from a cat with a normal electrophoretic pattern. Bottom tracing is from this patient.

QUESTIONS

1 What is your analysis of these findings?
2 What additional testing might be of benefit in this case?

CASE 123

An 11-month-old male Giant Schnauzer presented because of anorexia, lethargy and a failure to thrive.

HAEMATOLOGY

The thrombon and leucon are within reference interval.

Measurand (units)	Result	Reference Interval
RBC count (10^{12}/l)	**4.62**	5.5–8.5
Haemoglobin (g/l)	**103**	115–180
Haematocrit (l/l)	**0.31**	0.37–0.55
MCV (fl)	66.40	60–77
MCHC (g/l)	335	335–379

BIOCHEMISTRY

Analyte (units)	Result	Reference Interval
Cobalamin (pmol/l)	**13,948.2**	22,140–59,040
Folic acid (nmol/l)	24.47	9.06–27.31

QUESTIONS

1 How do you interpret the laboratory findings?
2 Describe the process from cobalamin ingestion to cobalamin absorption.
3 How do cobalamin and folate interact?

CASE 124

A 6-year-old male neutered Labrador Retriever presented because of a change in temperament in the last few months and constipation in the last few days.

HAEMATOLOGY

Unremarkable.

BIOCHEMISTRY

Analyte (units)	Result	Reference Interval
Total protein (g/l)	61	55–75
Albumin (g/l)	34	25–40
Globulins (g/l)	32	23–35
Glucose (mmol/l)	6.0	3.3–6.5
ALP (U/l)	112	0–130
ALT (U/l)	69	0–85
Urea (mmol/l)	7.8	3.3–8.0
Creatinine (µmol/l)	140	45–150
Sodium (mmol/l)	145	135–155
Chloride (mmol/l)	115	105–120
Potassium (mmol/l)	**5.3**	3.35–4.37
Total calcium (mmol/l)	**3.57**	2.30–2.80
Ionised calcium (mmol/l)	**1.48**	1.18–1.40
Phosphate (mmol/l)	**0.5**	0.78–1.41

BIOCHEMISTRY (few days later)

Analyte (units)	Result	Reference Interval
Total calcium (mmol/l)	**1.95**	2.30–2.80
Ionised calcium (mmol/l)	**1.09**	1.18–1.40

QUESTIONS

1 How would you explain the initial high calcium?
2 What additional test would you do?
3 What is your suspicion?
4 How would you explain the reduced calcium concentration after a few days?

CASE 125

A 2-year-old female neutered DSH cat presented for lethargy and anorexia of 2 days' duration.

HAEMATOLOGY

Measurand (units)	Result	Reference Interval
RBC count (10¹²/l)	**0.98**	5.5–8.5
Haemoglobin (g/l)	**21**	120–180
Haematocrit (l/l)	**0.06**	0.37–0.55
MCV (fl)	63.5	60–77
MCH (pg)	21.1	19.5–24.5
MCHC (g/l)	333	320–370
RDW (%)	**23.6**	13.2–17.8
Platelet count (10⁹/l)	195	175–500
WBC count (10⁹/l)	6.8	6–17
Neutrophils (10⁹/l)	4.7	3.0–11.5
Lymphocytes (10⁹/l)	2	1.0–4.8
Monocytes (10⁹/l)	**0.1**	0.2–1.5
Eosinophils (10⁹/l)	**0**	0.1–1.3

BLOOD FILM EVALUATION

RBCs: rare polychromatophils (0–1 polychromatophils/hpf, ×100); WBCs: within normal limits; platelets: no platelet clumps.

BIOCHEMISTRY

Unremarkable. Very slight and non-specific increase in ALT and AST.

SEROLOGY

Analyte	Result
FIV (SNAP test)	Negative
FeLV (SNAP test)	**Positive**

QUESTIONS

1 How would you describe this anaemia, and what are the possible causes?
2 What further investigation would you suggest?
3 Could FeLV infection be related to this?
4 What is your overall interpretation?

CASE 126

A 2-year-old female Basenji presented because of recurrent episodes of lethargy and weakness. Exercise intolerance was also noted. A diagnostic panel to exclude infectious disease was negative.

EXAMINATION FINDINGS

Hepatosplenomegaly and pale mucous membranes were found.

HAEMATOLOGY

Measurand (units)	Result	Reference Interval
RBC count (10¹²/l)	**2.1**	5.5–8.5
Haemoglobin (g/l)	**53**	74–112
Haematocrit (l/l)	**0.16**	0.37–0.55
MCV (fl)	76	60–77
MCH (pg)	**25.2**	12–15.1
MCHC (g/l)	**331.2**	196–221
NRBCs (%)	**72**	Rare
Platelet count (10⁹/l)	498	150–500
WBC count (10⁹/l)	15	6–17
Neutrophils (10⁹/l)	10.4	3.0–11.5
Lymphocytes (10⁹/l)	2.6	1.0–3.6
Monocytes (10⁹/l)	0.9	0.04–1.35
Basophils (10⁹/l)	0	0.0–0.4
Eosinophils (10⁹/l)	1.1	0.0–1.25

Technical comment: total WBC count corrected for NRBCs.

BLOOD SMEAR EVALUATION

No poikilocytosis of erythrocytes visible. Marked polychromasia.

QUESTIONS

1 Describe and discuss the haematological abnormalities.
2 Describe the underlying pathophysiology of the most likely cause of this dog's condition.
3 What other diagnostics can you perform to confirm your suspicion of disease?
4 What other breeds may have this disease?

CASE 127

A 17-year-old Warmblood gelding presented for repeated episodes of laminitis. Pituitary pars intermedia dysfunction (equine Cushing's disease) had been excluded previously by ACTH measurement.

EXAMINATION FINDINGS

There was an increased temperature of all the hooves, a strong pulse in the digital arteries and a reluctance to move. The horse is obese with abnormal fat deposits above the orbits, in the neck and crest, behind the shoulder and at the tail head.

HAEMATOLOGY

Measurand (units)	Result	Reference Interval
RBC count (10^{12}/l)	7.5	6.5–11.0
Haemoglobin (g/l)	132	100–180
Haematocrit (l/l)	0.37	0.32–0.53
MCV (fl)	50	37–55
Platelet count (10^9/l)	181	103–244
WBC count (10^9/l)	7	5–10
Neutrophils (10^9/l)	5.7	3–7
Lymphocytes (10^9/l)	**1**	1.5–4.0
Monocytes (10^9/l)	**0.7**	0.0–0.5
Eosinophils (10^9/l)	0.3	0.0–0.4

BIOCHEMISTRY AND ENDOCRINOLOGY

Analyte (units)	Result	Reference Interval
Total protein (g/l)	72	55–75
Total bilirubin (µmol/l)	15.39	11.97–53.01
ALP (U/l)	240	<350
AST (U/l)	**588**	<500

Analyte (units)	Result	Reference Interval
GLDH (U/l)	**24.7**	<13
GGT (U/l)	27.9	<30
LDH (U/l)	**570**	<450
CK (U/l)	**276**	<200
Triglycerides (mmol/l)	**0.78**	<0.57
Cholesterol (mmol/l)	**33.93**	10.36–31.08
Glucose (mmol/l)	**12.59**	3.05–5.27
Urea (mmol/l)	5.2	3.3–8.8
Creatinine (µmol/l)	61.88	<176.8
Calcium (mmol/l)	2.9	2.0–3.2
Phosphorus (mmol/l)	0.5	0.5–1.3
Magnesium (mmol/l)	0.7	0.7–1.2
Sodium (mmol/l)	133	126–157
Potassium (mmol/l)	4.3	3.5–4.5
Chloride (mmol/l)	**96**	98–107
Iron (µmol/l)	37.05	11.81–37.77
Insulin (µU/l)	**299**	5–36

QUESTIONS

1 What is the most likely cause for the lymphopaenia?
2 What is the presumptive clinical diagnosis?
3 What are the four biochemical findings that indicate this disease most consistently?
4 What calculated measurands can be used in addition to the measured ones?

CASE 128

A practitioner calls and needs help with a case. He regularly performs health checks on his patients and includes haematology examination and biochemistry as well as C-reactive protein (CRP). He uses CRP as it is extremely sensitive in the detection of acute-phase reactions and disease in an early state. In this dog the haematology and biochemistry findings were within reference intervals. The CRP results are:

Month	May	June	July	August
CRP (mg/l)	7.5	8.9	6.9	12.2
Reference interval	0–9.4			

The practitioner is worried that there may be an acute-phase reaction in the dog as the August CRP is above the upper limit of the reference interval. However, there are no clinical signs, fever or abnormalities in the leucocytes.

QUESTIONS

1 Is the CRP increase significant based on data on biological variation and reference change value (RCV)?
2 What is the index of individuality (IoI) for CRP, and how do you interpret it?

CASE 129

A group of six adult horses at pasture had been treated 3 days previously for dried/wilted red maple leaf ingestion. Two of the horses died. One horse appeared to be recovering, but on the third day he became lethargic, stopped eating and drinking and was observed to be passing only a small amount of urine.

HAEMATOLOGY

Measurand (units)	Result	Reference Interval
RBC count (10^{12}/l)	**3**	5.5–9.5
Haemoglobin (g/l)	**52**	80–140
Haematocrit (l/l)	**0.15**	0.24–0.45
MCV (fl)	50	40–56
MCHC (g/l)	346	340–380
Platelet count (10^9/l)	225	100–360
WBC count (10^9/l)	**14.98**	6–12
Neutrophils (10^9/l)	**12.3**	3.0–6.3
Band neutrophils (10^9/l)	0	0–0.17
Lymphocytes (10^9/l)	0.98	1.3–4.3
Monocytes (10^9/l)	**1.7**	0–1.0
Eosinophils (10^9/l)	0	0–1.0
Basophils (10^9/l)	0	0–0.3
Fibrinogen (g/l) (heat-precipitation method)	3	2–4

BLOOD FILM EVALUATION

No toxic changes in WBC observed. Platelet estimate adequate.

BIOCHEMISTRY

Analyte (units)	Result	Reference Interval
Total protein (g/l)	**80.4**	58–75
Albumin (g/l)	31.4	23–35
Globulins (g/l)	49	30–50
GGT (U/l)	19	13–44

Analyte (units)	Result	Reference Interval
GLDH (U/l)	2	1–12
AST (U/l)	**210**	258–554
CK (U/l)	**500**	150–385
Total bilirubin (µmol/l)	**55**	17–34
Urea (mmol/l)	**12.5**	2.5–8.3
Creatinine (µmol/l)	**225**	40–150
Calcium (mmol/l)	**2.4**	2.6–3.3
Phosphorus (mmol/l)	**3.9**	0.8–1.8

URINALYSIS

USG in a sample collected prior to institution of fluid therapy at this presentation is 1.015 (reference interval, >1.020). Haemoglobinuria was present at the initial presentation for toxicity, but had resolved.

QUESTIONS

1 What is your analysis of these results?
2 What are your differential diagnoses?
3 What abnormalities of Na^+, Cl^- and K^+ would you expect to find?

CASE 130

A 9-year-old female Boxer presented because of mild lethargy and a skin tumour on a hindlimb.

HAEMATOLOGY

Unremarkable except for several abnormal cells that were visible in the feathered edge and throughout a blood smear (**Fig. 130.1**).

BIOCHEMISTRY

Unremarkable.

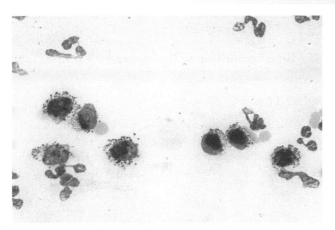

FIG. 130.1 Blood smear. Note the abnormal cells in the feathered edge and throughout the slide. May–Grünwald–Giemsa, ×50.

QUESTIONS

1 What are the granulated cells in the blood smear? What is your diagnosis?
2 What diseases can lead to this finding on a blood smear?
3 Briefly describe the hypersensitivity reaction of which these cells are a part.
4 Where do these cells originate from, and what stimuli lead to their final differentiation?
5 Several of the cells contain metachromatic granules. Why are these granules termed 'metachromatic'?
6 List the three metachromatic dyes.

CASE 131
A 20-year-old gelded Thoroughbred horse presented because of weight loss and diarrhoea.

HAEMATOLOGY

Measurand (units)	Result	Reference Interval
RBC count (10¹²/l)	**5.28**	7–11
Haemoglobin (g/l)	98	95–155
Haematocrit (l/l)	**0.28**	0.32–0.48
MCV (fl)	**53.2**	39–49
MCHC (g/l)	349	310–386
Platelet count (10⁹/l)	96	80–200
WBC count (10⁹/l)	**11.6**	5.8–11.0
Neutrophils (10⁹/l)	**9.28**	3.0–6.5
Lymphocytes (10⁹/l)	2.09	2–5
Monocytes (10⁹/l)	**0.12**	0.2–1.0
Eosinophils (10⁹/l)	0.12	0.1–0.5

Analyte (units)	Result	Reference Interval
ALP (U/l)	169	138–225
GGT (U/l)	7	0–53
AST (U/l)	260	256–369
Bile acids (µmol/l)	1.0	0–20
CK (U/l)	160	154–270
Urea (mmol/l)	7.0	3.0–7.5
Creatinine (µmol/l)	128	95–180
Sodium (mmol/l)	145	134–146
Chloride (mmol/l)	100	100–108
Potassium (mmol/l)	4.4	3.2–4.8
Total calcium (mmol/l)	3.4	2.9–3.4
Phosphate (mmol/l)	1.0	0.8–1.2

BLOOD FILM EVALUATION

RBCs: moderate rouleaux, proteinaceous background; WBCs: no morphological abnormalities; platelets: no platelet clumps, estimate 'adequate'.

BIOCHEMISTRY

Analyte (units)	Result	Reference Interval
Total protein (g/l)	**129**	58–67
Albumin (g/l)	**17**	32–40
Globulins (g/l)	**112**	22–40
Glucose (mmol/l)	5.3	3.3–6.5

QUESTIONS

1 How would you explain the presence of rouleaux?
2 How would you interpret the anaemia?
3 How would you explain the increase in total protein, and what tests would you recommend to further investigate this?
4 What are the main differential diagnoses?

CASE 132

A 12-year-old Connemara-cross gelding has been 'off colour' according to the owner.

EXAMINATION FINDINGS

No abnormality was detected on examination by the referring equine practitioner. He makes enquiries about urinary fractional excretion of electrolytes (UFEE) in horses and wants to know in what conditions this may be helpful.

QUESTIONS

1 What samples are required to perform UFEE?
2 What electrolytes are assessed?
3 What are typical reference intervals for UFEE?
4 In what conditions might UFEE be helpful?

CASE 133

The four coagulation tests described complement each other in the characterisation of coagulopathies.

QUESTION

1 Fill in the empty boxes in the Table with the expected findings (prolonged [time], decreased [concentration] or unaffected).

Condition/Treatment	PT	aPTT	Platelets	Buccal Mucosal Bleeding Time (BMBT)
Thrombocytopaenia				
DIC				
Warfarin treatment/poisoning or vitamin K deficiency				
Aspirin treatment				
von Willebrand's disease				
Haemophilia				
Uraemia				

CASE 134

A 3-year-old female neutered Labrador Retriever developed multiple ecchymotic areas on the ventral thorax 1 day post surgery for bite wounds in the neck region.

EXAMINATION FINDINGS

The dog is lethargic, febrile, tachypnoeic and has a weak femoral pulse with a rate of 220 bpm. A TEG analysis is performed (**Fig. 134.1**)

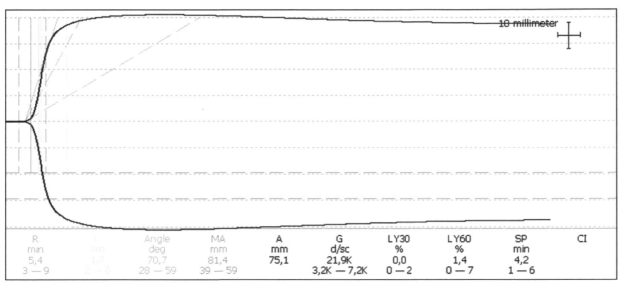

R min		Angle deg	MA mm	A mm	G d/sc	LY30 %	LY60 %	SP min	CI
5,4	1,7	70,7	81,4	75,1	21,9K	0,0	1,4	4,2	
3 — 9	2 — 8	28 — 59	39 — 59		3,2K — 7,2K	0 — 2	0 — 7	1 — 6	

FIG. 134.1 TEG tracing from this patient. R = 5.4 min (3–9 min); K = **1.7 min** (2–8 min); Angle = **70.7⁰** (28–59⁰); MA = **81.4 mm** (39–59 mm).

QUESTIONS

1 What is the likely complication?

2 Interpret the TEG results.

3 Explain the pathogenesis of the complication seen in this patient.

CASE 135
A 5-year-old male neutered cross-breed dog presented because of diarrhoea and muscle tremors.

HAEMATOLOGY

Measurand (units)	Result	Reference Interval
RBC count (10¹²/l)	**2.71**	5.5–8.5
Haemoglobin (g/l)	**72**	120–180
Haematocrit (l/l)	**0.28**	0.37–0.55
MCV (fl)	**104**	60–77
MCH (pg)	**26.6**	19.5–24.5
MCHC (g/l)	**250**	320–370
RDW (%)	16.8	13.2–17.8

Measurand (units)	Result	Reference Interval
Platelet count (10⁹/l)	191	175–500
WBC count (10⁹/l)	**17.4**	6–17
Neutrophils (10⁹/l)	**14.8**	3.0–11.5
Lymphocytes (10⁹/l)	**0.8**	1.0–4.8
Monocytes (10⁹/l)	1.5	0.2–1.5
Eosinophils (10⁹/l)	0.3	0.1–1.3

BLOOD FILM EVALUATION

Autoagglutination was observed macroscopically and was persistent with a saline agglutination test (saline dilution test). RBCs: marked anisocytosis, marked polychromasia, few NRBCs, moderate numbers of spherocytes (**Fig. 135.1**); WBCs: no significant morphological abnormalities; platelets: no platelet clumps observed.

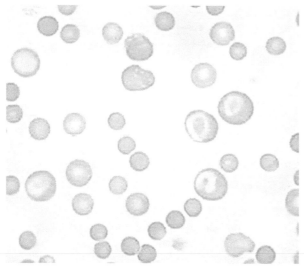

FIG. 135.1 Marked anisocytosis, high numbers of polychromatophils and spherocytes. Wright–Giemsa, ×100 (oil).

BIOCHEMISTRY

Analyte (units)	Result	Reference Interval
Total protein (g/l)	61	55–75
Albumin (g/l)	35	25–40
Globulins (g/l)	26	23–35
Glucose (mmol/l)	**6.9**	3.3–6.5
ALP (U/l)	125	0–130
ALT (U/l)	45	0–85
Urea (mmol/l)	8.0	3.3–8.0
Creatinine (μmol/l)	70	5–150
Sodium (mmol/l)	145	135–155
Chloride (mmol/l)	105	105–120
Potassium (mmol/l)	**4.4**	3.35–4.37
Total calcium (mmol/l)	**1.57**	2.3–2.8
Ionised calcium (mmol/l)	**0.77**	1.18–1.40
Phosphate (mmol/l)	**2.7**	1.78–1.41

QUESTIONS

1 How would you interpret this anaemia?
2 How would you interpret the mild leucocytosis observed?
3 How would you explain the low calcium, and what additional tests would you suggest?
4 Give a possible explanation for this case.

CASE 136
A 3-year-old male neutered Dachshund dog presents for pale mucous membranes, tachycardia and profound lethargy.

EXAMINATION FINDINGS

Haematology revealed a moderate, highly regenerative anaemia accompanied by a moderate number of spherocytes consistent with immune-mediated haemolytic anaemia (IMHA). One drop of blood was placed on a glass slide to evaluate autoagglutination (**Fig. 136.1**).

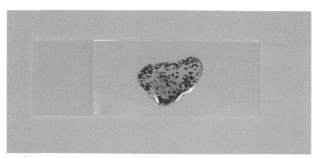

FIG. 136.1 Blood on a glass slide.

QUESTIONS

1 How do you interpret the finding visible in **Fig. 136.1**?
2 What additional test should be performed to confirm the finding?

CASE 137

A 5-year-old female Labrador Retriever is referred for surgery because of a possible bite wound, which keeps oozing blood after flushing and treatment with antibiotics (unspecified).

EXAMINATION FINDINGS

On initial examination the dog is slightly depressed, a clot is hanging from the wound surface and the removed bandage is soaked with blood. She is admitted to the hospital. Initial blood work is requested and further action is pending results. Three hours after admission the dog becomes severely depressed, acutely lame in the right hindlimb with massive swelling of the thigh area, and the PCV drops from 36% to 14%.

QUESTIONS

1 What abnormalities would you expect to find in blood work results if this dog has a coagulopathy secondary to angiostrongylosis (lungworm)?
2 What findings would you expect in a faecal examination, and what type of faecal testing is usually necessary to diagnose angiostrongylosis?
3 What is the prognosis for the coagulopathy in angiostrongylosis?

CASE 138

A 6-year-old female neutered Cocker Spaniel presented because it had been anorexic for 1 day.

EXAMINATION FINDINGS

The dog was quiet, alert and responsive with moderate petechiae on the oral mucous membranes and the inside of the ear pinnae.

HAEMATOLOGY

Unremarkable except for platelets of $3 \times 10^9/l$ (reference interval, 200–500).

BLOOD FILM EVALUATION

Erythrocyte morphology: no abnormality detected; leucocyte morphology: no abnormality detected; platelet estimate: markedly decreased, few clumps observed, few large-form platelets present.

QUESTIONS

1 What is your interpretation of these findings?
2 What is the relationship between the laboratory and clinical findings?
3 What other clinical findings are commonly observed with this laboratory abnormality?
4 Why is evaluation of the peripheral blood film critical?
5 What is the significance of the few large form platelets seen in the peripheral blood film?
6 What are your differential diagnoses?
7 What is the most likely clinical diagnosis, and why?

CASE 139
A 5-year-old female neutered diabetic cat is presented.

HAEMATOLOGY

A mild non-regenerative anaemia is noted (**Fig. 139.1**).

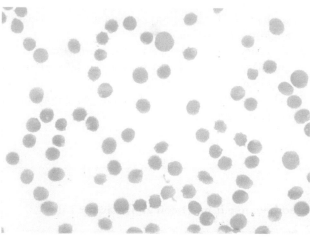

FIG. 139.1 Blood smear from this cat. May–Grünwald–Giemsa, ×100 (oil). (Courtesy Dr Ernst Leidinger)

QUESTIONS

1 Describe the erythrocytes and make a diagnosis.
2 How can you confirm your finding?
3 Briefly describe the pathophysiological changes leading to this condition, including possible causes.

CASE 140
The manufacturer of a biochemistry instrument claims that 18 out of 24 of the routine biochemistry analytes will achieve 6 sigma or better performance when using the manufacturer's reagents and commonly applied quality specifications for these analytes. Of the six analytes that do not obtain 6 sigma or better performance, the manufacturer claims that four of these have sigma metrics between 4 and 5 and two of them have sigma metrics between 3 and 4.

QUESTIONS

1 What is a sigma metric, and how is it calculated?
2 What is the relationship between the sigma metric and application of statistical quality control (QC)?
3 Why is knowing the sigma metric for a test important?

CASE 141

A 9-year-old male gelded Anglo-Arab endurance horse appeared stiff towards the end of a 20-mile ride and showed bilateral hindlimb lameness when trotted up for the post-ride veterinary inspection.

EXAMINATION FINDINGS

The gluteal muscles were slightly firm but the horse was bright and keen to eat and drink. Blood samples were collected 3 and 24 hours after the ride.

BIOCHEMISTRY

Analyte (units)	Result		Reference Interval
	3 Hours Post Exercise	24 Hours Post Exercise	
CK (U/l)	1,402	600	<80
AST (U/l)	320	720	<200
Calcium (mmol/l)	3.3	Not done	2.8–3.9
Phosphorus (mmol/l)	1.3	Not done	1.1–1.5

Three weeks later, the horse appeared normal and was back in full work. The urinary fractional excretion (FE) of electrolytes was calculated from the formula:

$$\text{FE (\%) of electrolyte} = \frac{U[e]}{S[e]} \times \frac{S[cr]}{U[cr]} \times 100$$

Where U[e] and U[cr] = urinary concentration of electrolyte and creatinine, respectively, and S[e] and S[cr] = serum concentration of electrolyte and creatinine, respectively.

The raw data is not shown, but the calculated results were as follows:

Analyte (units)	Result	Reference Interval
FE-Na (%)	0.6	0.02–1.0
FE-K (%)	10	15–65

QUESTIONS

1 Discuss the laboratory findings and their significance.
2 What would be differential diagnoses for increased FE-Na and FE-K in this horse?

CASE 142

A 1-year-old female Kuvasz dog has always been thin and has demonstrated a marked PU/PD (>2 litres/kg body weight). Weakness, vomiting and diarrhoea were observed 2 days prior to presentation.

EXAMINATION FINDINGS

Abnormalities included pale, dry mucous membranes, a dull hair coat and a bounding pulse.

HAEMATOLOGY

Measurand (units)	Result	Reference Interval
RBC count (10¹²/l)	1.66	5.5–8.5
Haemoglobin (g/l)	28	74–112
Haematocrit (l/l)	0.13	0.37–0.55
MCV (fl)	77.5	60–77
Platelet count (10⁹/l)	390	150–500
Reticulocytes (10⁹/l)	9.3	<60
WBC count (10⁹/l)	16	6–17
Neutrophils (10⁹/l)	11.25	3.0–11.5

Measurand (units)	Result	Reference Interval
Lymphocytes (10⁹/l)	3.16	1.0–3.6
Monocytes (10⁹/l)	0.34	0.04–1.35
Eosinophils (10⁹/l)	1.26	0.0–1.25
Basophils (10⁹/l)	0.01	0.0–0.04
Large unstained cells [LUCs] (10⁹/l)	0.02	0.0–0.04

LUCs: this variable is specific for the ADVIA 120/2120® Haematology System and includes plasma cells, reactive lymphocytes and lymphatic blasts.

BLOOD SMEAR EVALUATION

The majority of the erythrocytes are normocytic-normochromic. There is slight polychromasia of erythrocytes. Apart from a slight eosinophilia, leucocytes and platelets are normal in number and morphology.

BIOCHEMISTRY

Analyte (units)	Result	Reference Interval
Total protein (g/l)	57.3	55–70
Albumin (g/l)	**22.3**	30–37
Globulins (g/l)	35	23–36
Glucose (mmol/l)	6.16	3.3–6.5
Total bilirubin (µmol/l)	**4.37**	<3.6
Cholesterol (mmol/l)	8.39	3.3–8.6
Triglycerides (mmol/l)	0.63	<0.75
ALP (U/l)	97	<131
ALT (U/l)	**119**	<85
GLDH (U/l)	**18**	<10
Urea (mmol/l)	**104.02**	3.03–9.82
Creatinine (µmol/l)	**1,528**	53–123
Sodium (mmol/l)	150	147–152
Chloride (mmol/l)	**97**	102–110
Potassium (mmol/l)	4.1	3.35–4.37
Ionised calcium (mmol/l)	**0.9**	1.23–1.43
Phosphate (mmol/l)	**8.79**	0.79–2.1

URINALYSIS (cystocentesis)

Item	Result	Reference Interval
USG	**1.016**	>1.030
Dipstick evaluation		
pH	5	
Bilirubin	Negative	Negative
Blood	**+++**	Negative
Glucose	**+++**	Negative
Protein	**+**	Negative
UPCR	**1.9**	<0.2 (<1.0)
Sediment analysis		
Erythrocytes	**>5**	0–5/hpf
Leucocytes	**>5**	0–5/hpf
Epithelial cells	**>5**	0–5/hpf
Crystals	Negative	Variable
Casts	Negative	
Bacteria	**Numerous rods**	None

hpf: ×40 magnification.

Urine sediment

Several renal epithelial cells, several squamous epithelial cells, few transitional epithelial cells.

QUESTIONS

1 Describe and discuss the significant haematological and biochemistry findings as well as the urinalysis.
2 What diagnosis can be made based on the clinical and laboratory findings, and what is the prognosis for this patient?

CASE 143
A 6-month-old Doberman Pinscher presented because the owner wanted to have the dog neutered.

EXAMINATION FINDINGS

No abnormality detected. The pre-anaesthetic protocol in the clinic includes evaluation of buccal mucosal bleeding time (BMBT) in Doberman Pinschers:

Item (units)	Result	Reference Interval
BMBT (seconds)	**400**	<200

QUESTIONS

1 Is a congenital coagulation factor deficiency likely in this case?
2 What types of conditions can result in a prolonged BMBT?
3 Does a BMBT within normal limits rule out the possibility of von Willebrand's disease in a dog?

CASE 144

A 9-year-old male neutered DSH cat has been diagnosed previously with hyperthyroidism and is being treated with methimazole (felimazole) (2.5 mg tablet bid). He presented anorexic with weight loss and generalised muscle weakness including ventroflexion of the neck.

HAEMATOLOGY

Measurand (units)	Results	Reference Interval
RBC count (10^{12}/l)	7.14	5.5–10.0
Haemoglobin (g/l)	97	80–150
Haematocrit (l/l)	0.32	0.27–0.50
MCV (fl)	44.8	40–55
MCHC (g/l)	**303**	310–340
Platelet count (10^9/l)	Appears normal in the film	200–600
WBC count (10^9/l)	12.8	4–15
Neutrophils (10^9/l)	11.8	2.5–12.5
Band neutrophils (10^9/l)	0	0.0–0.3
Lymphocytes (10^9/l)	**0.9**	1.5–7.0
Monocytes (10^9/l)	0.1	0.0–0.8
Eosinophils (10^9/l)	0	0.0–1.5

BIOCHEMISTRY

Analyte (units)	Results	Reference Interval
Total protein (g/l)	66.2	54–78
Albumin (g/l)	31.5	21–39
Globulins (g/l)	34.7	15–57
ALP (U/l)*	**111**	0–40
GGT (U/l)*	2	0–27
ALT (U/l)*	**548**	0–20
GLDH (U/l)*	**290**	0–10
Total bilirubin (µmol/l)	**13.1**	0–10
Bile acids (µmol/l)	**35.2**	0–15
CK (U/l)*	**>10,000**	0–152
Cholesterol (mmol/l)	3.9	1.9–3.9

Analyte (units)	Results	Reference Interval
Triglycerides (mmol/l)	0.55	0.22–1.24
Glucose (mmol/l)	**6.7**	4.3–6.6
Urea (mmol/l)	9.5	6–10
Creatinine (µmol/l)	106	80–180
Sodium (mmol/l)	**159**	120–155
Potassium (mmol/l)	**2.6**	3.6–5.6
Chloride (mmol/l)	119	112–129
Calcium (mmol/l)	2.34	1.6–3.0
Phosphate (mmol/l)	1.52	1.4–2.6
TT4 (nmol/l)	17	15–40

*Assay performed at 37°C.

FOLLOW-UP TEST

Analyte (units)	Results	Reference Interval
Aldosterone (pmol/l)	**>3,300**	195–390

QUESTIONS

1 Describe the abnormalities and potential associations, and provide an interpretation.
2 Interpret the follow-up test result and discuss how you would distinguish between primary and secondary causes of this increase.
3 Give advice regarding the special laboratory tests that may be performed during work up of this condition.

CASE 145

A 6-year-old male mixed-breed dog was admitted with pain in the nasal region and depression after a brief escape in the wood.

EXAMINATION FINDINGS

Weakness, fever (39.8°C [103°F]); pale mucous membranes. Slight discomfort during abdominal palpation.

HAEMATOLOGY

Leucon and thrombin unremarkable.

Measurand (units)	Result	Reference Interval
RBC count (10¹²/l)	**3.01**	5.70–8.56
Haemoglobin (g/l)	**75**	141–212
Haematocrit (l/l)	**0.20**	0.39–0.59
MCV (fl)	68	63.1–72.6
MCH (pg)	25	21.8–25.4
MCHC (g/l)	**369**	333–368
RDW (%)	12.6	11.6–14.7
NRBCs/100 WBCs	0	0

BLOOD SMEAR EVALUATION

The most relevant morphological changes are shown (**Fig. 145.1**).

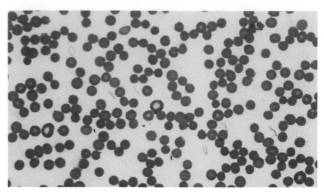

FIG. 145.1 Red blood cells in the smear. Giemsa, ×50.

QUESTIONS

1 What are the round structures besides the erythrocytes represented in the smear?
2 What is the most probable pathogenic mechanism of formation?
3 What other cells are associated with these structures?

CASE 146

An 8-year-old Quarter horse gelding presented because red urine was observed when the horse urinated prior to running in a barrel race the day before.

EXAMINATION FINDINGS

Unremarkable.

URINALYSIS (free catch)

Item	Result	Reference Interval
Colour	Dark yellow	Light to dark yellow
Transparency	Cloudy	Clear to cloudy
USG	1.030	≥1.025
Dipstick evaluation		
pH	8	Alkaline
Protein	Negative	Negative to trace
Glucose	Negative	Negative
Ketone bodies	Negative	Negative
Bilirubin	Negative	Negative
Blood	**++**	Negative
Sediment analysis		
Erythrocytes	**40–50/hpf**	<5/hpf

Item	Result	Reference Interval
Leucocytes	<5/hpf	<5/hpf
Epithelial cells	Few	None to moderate
Casts	Negative	None to few
Crystals	Numerous calcium carbonate; moderate calcium oxalate dihydrate	Variable

QUESTIONS

1 What number of RBCs is usually needed to see gross discolouration of the urine?
2 Why is cloudy urine within expected limits in the horse?
3 Why might additional knowledge about when during urination the haemorrhage is observed be of benefit?
4 What are the differential diagnoses for discoloured urine in the horse, and what clinical and/or pathological findings may be helpful in their differentiation?

CASE 147

A 5-year-old male cross-breed dog presented for evaluation of decreased activity.

EXAMINATION FINDINGS

Unremarkable.

HAEMATOLOGY

Unremarkable.

BIOCHEMISTRY

Analyte (units)	Result	Reference Interval
Total protein (g/l)	**73.1**	55.3–69.84
Albumin (g/l)	30.8	29.6–37.01
Globulins (g/l)	**42.3**	22.9–35.6
Glucose (mmol/l)	5.99	3.3–6.53
Total bilirubin (µmol/l)	2.16	0–3.6
Cholesterol (mmol/l)	6.53	3.3–6.53
Triglycerides (mmol/l)	0.6	0.08–0.75
ALP (U/l)	123	0–130
ALT (U/l)	50	0–85
GLDH (U/l)	8	0–9.9
CK (U/l)	77	<143

Analyte (units)	Result	Reference Interval
Urea (mmol/l)	7.93	3.3–9.82
Creatinine (µmol/l)	95	53–122
Sodium (mmol/l)	145	141–146
Chloride (mmol/l)	108	104–112
Potassium (mmol/l)	3.9	3.35–4.37
Ionised calcium (mmol/l)	**2.13**	1.23–1.43
Phosphorus (mmol/l)	0.92	0.79–2.1
Ionised magnesium (mmol/l)	**0.41**	0.47–0.63

OTHER TESTS

USG = 1.045; **PTH = 50** pg/ml (reference interval, 8–45).

QUESTIONS

1 What is the most likely diagnosis?
2 What are the most frequent clinical signs associated with this diagnosis?
3 What are the causes of this diagnosis?

CASE 148

An 11-year-old female neutered Siamese cat was presented to a small animal practice for routine vaccination.

HAEMATOLOGY

Measurand (units)	Result	Reference Interval
Spun PCV (%)	**18**	24–45

BIOCHEMISTRY

Within normal limits.

Because of the low PCV, the patient was referred to a larger clinic nearby to investigate the cause of the anaemia. A full haematology examination was performed.

HAEMATOLOGY (in clinic)

Measurand (units)	Result	Reference Interval
RBC count (10^{12}/l)	8.41	5–10
Haemoglobin (g/l)	135	130–195
Haematocrit (l/l)	0.37	0.24–0.45
MCV (fl)	41.4	40–55

Measurand (units)	Result	Reference Interval
Platelet count (10^9/l)	398	180–550
WBC count (10^9/l)	7.08	6–18
Neutrophils (10^9/l)	4.55	2.5–12.5
Lymphocytes (10^9/l)	**1.4**	1.5–7.0
Monocytes (10^9/l)	0.15	0.04–0.85
Eosinophils (10^9/l)	0.08	<1.50
Basophils (10^9/l)	0	<0.04

QUESTIONS

1 There is a discrepancy between the spun PCV performed initially and the haematocrit performed in the clinic. Summarise the pre-analytical, analytical or post-analytical reasons that may influence the result of the microhaematocrit method (spun PCV).
2 Does sample ageing influence the spun PCV?

CASE 149

A 5-year-old female Jack Russell Terrier was unwell, mildly pyrexic and vomiting. There was no travel history. The dog lives in a countryside environment and has not been regularly vaccinated. Her last oestrous cycle was 4 months ago.

HAEMATOLOGY

Analyte (units)	Result	Reference Interval
RBC count (10^{12}/l)	5.91	5.5–8.5
Haemoglobin (g/l)	223	193–290
Haematocrit (l/l)	0.41	0.37–0.55
MCV (fl)	68.9	60–77
MCH (pg)	23.4	19.5–25.5
MCHC (g/l)	341	300–380
Platelet count (10^9/l)	193	200–500
WBC count (10^9/l)	15.42	6–15
Neutrophils (10^9/l)	14.49	3.0–11.5
Lymphocytes (10^9/l)	0.62	1.0–4.8
Monocytes (10^9/l)	0.31	0.2–1.4
Eosinophils (10^9/l)	0	0.1–1.2
Basophils (10^9/l)	0	0.0–0.1

Analyte (units)	Result	Reference Interval
Total protein (g/l)	60	54–77
Albumin (g/l)	27	25–40
Globulins (g/l)	33	23–45
Glucose (mmol/l)	7.1	3.3–5.8
ALP (U/l)	647	14–105
ALT (U/l)	124	13–88
AST (U/l)	157	13–60
GGT (µmol/l)	18	0–10
Total bilirubin (µmol/l)	23	0–16
CK (U/l)	1,510	0–190
Urea (mmol/l)	37.6	2.5–7.4
Creatinine (µmol/l)	661	40–145
Sodium (mmol/l)	137	139–154
Chloride (mmol/l)	98	105–122
Potassium (mmol/l)	4.8	3.4–5.6
Total calcium (mmol/l)	2.6	2.1–2.8
Phosphate (mmol/l)	3	0.6–1.4

BLOOD SMEAR EVALUATION

RBCs show mild anisocytosis and are normochromic. The morphology of the leucocytes is unremarkable. Platelets are consistent with the automated count and no clumps are seen. They show mild anisocytosis.

BIOCHEMISTRY

The sample was mildly icteric and mildly haemolysed.

QUESTIONS

1 What is the most likely explanation for the laboratory abnormalities?
2 What further test would you perform to confirm your diagnosis?
3 What is the pathophysiology behind the biochemistry changes?

CASE 150

A 3-month-old male Miniature Schnauzer-cross presented with intermittent anorexia and lethargy with marked PU/PD. USG ranged from 1.003 to 1.025; the latter was obtained with water restriction according to water intake required for body weight.

HAEMATOLOGY

Measurand (units)	Result	Reference Interval
RBC count (10^{12}/l)	7.6	5.5–8.0
Haemoglobin (g/l)	129	120–180
Haematocrit (l/l)	0.42	0.37–0.55
MCV (fl)	**55**	60–72
MCHC (g/l)	**307**	340–380
Platelet count (10^9/l)	220	150–900
WBC count (10^9/l)	14.8	6–17
Neutrophils (10^9/l)	**12.6**	3.0–11.5
Band neutrophils (10^9/l)	0	0.0–0.31
Monocytes (10^9/l)	1.3	0.1–1.3
Lymphocytes (10^9/l)	**0.9**	1.0–4.8
Eosinophils (10^9/l)	**0**	0.12–1.5
Plasma protein (g/l) (refractometer)	**48**	60–80

BLOOD FILM EVALUATION

Erythrocytes show a mild microcytosis; occasional hypochromasia is present.

BIOCHEMISTRY

Analyte (units)	Result	Reference Interval
Total protein (g/l)	**44**	54–74
Albumin (g/l)	**22**	27–45
Globulins (g/l)	22	19–34
Total bilirubin (µmol/l)	1.0	0–6.8
Cholesterol (mmol/l)	**2.6**	3.4–9.6
Glucose (mmol/l)	**6.4**	3.5–6.0
ALT (U/l)	**400**	10–120
ALP (U/l)	**312**	35–280
AST (U/l)	120	35–280
Creatinine kinase (U/l)	200	74–385
Amylase (U/l)	**1,296**	50–1,250
Lipase (U/l)	420	30–560
Fasting (pre-prandial) bile acids (µmol/l)	**115**	0–5

Analyte (units)	Result	Reference Interval
Post-prandial bile acids (µmol/l)	**163**	<30
Urea (mmol/l)	**1.8**	2.5–10.0
Creatinine (µmol/l)	**55**	80–150
Calcium (mmol/l)	**2.95**	2.25–2.80
Phosphorus (mmol/l)	**5.5**	2.8–5.2
Sodium (mmol/l)	146	145–158
Potassium (mmol/l)	4.5	4.1–5.5
Chloride (mmol/l)	108	106–127

URINALYSIS (free flow)

Item	Result	Reference Interval
Colour	**Pale yellow**	Yellow
Transparency	Clear	Clear
USG	**1.003**	>1.030
Dipstick evaluation		
pH	6.0	
Bilirubin	Negative	Negative to trace
Blood	Negative	Negative
Glucose	Negative	Negative
Ketone bodies	Negative	Negative
Protein	Negative	Negative
Sediment analysis		
Erythrocytes	0	0–5/hpf
Leucocytes	0	0–5/hpf
Epithelial cells	None	None
Crystals	**Rare ammonium biurate**	Variable/lpf
Casts	None	None
Bacteria	None	None/lpf

QUESTIONS

1 Summarise and interpret the abnormalities in these laboratory results.
2 Discuss any additional tests you could perform in order to confirm or exclude the possible diagnosis.

CASE 151

A 4-year-old female neutered Labrador Retriever presented because she tires easily, is depressed, has a decreased appetite, is vomiting and is passing brown urine.

EXAMINATION FINDINGS

T = 40.8°C (105.4°F), pale mucous membranes, bilateral epistaxis.

HAEMATOLOGY

Measurand (units)	Result	Reference Interval
RBC count (10^{12}/l)	4.85	5.5–8.0
Haemoglobin (g/l)	116	120–180
Haematocrit (l/l)	0.32	0.37–0.55
MCV (fl)	68	60–77
Reticulocytes (10^9/l)	26	28–80
Platelet count (10^9/l)	31	200–500
WBC count (10^9/l)	4.2	6–15
Neutrophils (10^9/l)	3.1	3.6–10.5
Lymphocytes (10^9/l)	0.6	1.0–3.6
Monocytes (10^9/l)	0.4	0.0–1.2
Eosinophils (10^9/l)	0.1	0.0–0.5
Comment: platelet estimate on smear confirms count.		

BLOOD SMEAR EVALUATION

See **Fig. 151.1**.

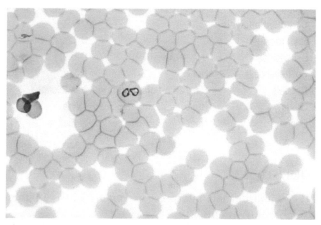

FIG. 151.1 Blood smear. Wright–Giemsa, ×100 (oil).
(Courtesy Dr Emma Hooijberg)

BIOCHEMISTRY

Analyte (units)	Result	Reference Interval
Total protein (g/l)	78	60–75
Albumin (g/l)	21	23–35
Globulins (g/l)	57	37–45
Urea (mmol/l)	10.32	3.3–8.9
Creatinine (µmol/l)	159.1	70.7–106.1

QUESTIONS

1 How would you classify the anaemia?
2 What is your diagnosis based on the haematology and the blood smear?
3 Where on the blood smear would you look for the organisms causing the anaemia?
4 Would a serology test (immunoflourescence) or a PCR be useful for further confirmation?
5 What is the most frequent change in the FBC in this infection?
6 What does the biochemistry profile indicate?

CASE 152

A 6-year-old Labrador Retriever is overweight and lethargic and his owner is concerned that he no longer wants to go on walks and that his coat is dull.

HAEMATOLOGY

Measurand (units)	Results	Reference Interval
RBC count (10^{12}/l)	**4.3**	5.0–8.5
Haemoglobin (g/l)	**112**	120–180
PCV (l/l)	**0.36**	0.37–0.55
MCV (fl)	70.9	60–80
MCH (pg)	**24.2**	19–23
MCHC (g/l)	**341**	310–340
Reticulocytes (10^9/l)	40	60–80
Platelet count (10^9/l)	220	200–500
WBC count (10^9/l)	11.9	6–15
Neutrophils (10^9/l)	**14.4**	3.0–11.5
Lymphocytes (10^9/l)	**0.7**	1.0–4.8
Monocytes (10^9/l)	0.7	0.0–1.3
Eosinophils (10^9/l)	0.1	0.1–1.3

Analyte (units)	Result	Reference Interval
CK (U/l)*	124	0–190
Glucose (mmol/l)	5.6	3.8–7.0
Amylase (U/l)*	850	100–900
Lipase (U/l)*	171	0–250
Urea (mmol/l)	6	1.7–7.4
Creatinine (µmol/l)	82	0–106
Sodium (mmol/l)	146	139–154
Potassium (mmol/l)	**12**	3.6–5.6
Chloride (mmol/l)	111	105–122
Calcium (mmol/l)	**0.2**	2.3–3.0
Phosphate (mmol/l)	**2**	0.8–1.6
Total T4 (nmol/l)	**13**	15–40
TSH (ng/mL)	0.14	0.01–0.60

* Analysis performed at 37°C.

BLOOD FILM EVALUATION

Confirms the platelet count.

BIOCHEMISTRY

Analyte (units)	Result	Reference Interval
Total protein (g/l)	57.7	54–77
Albumin (g/l)	30.3	25–37
Globulins (g/l)	27.4	23–52
ALP (U/l)*	20	0–50
ALT (U/l)*	**35**	0–25
GGT (U/l)*	2	0–27
GLDH (U/l)*	5	0–10
Cholesterol (mmol/l)	**9.6**	3.8–7.0
Total bilirubin (µmol/l)	2.9	0–16
Bile acids (µmol/l)	4	0–10

QUESTIONS

1 Identify and list the abnormalities and explain their associations.
2 What further tests would you recommend?
3 Discuss the mechanisms by which EDTA contamination of a serum sample produces marked hyperkalaemia and hypocalcaemia.
4 What other parameter will have been affected by the problem in this profile, and explain why a change is not obvious on evaluation of the profile.
5 When collecting blood into multiple different types (plain and anticoagulants) of blood vacutainers, in which order should they be collected?

CASE 153

A 2-year-old female neutered Cavalier King Charles Spaniel (CKCS) presents for a routine health check.

EXAMINATION FINDINGS

No abnormalities noted.

HAEMATOLOGY

The erythron and leucon are within normal limits. The platelet count is $70 \times 10^9/l$ (reference interval, $150–500 \times 10^9/l$).

BLOOD SMEAR EVALUATION

Normocytic-normochromic erythrocytes with physiological anisocytosis, slight poikilocytosis with occasional codocytes. Platelets are predominantly present as macroplatelets. No platelet clumps are visible.

QUESTIONS

1 Discuss the haematological abnormalities.
2 Describe the underlying pathophysiology.

CASE 154

An 8-year-old female neutered Bichon Frise is presented with a history of lethargy, depression and anorexia, PU/PD and a slightly pendulous abdomen.

HAEMATOLOGY

Measurand (units)	Result	Reference Interval
RBC count ($10^{12}/l$)	**8.6**	5.5–8.0
Haemoglobin (g/l)	**190**	120–180
Haematocrit (l/l)	**0.58**	0.37–0.55
MCV (fl)	68	60–72
MCHC (g/l)	**328**	340–380
Platelet count ($10^9/l$)	180	150–900
WBC count ($10^9/l$)	16.5	6–17
Neutrophils ($10^9/l$)	**14.2**	3.0–11.5
Band neutrophils ($10^9/l$)	0.1	0–0.31
Monocytes ($10^9/l$)	**1.4**	0.1–1.3
Lymphocytes ($10^9/l$)	**0.8**	1.0–4.8
Plasma protein (g/l) (refractometer)	72	60–80

BIOCHEMISTRY

Analyte (units)	Result	Reference Interval
Total protein (g/l)	69	54–74
Albumin (g/l)	38	27–45
Globulins (g/l)	31	19–34
Total bilirubin (µmol/l)	4.3	0–6.8
Cholesterol (mmol/l)	**11.2**	3.4–9.6
Glucose (mmol/l)	**7.3**	3.5–6.0
ALT (U/l)	**165**	10–120
AST (U/l)	**55**	16–40
ALP (U/l)	**2,252**	35–280
Amylase (U/l)	1,098	50–1,250
Lipase (U/l)	420	30–560
Urea (mmol/l)	6.8	2.5–10.0
Creatinine (µmol/l)	135	80–150
Calcium (mmol/l)	2.5	2.25–2.80

Analyte (units)	Result	Reference Interval
Phosphorus (mmol/l)	1	0.85–1.95
Sodium (mmol/l)	**160**	145–158
Potassium (mmol/l)	**4.0**	4.1–5.5
Chloride (mmol/l)	115	106–127
TCO$_2$ (mmol/l)	18	14–27

URINALYSIS (catheterised)

Item	Result	Reference Interval
Colour	Yellow	Yellow
Transparency	**Turbid +**	Clear
USG	**1.015**	>1.030
Dipstick evaluation		
pH	7.0	Acidic
Protein	**1+**	Negative to trace
Glucose	Negative	Negative
Bilirubin	Negative	Negative to trace
Blood	Negative	Negative
Sediment analysis		
Leucocytes	7	<10/hpf
Erythrocytes	6	<10/hpf
Epithelial cells	4	Rare/lpf
Crystals	Negative	
Casts	Negative	Variable/lpf
Bacteria	**2+**	Negative

QUESTIONS

1 Summarise and interpret the abnormalities in these laboratory results.
2 What additional tests could you perform in order to confirm or exclude the possible diagnosis?

CASE 155

A 3-year old female American Staffordshire Terrier had been lethargic and polydipsic for the last 24 hours and was moderately dehydrated. The owner mentioned that the dog "probably ate something".

EXAMINATION FINDINGS

There was an elevated temperature of 32.2°C (108°F).

HAEMATOLOGY

Measurand (units)	Result	Reference Interval
RBC count (10¹²/l)	**9.3**	5.5–8.0
Haemoglobin (g/l)	**210**	120–180
Haematocrit (l/l)	**0.62**	37–55
MCV (fl)	64	60–77
Platelet count (10⁹/l)	**122**	200–500
Leucocytes (10⁹/l)	**20**	6–15
Neutrophils (10⁹/l)	**17.1**	3.6–10.5
Lymphocytes (10⁹/l)	**0.6**	1.0–3.6
Monocytes (10⁹/l)	**1.6**	0.0–1.2
Eosinophils (10⁹/l)	0.5	0.0–0.5
NRBCs	**Few** (<5%)	None

BLOOD SMEAR EVALUATION

Erythrogram: haemoconcentration/polycythaemia, isolated normoblasts; leucogram: mature neutrophilia, lymphopaenia, monocytosis.

BIOCHEMISTRY

Analyte (units)	Result	Reference Interval
Total protein (g/l)	**91**	60–75
Albumin (g/l)	**50**	23–35
Urea (mmol/l)	**32.84**	7.14–19.28
Creatinine (µmol/l)	**238.68**	<106.08
Calcium (mmol/l)	**2.1**	2.3–2.9
Phosphorus (mmol/l)	1.4	<1.6
Sodium (mmol/l)	**160**	140–152
Potassium (mmol/l)	5.4	3.6–5.6

URINALYSIS

Item	Result	Reference Interval
Colour	Light yellow	
Turbidity	**Cloudy**	Clear
USG	**1.010**	>1.035
Dipstick evaluation		
pH	5.5	
Protein	1+	Negative to trace

There is isosthenuria. Sediment analysis showed granular casts and many calcium oxalate dihydrate crystals.

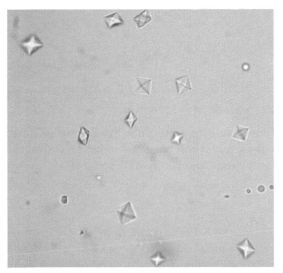 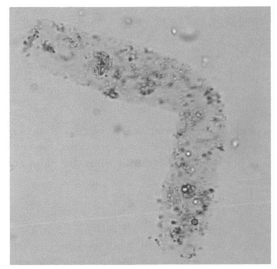

FIG. 155.1 Left: unstained sediment. Wet-drop preparation, ×40. Right: methylene blue-stained sediment. Wet-drop preparation, ×10. (Courtesy Dr Judith Leidinger)

QUESTIONS

1 What does the FBC tell you?
2 What might the finding of NRBCs indicate?
3 What does the urinalysis indicate?

CASE 156

A 15-year-old male Yorkshire Terrier presented for re-assessment of chronic renal failure. Biochemistry revealed marked azotaemia.

ACID-BASE AND BLOOD GAS DATA

Analyte (units)	Result	Reference Interval
Arterial pH	7.44	7.36–7.44
PaCO$_2$ (mmHg)	**20**	36–44
PaO$_2$ (mmHg)	**100**	85–95
Plasma HCO$_3^-$ (mmol/l)	**13**	18–26
Sodium (mmol/l)	145	145–155
Potassium (mmol/l)	**3.5**	4–5
Chloride (mmol/l)	115	105–115
Anion gap	20.5	15–25

QUESTIONS

1 What is your assessment of the arterial pH?
2 What is your assessment of the likely underlying aetiology for this arterial pH?
3 Is there appropriate compensation for this condition, and what does it suggest?
4 What might be underlying causes for this condition?

CASE 157

The International Renal Interest Society (IRIS) recommends staging of chronic renal disease based initially on fasting plasma creatinine, assessed on at least two occasions in the stable patient. The patient is then substaged based on proteinuria and blood pressure.

QUESTION

1 Based on what is known about biological variation in creatinine in dogs, are two samples adequate to estimate the homeostatic setting point for creatinine within an individual dog (assuming chronic stable renal disease)?

CASE 158

A Shorthorn-cross heifer is one of two heifers on a smallholding with poor quality upland pasture. The farmer has not checked these cows for several days, but when checked today he found this one with incoordination, bleeding from the anus and a serosanguineous nasal discharge.

EXAMINATION FINDINGS

Petechiae are present on the oral mucous membranes. Incoordination, lethargy and fever are present. The body condition is poor (owner reports that the weight loss has occurred rapidly and recently). Red urine is observed when the heifer urinates while in the stocks for clinical examination. No clinical signs or poor condition are observed in the other heifer and or in two older cows on the same pasture.

HAEMATOLOGY

Measurand (units)	Result	Reference Interval
RBC count (10¹²/l)	**4.82**	5.0–7.2
Haemoglobin (g/l)	**69**	87–124
Haematocrit (l/l)	**0.20**	0.25–0.33
MCV (fl)	42.1	38–51
MCH (pg)	14.3	14–19
MCHC (g/l)	340	340–380
Platelet count (10⁹/l)	**20**	252–724
WBC count (10⁹/l)	**5.34**	5.9–14.0
Neutrophils (10⁹/l)	**1.02**	1.8–7.2
Lymphocytes (10⁹/l)	3.83	1.7–7.5
Monocytes (10⁹/l)	0.49	0.0–0.9
Eosinophils (10⁹/l)	0	0.0–1.3
Basophils (10⁹/l)	0	0.0–0.3

Measurand (units)	Result	Reference Interval
Fibrinogen (g/l) (heat precipitation method)	4	2–4
Plasma protein (g/l) (refractometer)	**50**	55–80
Fibrinogen:total protein ratio	8	<10

BLOOD FILM EVALUATION

No polychromasia noted. No platelet clumps seen. Platelet estimate = markedly decreased. No blood parasites seen.

QUESTIONS

1 What is your assessment of these findings?
2 What are your differential diagnoses?

CASE 159

A 5-year-old Bernese Mountain Dog presented for intermittent lameness. As the owners are living in an endemic area for *Borrelia burgdorferi* (Lyme disease), the dog was vaccinated against the disease. They are now concerned that he may be suffering from Lyme borreliosis despite the vaccination. Rarely, ticks have been noted.

ELISA SNAP TEST

Positive.

QUESTIONS

1 What does the ELISA SNAP Test detect?
2 How do you interpret the result of the ELISA?
3 Might the test be positive owing to previous vaccination?

CASE 160

A 2-year-old male neutered DSH presented for a routine health check.

HAEMATOLOGY AND BIOCHEMISTRY

Unremarkable.

URINALYSIS

Item	Result	Reference Interval
USG	1.042	>1.035
Dipstick evaluation		
pH	7.0	Acidic
Leucocyte esterase	**++**	Negative
Nitrite	Negative	Negative
Protein	Negative	Negative to trace
Glucose	Negative	Negative
Ketone bodies	Negative	Negative
Bilirubin	**+**	Negative to trace
Blood	Negative	Negative
Sediment analysis		
Erythrocytes	Negative	<5/ hpf
Leucocytes	Negative	<5/ hpf

Item	Result	Reference Interval
Squamous epithelial cells	Negative	
Transitional epithelial cells	Rare	
Crystals	Negative	

QUESTIONS

1 The nurse comes to you with a urine specimen that is testing 2+ positive for leucocyte esterase on dipstick analysis, but no neutrophils are seen in the urine sediment examination. She is concerned that one of these results is in error. What can you tell the nurse regarding this situation in a cat?
2 What if this urine specimen were from a dog?
3 What other test pad results available on some dipsticks may be unreliable or of limited use in dogs and/or cats?
4 What urine dipstick tests may be of different significance in the dog and cat?

CASE 161

A 3-year-old Thoroughbred-cross gelding is newly acquired and exhibits 'stud-like' behaviour (wants to mount mares in pasture).

QUESTIONS

1 What test can be used for evaluation for possible cryptorchidism in this horse?

2 What recommendations would you make for detection of cryptorchidism in a dog or a cat?

CASE 162

A 10-year-old male neutered DSH presented with a history of weight loss.

HAEMATOLOGY

Measurand (units)	Result	Reference Interval
Haematocrit (l/l)	**0.21**	0.29–0.36
Platelet count (10^9/l)	414	250–800
WBC count (10^9/l)	5.77	5.5–19.5
Neutrophils (10^9/l)	4.96	2.5–12.5
Lymphocytes (10^9/l)	0.23	1.5–7.0
Monocytes (10^9/l)	0.35	0.0–1.0
Eosinophils (10^9/l)	0.10	0.0–0.1
Basophils (10^9/l)	**0.17**	0.0–0.1
Atypical cells (10^9/l)	**0.1**	<0.01

BLOOD FILM EVALUATION

The monolayer of the blood film is thin, thus supporting the anaemia. The erythrocytes show moderate poikilocytosis and are normochromic. The leucocytes are morphologically unremarkable. Low numbers of atypical cells are found in the feathered edge or, occasionally, in the monolayer (**Fig. 162.1**). Platelets are consistent with the analyser count and are morphologically unremarkable.

BIOCHEMISTRY

Unremarkable.

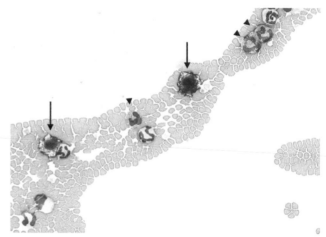

FIG. 162.1 A section of the feathered edge of the blood film of this patient. The long arrows indicate the cells classified as atypical during the differential cell count. May–Grünwald–Giemsa, ×50.

QUESTIONS

1 What are the cells shown (long arrows and arrow heads)?
2 What is the significance of this finding, and what further test would you perform?
3 What are the differential diagnoses for the anaemia?

CASE 163

A 13-year-old male neutered DSH cat presents for anorexia and polydipsia. The owner reports that the cat has blood in its urine.

URINALYSIS

Item	Result	Reference Interval
Colour	**Orange–brown (163.1)**	Yellow
Transparency	Clear	Clear
USG	1.036	1.020–1.045
Dipstick evaluation		
pH	6.5	Acidic
Leucocyte esterase	+++	Negative
Nitrite	Negative	Negative
Protein	++	Negative to trace
Protein (SSA)	++	Negative to trace
Glucose	Negative	Negative
Ketone bodies	Negative	Negative
Bilirubin	+++	Negative
Blood	+	Negative
Sediment analysis		
Amount	Increased	
Squamous epithelial cells	Sparse	
Transitional epithelial cells	Negative	
Erythrocytes	Negative	Negative
Leucocytes	Negative	Negative
Crystals	Moderate	

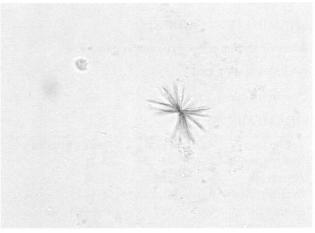

FIG. 163.2 Crystal found in an unstained urine sediment. Wet-drop preparation, ×40. (Courtesy Dr Judith Leidinger)

QUESTIONS

1 What is the significance of: (a) the +++ positive leucocyte esterase reaction; (b) the ++ positive protein reaction; (c) the + positive blood?
2 Which crystal is shown in **Fig. 163.2**?
3 What is the next step in a cat with this finding?

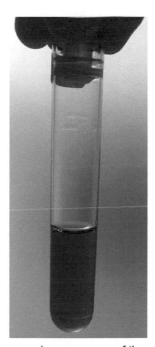

FIG. 163.1 Macroscopic appearance of the urine sample. (Courtesy Dr Judith Leidinger)

CASE 164

An 11-year-old female mongrel dog had surgery 1 month ago for a thyroid carcinoma. She is now being treated with levothyroxine tablets. Since yesterday, the owner has noted frequent vomiting and lethargy.

EXAMINATION FINDINGS

Anterior abdominal palpation was painful.

HAEMATOLOGY

Unremarkable.

BIOCHEMISTRY

Analyte (units)	Result	Reference Interval
Total protein (g/l)	**75**	54–71
Albumin (g/l)	**33.5**	26–33
Globulins (g/l)	41.5	27–44
Glucose (mmol/l)	5.63	3.66–6.31
Total bilirubin (µmol/l)	**3.97**	0–3.4
Cholesterol (mmol/l)	**9.14**	3.5–7.0
Triglycerides (mmol/l)	0.83	0.29–3.88
ALP (U/l)	**244**	0–97
ALT (U/l)	**58**	0–55

Analyte (units)	Result	Reference Interval
GLDH (U/l)	0	0–12
Amylase (U/l)	**8,086**	0–2,535
Lipase (U/l)	**1,532**	0–348
Urea (mmol/l)	4.35	3.57–8.57
Creatinine (µmol/l)	87	35–106
Sodium (mmol/l)	149	141–152
Chloride (mmol/l)	104	100–120
Potassium (mmol/l)	3.9	3.6–5.35
Ionised calcium (mmol/l)	**1.0**	1.16–1.31
Phosphate (mmol/l)	1.1	0.7–1.6

QUESTIONS

1 Describe and discuss the biochemistry changes.
2 What further analyses would you recommend to confirm your diagnosis?

CASE 165

Capillary zone electrophoresis is an extremely useful tool to separate and gain more insight into the patient's proteins. Knowing which entities can be identified using this method is crucial in deciding if performing this analysis represents value for money.

QUESTION

1 What types of gammopathy can be identified on serum protein electrophoresis using capillary zone electrophoresis?

CASE 166

A 6-year-old female neutered Golden Retriever presents for lethargy, fever and intermittent lameness. The dog is vaccinated against *Borrelia burgdorferi*. The owners had been told to apply tick preventive medication but did not do so and frequently ticks have been found on the dog. To rule out Lyme borreliosis, an ELISA rapid in-house test was performed.

ELISA RAPID IN-HOUSE TEST

Positive.

QUESTIONS

1 How do you interpret the result of the ELISA?
2 How would you proceed with this dog with regard to additional laboratory testing?

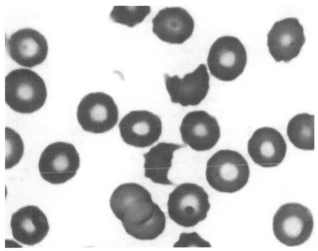

CASE 167
An 11-year-old female neutered Jack Russell Terrier presented following a few days of vomiting, diarrhoea and oliguria.

HAEMATOLOGY

Measurand (units)	Result Day 1	Result Day 3	Reference Interval
RBC count (10¹²/l)	5.05	3.52	5.5–8.5
Haemoglobin (g/l)	119	61	120–180
Haematocrit (l/l)	33.8	27.9	37–55
MCV (fl)	66.9	79.2	60–77
MCH (pg)	23.6	17.3	19.5–24.5
MCHC (g/l)	352	218	320–370
RDW (%)	13.3	19.4	13.2–17.8
Reticulocytes (%)	1.03	4.25	0–1.5
Reticulocytes (10⁹/l)	52.0	149.6	0–70
Platelet count (10⁹/l)	12	8	175–500
WBC count (10⁹/l)	31.78	30.42	6–17
Neutrophils (10⁹/l)	26.38	24.88	3.0–11.5
Lymphocytes (10⁹/l)	1.6	2.5	1.0–4.8
Monocytes (10⁹/l)	2.86	1.84	0.2–1.5
Eosinophils (10⁹/l)	0.95	1.23	0.1–1.3

BIOCHEMISTRY

Analyte (units)	Day 1	Day 2	Day 3	Day 4	Reference Interval
Total protein (g/l)	44	40	38	42	55–77
Albumin (g/l)	19	17	16	16	25–41
Globulins (g/l)	25	23	22	26	24–47
ALT (U/l)	63	n.d.	60	68	14–67
AST (U/l)	377	n.d.	n.d.	n.d.	12–49
CK (U/l)	822	n.d.	n.d.	n.d.	42–206
GGT (U/l)	0.7	n.d.	n.d.	n.d.	0–10
ALP (U/l)	107	n.d.	85	86	26–107
Bilirubin (µmol/l)	5.7	n.d.	n.d.	n.d.	0–12
Cholesterol (mmol/l)	6.72	n.d.	n.d.	n.d.	3.3–6.5
Triglycerides (mmol/l)	1.0	n.d.	n.d.	n.d.	0.4–1.3
Glucose (mmol/l)	4.6	n.d.	5.7	5.6	3.4–5.6
Amylase (U/l)	1,541	n.d.	n.d.	n.d.	256–1,609
Lipase (U/l)	417.3	n.d.	n.d.	n.d.	0–200
Urea (mmol/l)	598	586	514	458	60–77
Creatinine (µmol/l)	1,208	1,173	1,110	1,094	34–136
Calcium (mmol/l)	2.96	2.66	2.62	2.61	2.2–2.9
Phosphate (mmol/l)	5.95	5.13	4.07	3.48	0.8–1.73
Sodium (mmol/l)	143	145	147	146	135–155
Potassium (mmol/l)	6.1	6.2	6.2	5.5	3.6–5.7
Chloride (mmol/l)	119	116	116	115	103–120

n.d. = not done.

BLOOD FILM EXAMINATION – DAY 3

Moderately haemolysed. RBCs: see **Fig. 167.1**. Leucocytes: unremarkable morphology. Platelets: no platelet clumps, consistent with count.

FIG. 167.1 Day 3, blood film. Modified Wright–Giemsa, ×100 (oil).

URINALYSIS (performed at day 1: free catch)

Item	Result	Reference Interval
Appearance	Slightly red	Clear
USG	1.012	>1.025
Dipstick evaluation		
pH	5.0	Acidic to neutral
Protein	5.0	Negative
Glucose	1+	Negative
Ketone bodies	Negative	Negative
Bilirubin	Negative	Negative
Blood	++++	Negative
Sediment analysis	Inactive sediment	
Leucocytes	<5	0–5/hpf
Erythrocytes	<5	0–5/hpf
Protein: creatinine ratio	17.2	<0.5

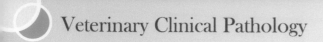

QUESTIONS

1 How would you classify this anaemia, and what are possible causes?
2 What RBC morphological abnormalities can be observed in the blood film?
3 How would you classify the azotaemia in this patient?
4 What would be your main differential for a dog with acute onset of haemolytic anaemia, thrombocytopaenia and azotaemia?

CASE 168
A 10-year-old male neutered mixed-breed dog shows slight weight loss, is lethargic, is 'not himself' and is slightly dehydrated.

HAEMATOLOGY

A slight non-responding anaemia is present, with no abnormalities in the leucon or thrombon.

BIOCHEMISTRY

Analyte (units)	Result			Reference Interval
	Day 1	Day 15	Day 30	
Total protein (g/l)	60	**50**	**48**	55–75
Albumin (g/l)	25	**20**	**19**	25–40
Globulins (g/l)	35	30	29	23–35
Glucose (mmol/l)	**6.9**	6.5	6.3	3.3–6.5
ALP (U/l)	**1,450**	**1,010**	**876**	0–130
ALT (U/l)	**245**	**196**	**178**	0–85
Urea (mmol/l)	**12.0**	7.5	7.8	3.3–8.0
Creatinine (µmol/l)	**240**	120	100	45–150
Sodium (mmol/l)	145	150	155	135–155
Chloride (mmol/l)	105	108	105	105–120
Potassium (mmol/l)	3.37	4.2	4.1	3.35–4.37
Phosphorus (mmol/l)	**2.7**	1.29	1.28	0.78–1.41
Total calcium (mmol/l)	2.79	2.37	2.35	2.3–2.8

ADDITIONAL INFORMATION

The initial evaluation of the day 1 laboratory findings was that the increases in urea, creatinine and phosphorus were likely due to dehydration, since a small urine specimen obtained by catheterisation had a USG of 1.050. The slight increase in glucose was thought to be due to 'stress'. There was no glucosuria on dipstick evaluation. The marked increase in ALP with moderate increase in ALT was considered likely to represent cholestasis and hepatocellular injury. Steroid induction of these enzymes was considered less likely because of the concentrated USG. Because of limited finances, the owners elected to try hepatic support measures, including ursodeoxycholic acid (Destolit) and SAMe.

At days 15 and 30, the patient was re-assessed and the hydration status was found to be within normal limits and the owners reported that the dog was eating well and had normal energy levels and attitude.

QUESTIONS

1 What is your assessment of the biochemistry findings at day 15 and day 30 following the institution of treatment?
2 Based on your knowledge of biological variation in the dog, index of individuality and reference change value, what findings do you consider likely to be statistically 'significant' or 'highly significant'?
3 Do you feel that these results are also of clinical significance? If so, why?
4 What additional testing would you recommend?

CASE 169

A 5-year-old Luing cow presents for lethargy, pale mucous membranes and partial anorexia.

HAEMATOLOGY

Measurand (units)	Result	Reference Interval
RBC count (10^{12}/l)	**2.85**	5.0–7.5
Haemoglobin (g/l)	**55**	85–132
Haematocrit (l/l)	**0.15**	0.24–0.36
MCV (fl)	52.6	37.8–56.0
MCH (pg)	19.3	14.2–20.1
MCHC (g/l)	367	317–404
Platelet count (10^9/l)	334	220–640
WBC count (10^9/l)	**11.2**	3.8–11.0
Neutrophils (10^9/l)	**6.5**	0.7–4.9
Lymphocytes (10^9/l)	4.6	1.0–5.8
Monocytes (10^9/l)	0.2	0.0–0.9
Eosinophils (10^9/l)	0	0.0–1.9
Basophils (10^9/l)	0	0.0–0.1
Fibrinogen (g/l) (heat precipitation method)	0.6	0.2–0.6

BLOOD SMEAR EVALUATION

WBC morphology within expected limits. Platelet estimate adequate. RBCs show moderate polychromasia and slight anisocytosis with moderate basophilic stippling and occasional acanthocytes. Clumping of erythrocytes in the smears suggestive of autoagglutination, but no autoagglutination visible in the tube macroscopically.

BIOCHEMISTRY

Slight hyperbilirubinaemia (16.93 µmol/l; reference interval: 0.17–8.55) with the rest of analytes in the comprehensive profile within reference intervals.

QUESTIONS

1 What is your assessment of these findings?
2 What is the most likely clinical diagnosis?
3 What are the differential diagnoses, and what other tests should be considered in this case?

CASE 170

A 10-day-old female Arabian foal was admitted following a seizure a few hours previously. There was normal foaling and behaviour prior to observation of the seizure. The foal was nursing normally and frequently, with good milk production by the mare.

EXAMINATION FINDINGS

Intermittent sweating, menace reflex absent, no further recurrence of seizure between the time of first observation and arrival at the clinic. There was intermittent, slight muscle fasciculation over the flanks.

HAEMATOLOGY

Slight leucocytosis with slight neutrophilia and monocytosis, attributed to 'stress' associated with the seizure.

BIOCHEMISTRY

Analyte (units)	Result	Reference Interval (foals 1–3 weeks old)
Total protein (g/l)	55	40–60
Albumin (g/l)	27	26–37
Globulins (g/l)	28	15–35
SAA (mg/l)	2.5	0–5.5
ALP (U/l)	2,220	1,195–3,500
AST (U/l)	**200**	250–357
CK (U/l)	**1,500**	200–350

Analyte (units)	Result	Reference Interval (foals 1–3 weeks old)
Total bilirubin (µmol/l)	39	15–84
Glucose (mmol/l)	**9.5**	3.2–6.5
Urea (mmol/l)	3.7	2.9–7.5
Creatinine (µmol/l)	102	95–140
Total calcium (mmol/l)*	**1.2**	2.9–3.2
Phosphorus (mmol/l)	**2.9**	1.8–2.5
Sodium (mmol/l)	139	135–142
Chloride (mmol/l)	95	95–103
Magnesium (mmol/l)	0.9	0.7–1.0
Total T4 (nmol/l)	120	60–380

* Confirmed by repeat evaluation of the serum specimen.

QUESTIONS

1 What is your assessment of these results?
2 What additional tests would be needed to confirm the likely diagnosis in this case?
3 What are the pathophysiological bases for the observed abnormalities?

CASE 171
A 3-month-old male neutered mixed-breed dog presented with seizures and hypersalivation.

EXAMINATION FINDINGS

Lethargy, fever, presence of papulae and small yellow vesicles on the skin of the abdomen.

HAEMATOLOGY

Measurand (units)	Result	Reference Interval
RBC count (10^{12}/l)	5.78	5.70–8.56
Haemoglobin (g/l)	**116**	120–180
Haematocrit (l/l)	**0.38**	0.39–0.59
MCV (fl)	66.1	63.1–72.6
MCH (pg)	**20.0**	21.8–25.4
MCHC (g/l)	**303**	333–368
RDW (%)	**16.0**	11.6–14.7
Platelet count (10^9/l)	259	176–479
WBC count (10^9/l)	6.91	5.45–12.98
Neutrophils (10^9/l)	5.4	3.5–9.3
Lymphocytes (10^9/l)	**0.5**	1.1–3.8
Monocytes (10^9/l)	**0.8**	0.1–0.7
Eosinophils (10^9/l)	0.06	0–0.1

BLOOD SMEAR EVALUATION

The most relevant morphological changes on the blood smear are shown (**Fig. 171.1**).

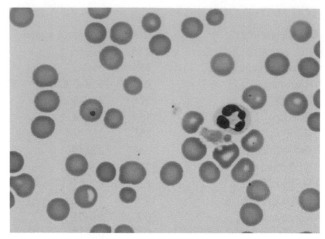

FIG. 171.1 Blood smear. Giemsa, ×100 (oil).

QUESTIONS

1 What is the pink inclusion in the cytoplasm of the erythrocyte?
2 How long would you expect inclusions to be observed in blood smears?
3 How can the disease be confirmed?

CASE 172
A veterinary practitioner dealing mostly with race horses asks you which laboratory analysis he can use to exclude inflammation in the horse besides leucocytes, as these are also influenced by stress.

QUESTIONS

1 Discuss which panel of laboratory markers you would recommend.

2 What actions does serum amyloid A (SAA) contribute to an inflammatory reaction?

CASE 173

A 6-year-old female neutered Great Dane presented with vomiting that had increased in frequency over the past 4–5 days. The dog was depressed and had diarrhoea on the day of presentation.

EXAMINATION FINDINGS

Largely unremarkable except for a temperature of 39.8°C (103.6°F), slight abdominal discomfort and possible scleral jaundice.

HAEMATOLOGY

Measurand (units)	Result	Reference Interval
RBC count (10¹²/l)	7.65	5.4–8.5
Haemoglobin (g/l)	180	120–180
Haematocrit (l/l)	0.54	0.37–0.56
MCV (fl)	70.5	65–75
MCHC (g/l)	350	310–350
Platelet count (10⁹/l)	**180**	200–900
WBC count (10⁹/l)	13.0	5–18
Neutrophils (10⁹/l)	10.27	3.7–13.32
Band neutrophils (10⁹/l)	0	0–0.54
Lymphocytes (10⁹/l)	2.73	1.00–3.60
Monocytes (10⁹/l)	0	0.00–0.72
Eosinophils (10⁹/l)	0	0.00–1.25

BLOOD FILM EVALUATION

Normocytic-normochromic erythrocytes. Platelet clumping.

BIOCHEMISTRY

Analyte (units)	Result	Reference Interval
Total protein (g/l)	65	55–75
Albumin (g/l)	33	29–35
Globulins (g/l)	32	18–38
ALP (U/l)	**1,289**	0–135
ALT (U/l)	**3,270**	0–40
GGT (U/l)	**20**	0–14
Total bilirubin (µmol/l)	**46.8**	0–5.0
Cholesterol (mmol/l)	7.3	3.8–7.9
Bile acids (µmol/l)	**>150**	0–30 (fasting)
Glucose (mmol/l)	4.2	3.0–5.5
Urea (mmol/l)	5.5	3.5–7.0
Creatinine (µmol/l)	113	0–130
Calcium (mmol/l)	2.4	2.3–3.0
Phosphorus (mmol/l)	1.2	0.9–1.6
Sodium (mmol/l)	149	135–150
Potassium (mmol/l)	4.4	3.5–5.6
Sodium:potassium ratio	34:1	>27:1
Canine PLI* (µg/l)	<30	>400 suggests pancreatitis

* Canine pancreatic lipase immunoreactivity.

QUESTIONS

1 What is your interpretation of the profile results, and what are the possible aetiologies?
2 How might you investigate further?

CASE 174

A male neutered mongrel dog of unknown age has been imported from Italy and immediately taken to a veterinarian.

EXAMINATION FINDINGS

Ticks are found on the dog. To exclude *Ehrlichia canis* infection, a rapid in-house test is performed. The test is negative.

QUESTIONS

1 How do you interpret the negative result of the rapid in-house test?
2 How would you proceed with this patient?

CASE 175

Case 157 looked at the critical number of test samples needed to obtain an estimate of the homeostatic setting point of creatinine in an individual dog. The International Renal Interest Society (IRIS) recommends staging of chronic renal disease based initially on fasting plasma creatinine, assessed on at least two occasions in the stable patient.

QUESTION

1 Would there be any benefit in analysing the two patient samples in duplicate in order to estimate the homeostatic setting point for creatinine in an individual dog with chronic stable renal disease?

CASE 176

A 5-year-old male German Shepherd Dog presented because of lethargy and exercise intolerance.

EXAMINATION FINDINGS

Unremarkable, as were the results of the blood biochemistry.

HAEMATOLOGY

Measurand (units)	Result	Reference Interval
RBC count (10^{12}/l)	5.85	5.5–8.5
Haemoglobin (g/l)	132	120–180
Haematocrit (l/l)	0.42	0.37–0.55
MCV (fl)	71.1	60–77
MCH (pg)	22.1	19.5–24.5
MCHC (g/l)	306	290–340
Reticulocytes (10^9/l)	**80.43**	0–60
Platelet count (10^9/l)	465	150–500
WBC count (10^9/l)	12.35	6–17
Neutrophils (10^9/l)	8.2	3.0–11.5
Lymphocytes (10^9/l)	2.8	1.0–3.6
Monocytes (10^9/l)	1.0	0.04–1.35
Eosinophils (10^9/l)	0.35	0.0–1.25
Basophils (10^9/l)	0.0	0.0–0.4

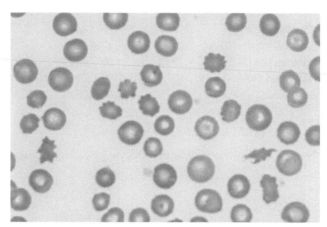

FIG. 176.1 RBCs in a blood film. May–Grünwald–Giemsa, ×100.

QUESTIONS

1 Describe the haematological abnormalities. What do you see on the blood smear? State the underlying pathophysiological mechanism.
2 How would you proceed with this patient?

CASE 177

A 13-month-old male Beagle presented with a long, vague history of intermittent lethargy, depression, possible PU/PD and occasional diarrhoea. The dog was fully vaccinated and had been dewormed regularly. According to the owner, he has never shown the exuberance of a normal puppy.

EXAMINATION FINDINGS

There was a slight bradycardia.

HAEMATOLOGY

Measurand (units)	Result	Reference Interval
RBC count (10^{12}/l)	5.3	5.5–8.0
Haemoglobin (g/l)	118	120–180
Haematocrit (l/l)	0.34	0.37–0.55
MCV (fl)	64	60–72
MCHC (g/l)	347	340–380
Reticulocyte count (10^9/l)	35	<80
Platelet count (10^9/l)	298	150–900
WBC count (10^9/l)	22	6–17
Neutrophils (10^9/l)	13.3	3.0–11.5
Band neutrophils (10^9/l)	0	0.0–0.31
Monocytes (10^9/l)	1.4	0.1–1.3
Lymphocytes (10^9/l)	4.9	1.0–4.8
Eosinophils (10^9/l)	2.4	0.12–1.5
Plasma protein (g/l) (refractometer)	84	60–80

BIOCHEMISTRY

Analyte (units)	Result	Reference Interval
Total protein (g/l)	79	54–74
Albumin (g/l)	48	27–45
Globulins (g/l)	31	19–34
Total bilirubin (µmol/l)	4.3	0–6.8
Cholesterol (mmol/l)	8.8	3.4–9.6
Glucose (mmol/l)	5.3	3.5–6.0
ALT (U/l)	111	10–120
AST (U/l)	34	35–280
ALP (U/l)	225	35–280
Amylase (U/l)	1,098	50–1,250
Lipase (U/l)	410	30–560
Urea (mmol/l)	59	2.5–10.0
Creatinine (µmol/l)	357	80–150
Calcium (mmol/l)	3.3	2.25–2.80

Analyte (units)	Result	Reference Interval
Phosphorus (mmol/l)	6.2	2.8–5.2
Sodium (mmol/l)	130	145–158
Potassium (mmol/l)	7.9	4.1–5.5
Chloride (mmol/l)	98	106–127
TCO_2^- (mmol/l)	11	14–27
Anion gap	29	8–25
Na:K ratio	16.5:1	

URINALYSIS (free catch)

Item	Result	Reference Interval
Colour	Light yellow	Yellow
Transparency	Clear	Clear
USG	1.022	>1.030
Dipstick evaluation		
pH	6.5	Acidic
Bilirubin	Negative	Negative to trace
Blood	Negative	Negative
Glucose	Negative	Negative
Ketone bodies	Negative	Negative
Protein	Negative	Negative to trace
Sediment examination		
Erythrocytes	2	0–5/hpf
Leucocytes	0	0–5/hpf
Epithelial cells	2	Variable/lpf
Crystals	None	Variable/lpf
Casts	None	None
Bacteria	None	None/lpf

QUESTIONS

1 Summarise and interpret the abnormalities in these laboratory results.
2 What additional tests could you perform in order to confirm or exclude the possible diagnosis?

Veterinary Clinical Pathology

CASE 178

You have looked at your biochemistry analyser performance and determined sigma metrics for a variety of the analytes. There are several analytes that have a sigma metric <5.

QUESTION

1 What can you do to determine the underlying cause for this lower than desirable level of performance capability?

CASE 179

A 5-year-old male gelded Thoroughbred steeplechaser was showing reduced performance but was normal on clinical examination. The trainer routinely carried out haematology on his horses "to monitor fitness" and this case gave the following results.

HAEMATOLOGY

Measurand (units)	Result	Reference Interval
RBC count (10^{12}/l)	**7.8**	8–12
Haemoglobin (g/l)	**98**	100–180
Spun PCV (%)	**34**	35–50
MCV (fl)	44	36–49
MCHC (g/l)	**290**	300–370
WBC count (10^9/l)	**3.9**	5.5–12.5
Neutrophils (10^9/l)	**2.1**	2.6–6.7
Lymphocytes (10^9/l)	**1.0**	1.5–5.5

Measurand (units)	Result	Reference Interval
Monocytes (10^9/l)	0.5	0–1
Eosinophils (10^9/l)	0.3	0–1
Basophils (10^9/l)	0	0.0–0.2

QUESTIONS

1 Discuss the laboratory findings and their significance.
2 What is your interpretation, and what are your recommendations?

CASE 180

An 8-month-old male neutered Jack Russell Terrier-cross presented for thin body condition, muscle tremors, rough hair coat with variable appetite and occasional diarrhoea.

HAEMATOLOGY

Measurand (units)	Result	Reference Interval
RBC count (10^{12}/l)	6.2	5.5–8.5
Haemoglobin (g/l)	**112**	120–180
Haematocrit (l/l)	**0.32**	0.37–0.55
MCV (fl)	**52**	60–77
MCH (pg)	**18.1**	19.5–24.5
MCHC (g/l)	350	320–370
RDW (%)	16.8	13.2–17.8
Platelet count (10^9/l)	191	175–500
WBC count (10^9/l)	**20**	6–17

Measurand (units)	Result	Reference Interval
Neutrophils (10^9/l)	**13.5**	3.0–11.5
Lymphocytes (10^9/l)	4.5	1.0–4.8
Monocytes (10^9/l)	**1.7**	0.2–1.5
Eosinophils (10^9/l)	0.3	0.1–1.3

BLOOD FILM EVALUATION

Erythrocyte, leucocyte and platelet morphology within normal limits. Platelet estimate adequate.

BIOCHEMISTRY

Analyte (units)	Result	Reference Interval
Total protein (g/l)	61	55–75
Albumin (g/l)	**22**	25–40
Globulins (g/l)	**39**	23–35
Glucose (mmol/l)	3.3	3.3–6.5
ALP (U/l)	**185**	0–130
ALT (U/l)	**125**	0–85
Pre-prandial bile acids (µmol/l)	**40**	<15
Post-prandial bile acids–2 hours (µmol/l)	**250**	<25
Urea (mmol/l)	3.5	3.3–8.0
Creatinine (µmol/l)	**40**	45–150
Sodium (mmol/l)	145	135–155
Chloride (mmol/l)	105	105–120
Potassium (mmol/l)	**4.4**	3.35–4.37
Total calcium (mmol/l)	**1.57**	2.3–2.8
Protein C (% activity)	**48**	≥70

QUESTIONS

1 What is your assessment of these findings?
2 What does the low protein C result support as a likely underlying cause?
3 What other biochemistry alterations are common with this suspected condition?
4 What might you expect to see on urinalysis?

CASE 181

An 11-year-old female neutered Jack Russell Terrier presented because of episodes of collapsing.

HAEMATOLOGY

Measurand (units)	Result	Reference Interval
RBC count (10^{12}/l)	**13.54**	5.5–8.5
Haemoglobin (g/l)	**261**	120–180
Haematocrit (l/l)	**0.788**	0.37–0.55
MCV (fl)	68	60–77
MCH (pg)	22.6	19.5–24.5
MCHC (g/l)	330	320–370
RDW (%)	**20.6**	13.2–17.8
Platelet count (10^9/l)	344	175–500
WBC count (10^9/l)	13.54	6–17
Neutrophils (10^9/l)	10.1	3.0–11.5
Lymphocytes (10^9/l)	2.8	1.0–4.8
Monocytes (10^9/l)	0.4	0.2–1.5
Eosinophils (10^9/l)	0.2	0.1–1.3

BLOOD SMEAR EVALUATION

RBCs: occasional NRBCs, moderate numbers of polychromatophils; WBCs: normal leucocyte morphology; platelets: no platelet clumps, consistent with count.

BIOCHEMISTRY

Unremarkable.

QUESTIONS

1 How would you distinguish relative from absolute erythrocytosis?
2 How would you distinguish primary from secondary absolute erythrocytosis?
3 What further investigations would you suggest, and what is your suspicion?

CASE 182

An equine practitioner calls and says he has a client who has a horse that is not performing well. It shows some reluctance to move and wrings its tail when asked to engage its hind end and move forward strongly. He is unsure whether this is a problem with tying up, a kidney stone or a sore back. He wants to know what laboratory test might be of benefit for diagnosis of tying up.

QUESTIONS

1 What laboratory test would you recommend?
2 How do you interpret your recommended test?

CASE 183
An 11-year-old female neutered mixed-breed dog presented for cystitis. Urine was obtained by catheterisation and submitted for evaluation after antibiotic treatment for the cystitis.

URINALYSIS

Item	Result	Reference Interval
Colour	Yellow	Yellow
Transparency	Clear	Clear
USG	1.032	1.020–1.045
Dipstick evaluation		
pH	6.0	Acidic
Leucocyte esterase	Negative	Negative
Nitrite	Negative	Negative
Protein	Negative	Negative to trace
Protein (SSA)	Negative	Negative to trace
Glucose	Negative	Negative
Ketone bodies	Negative	Negative
Bilirubin	**Positive +**	Negative to trace
Blood	Negative	Negative
Sediment analysis		
Amount	**Increased**	
Squamous epithelial cells	Negative	Variable/lpf
Tansitional epithelial cells	**Many**	Rare/lpf
Erythrocytes	Negative	Rare
Leucocytes	Negative	Rare
Crystals	Negative	Variable/lpf

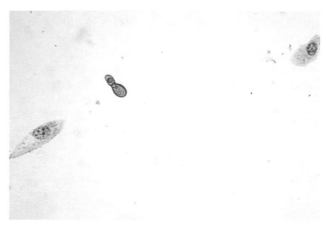

FIG. 183.2 Findings in the urine sediment. Methylene blue, ×40. (Courtesy Dr Judith Leidinger)

QUESTIONS

1 What cells can be seen in **Fig. 183.1**?
2 Is there evidence of neoplasia?
3 What is the pinkish structure in **Fig. 183.2**?

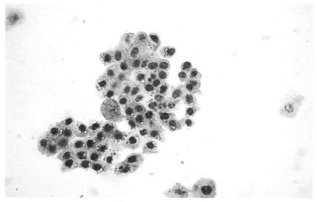

FIG. 183.1 Findings in the urine sediment. Methylene blue, ×10. (Courtesy Dr Judith Leidinger)

CASE 184

A 48-hour-old female Thoroughbred foal is presented for lethargy and poor suckling. The birth was attended and reported to be normal, with good suckling following foaling.

EXAMINATION FINDINGS

The mucous membranes are icteric.

INITIAL LABORATORY FINDINGS

Analyte (units)	Result	Reference Interval
Spun PCV (%)	10	30–50 (adult horse)
Total protein (g/l) (refractometer)	54	50–70 (adult horse)

RAPID FOAL-SIDE TEST FOR IMMUNOGLOBULINS

No demonstration of failure of passive transfer of maternal antibodies.

QUESTIONS

1 What tests would you recommend for this patient?
2 What is your interpretation of these tests?

CASE 185

An adult mongrel dog (age unknown) was imported from Spain recently. An ELISA in-house test was performed to rule out *Ehrlichia canis* infection. The test was positive. To exclude a false-positive result, a confirmatory PCR was added, which was negative.

QUESTIONS

1 How do you explain the positive result of the ELISA in-house test and the negative result of the PCR?

2 Which organism transmits *Ehrlichia* spp., and what other infectious agents may it carry?

CASE 186

A 12-year-old gelded Anglo-Arab horse presented with multiple skin lesions (peeling in the area of white blaze and white sock), hepatomegaly and bile duct distension on abdominal ultrasound.

HAEMATOLOGY

Unremarkable.

BIOCHEMISTRY

Analyte (units)	Result			Reference Interval
	Day 1	Day 30	Day 60	
Total protein (g/l)	**75**	69	69	55–75
Albumin (g/l)	**38**	**38**	**39**	26–37
Globulins (g/l)	38	31	30	24–45
Glucose (mmol/l)	5.1	6.4	5.3	3.4–6.4
AST (U/l)	**642**	**550**	430	183–497
CK (U/l)	**410**	**388**	331	113–333
GGT (U/l)	**663**	**245**	50	<50
ALP (U/l)	**460**	187	235	153–311
GLDH (U/l)	**43.9**	14.2	13.6	2.7–14.1
Bile acids (µmol/l)	15	15	14	0–15
Total bilirubin (µmol/l)	16.8	20.3	20.3	0–34

Analyte (units)	Result			Reference Interval
	Day 1	Day 30	Day 60	
Direct bilirubin (µmol/l)	5.0	5.3	6.2	<7
Urea (mmol/l)	3.6	4.0	3.9	3.3–6.7
Creatinine (µmol/l)	77	86	86	77–145
Sodium (mmol/l)	135	137	138	135–155
Potassium (mmol/l)	4.3	3.7	3.2	2.7–5.5
Chloride (mmol/l)	**93**	99	105	98–106
Calcium (mmol/l)	3.17	3.17	3.17	2.5–3.5
Phosphate (mmol/l)	0.91	1.20	1.50	0.9–1.6

QUESTIONS

1 How would you interpret the changes in liver enzymes?
2 According to the history, what are your main differentials?
3 What further investigations would you suggest?

CASE 187

A 2.5-year-old male hunting dog (breed not specified) presented with a history of poor stamina when hunting despite high enthusiasm early in the day. An episode of discoloured (red–brown) urine was observed on the way home.

HAEMATOLOGY

Measurand (units)	Result	Reference Interval
Spun haematocrit (PCV) (%)	15	35–55

BLOOD SMEAR EVALUATION

WBC count and platelet estimates and morphology are within normal limits. The erythrocytes are normocytic and normochromic.

QUESTIONS

1 What condition do you suspect may be present based on the clinical findings and/or the severe anaemia?
2 What is the pathophysiology underlying the suspected condition?
3 Are there any potential differential diagnoses, and what tests would you run to determine if these are likely?

CASE 188

An 8-year-old female Airedale Terrier presents because she tires easily, is depressed, has a decreased appetite and is vomiting.

EXAMINATION FINDINGS

T = 39.2°C (102.6°F), pale mucous membranes, bilateral epistaxis.

HAEMATOLOGY

Measurand (units)	Result	Reference Interval
RBC count (10^{12}/l)	3.30	5.5–8.0
Haemoglobin (g/l)	95	120–180
Haematocrit (l/l)	0.28	0.37–0.55
MCV (fl)	85	60–77
Reticulocytes (10^9/l)	33	28–80
Platelet count (10^9/l)	40	200–500
WBC count (10^9/l)	20.2	6–15
Neutrophils (10^9/l)	18.2	3.6–10.5
Lymphocytes (10^9/l)	0.8	1.0–3.6
Monocytes (10^9/l)	0	0.0–1.2
Eosinophils (10^9/l)	0	0.0–0.5

BLOOD SMEAR EVALUATION

See **Fig. 188.1**.

SEROLOGY

Infectious agent	Result	Borderline Titre
Borrelia burgdorferi (IgG, IFAT)	Negative	1:64
Babesia canis (IgG, IFAT)	Negative	1:40
Ehrlichia canis (IgG, IFAT)	Negative	1:40
Anaplasma phagocytophilum (IgG, IFAT)	Negative	1:80
Tick-borne encephalitis (TBE, ELISA)	Negative	1:100

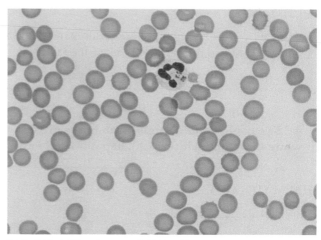

FIG. 188.1 Blood smear. Wright–Giemsa, ×100 (oil). (Courtesy Dr Georges Kirtz)

QUESTIONS

1 How would you classify the anaemia?
2 What is your diagnosis based on the haematology and serology results and the blood smear?
3 Why are antibodies to the organism causing this anaemia not detectable here?
4 What is the most frequent change in the FBC in this infection?

CASE 189

When a sigma metric <6 is determined for a laboratory test, further investigation should be considered in order to determine why 'world class' performance (reflected by ≥6 sigma) cannot be achieved. One tool for this is the Quality Goal Index (QGI) developed by Dr David Parry (St. Boniface General Hospital, Winnipeg).

$$QGI = Bias/1.5(CV)$$

CV = coefficient of variation for the individual test.

Derivation of this expression is based on mathematical reduction of the ratio (Bias/Accuracy Goal)/(CV/ Precision Goal). The QGI ratio represents the relative extent to which both bias and precision meet their respective quality goals, calculated using Total Allowable Error (TE_a). The quality goals chosen for use in this expression are $1.5 \times TE_a/6$ for bias and $TE_a/6$ for precision based on their widespread use in 6 sigma methodology literature.

QGI INTERPRETATION

Quality Goal Index	Likely Cause For <6 Sigma Performance
<0.8	Imprecision.
0.8–1.2	Imprecision and inaccuracy.
>1.2	Inaccuracy.

Below are some data regarding the performance of several tests on two different analysers used within the same laboratory.

Test	Instrument	TE_a (%)	Bias (%)	CV (%)	Sigma Metric
A	1	10	2.0	2.2	3.64
A	2	10	3.5	1.5	4.33
B	1	25	6.0	4.0	4.75
B	2	25	5.0	5.0	4.00

QUESTIONS

1 What are the QGIs associated with each of these test/ instrument combinations and the interpretations of the most likely reason for the <6 sigma performance?
2 What can be done to help improve inaccuracy and/or imprecision for a particular test?

CASE 190

A 2-year-old male English Bulldog presented to the referring veterinarian for clustering of seizures.

EXAMINATION FINDINGS

Physical examination was normal. Neurological examination revealed hindlimb ataxia.

HAEMATOLOGY

Unremarkable.

BIOCHEMISTRY

Sample quality: serum clear.

Analyte (units)	Result	Reference Interval
Total protein (g/l)	58	54–77
Albumin (g/l)	27	25–40
Globulins (g/l)	31	23–45
Glucose (mmol/l)	4.5	3.3–5.8
ALP (U/l)	57	14–105
ALT (U/l)	62	13–88
CK (U/l)	89	0–190
Urea (mmol/l)	**1.8**	2.8–8.3

Analyte (units)	Result	Reference Interval
Creatinine (µmol/l)	74	40–120
Sodium (mmol/l)	**123**	137–155
Chloride (mmol/l)	**85**	100–115
Potassium (mmol/l)	3.8	3.4–5.6
Na:K ratio	32.3	>27
Phosphate (mmol/l)	0.8	0.6–1.4

URINALYSIS

USG = 1.006; inactive sediment; protein:creatinine ratio = 0.2 (reference interval, <0.2).

QUESTIONS

1 What are the main differential diagnoses for the hyponatraemia?
2 What is the diagnostic approach to these changes?

CASE 191

A 17-year-old Cob mare presented because it had severe diarrhoea for the past 3 days.

HAEMATOLOGY

Blood was obtained following IV fluid therapy.

Analyte (units)	Result	Reference Interval
RBC count (10^{12}/l)	7.82	7.8–11.0
Haemoglobin (g/l)	138	130–170
Haematocrit (l/l)	0.40	0.34–0.46
MCV (fl)	**51.5**	38–49
MCH (pg)	17.6	14–19
MCHC (g/l)	342	310–390
Platelet count (10^9/l)	124	100–350
WBC count (10^9/l)	**3.6**	5–12
Neutrophils (10^9/l)	**2.23**	2.5–7.5
Lymphocytes (10^9/l)	**0.94**	1.5–4.0
Monocytes (10^9/l)	0.4	<0.5
Eosinophils (10^9/l)	0.04	0.0–0.5
Basophils (10^9/l)	0	<0.01
Fibrinogen (g/l) (heat precipitation method)	4	1–4

BLOOD FILM EVALUATION

Platelet clumping is present; true count probably higher than indicated. Platelet estimate adequate. No abnormal cells seen.

BIOCHEMISTRY

Analyte (units)	Result	Reference Interval
Total protein (g/l)	59.3	50–70
Albumin (g/l)	**15**	25–41
Globulins (g/l)	**44.3**	19–36
A:G ratio	**0.34**	0.6–2.0
ALP (U/l)	268	50–270
GGT (U/l)	40	10–45
AST (U/l)	259.4	100–370
Total bilirubin (µmol/l)	37	9–50
CK (U/l)	**461.3**	20–225
LDH (U/l)	863.2	130–1,085
GLDH (U/l)	**23.9**	0–11
Bile acids (µmol/l)	**34.1**	0.5–10.0
Cholesterol (mmol/l)	2.2	2.0–3.6
Urea (mmol/l)	5.4	3.3–7.4
Sodium (mmol/l)	136.2	132–146
Potassium (mmol/l)	4.3	3.3–5.4
Na:K ratio	31.67	28–40
Chloride (mmol/l)	97.7	89–108
Phosphorus (mmol/l)	**0.58**	0.9–1.8
Calcium (mmol/l)	**2.37**	2.5–3.6

SERUM PROTEIN ELECTROPHORESIS

Fraction (g/l)	Result	Reference Interval
Albumin	**18.5**	24–41
Alpha-1 globulin	1.05	0.5–3.0
Alpha-2 globulin	**10.6**	2–10
Beta-1 globulin	**11.86**	3–10
Beta-2 globulin	7.44	3–8
Gamma globulins	10.24	5–14

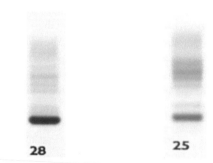

28   25

FIG. 191.1 Stained agarose gel electrophoresis. Albumin band is at the bottom of the gel. Left gel (28) is from a horse that is within normal limits. Right gel (25) is from this patient.

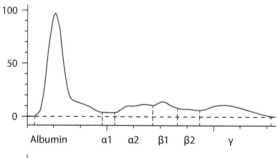

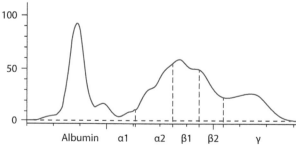

FIG. 191.2 Densitometry tracing of agarose gel. Top tracing is from a horse that is within normal limits. Bottom tracing is from this patient.

QUESTIONS

1 What is your analysis of these findings?
2 What additional testing may be of benefit in this case?

CASE 192

A 2-year-old male Miniature Schnauzer presented for occasional vomiting, mild diarrhoea and lethargy. A skin nodule over the left scapula proved to be a cutaneous xanthoma, based on fine needle aspiration and cytological examination.

HAEMATOLOGY

Unremarkable.

BIOCHEMISTRY

Analyte (units)	Result	Reference Interval
Total protein (g/l)	62.9	54.7–78.0
Albumin (g/l)	29.8	21–33
Globulins (g/l)	33.1	26–51
Glucose (mmol/l)	4.98	3.89–6.11
Cholesterol (mmol/l)	**11.5**	3.8–8.6
Triglycerides (mmol/l)	**5.4**	0.08–0.75
ALP (U/l)	**145**	0–39.7
ALT (U/l)	**206**	0–70
Urea (mmol/l)	**4.19**	7.14–10.7
Creatinine (μmol/l)	104	0–168
Sodium (mmol/l)	147	147–156
Chloride (mmol/l)	116	115–130
Potassium (mmol/l)	3.98	3.6–4.8
Ionised calcium (mmol/l)	1.29	1.17–1.32
Phosphate (mmol/l)	1.9	0.8–1.9

QUESTIONS

1 Considering the breed, what is the most likely diagnosis in this patient?
2 What differential diagnoses should you consider?
3 Which disease is often associated with hyperlipidaemia, also in Miniature Schnauzers?

CASE 193

A 1-year-old female Segugio Italiano dog presented for lethargy. She was used recently for hunting wild game.

EXAMINATION FINDINGS

Examination revealed hyperthermia (39.4°C [102.9°F]). No additional clinical signs were observed.

HAEMATOLOGY

Measurand (units)	Result	Reference Interval
RBC count (10^12/l)	7.05	5.9–8.1
Haemoglobin (g/l)	168	140–195
Haematocrit (l/l)	0.47	0.38–0.54
MCV (fl)	67.1	61–72
MCH (pg)	23.9	22–26
MCHC (g/l)	356	340–380
CHCM (g/l)	356	320–370
RDW (%)	13.3	12.2–15.0
Platelet count (10^9/l)	223	160–400
WBC count (10^9/l)	**18.3**	6.2–14.0
Neutrophils (10^9/l)	**9.42**	3.8–8.8

Measurand (units)	Result	Reference Interval
Band neutrophils (10^9/l)	**3.28**	0–3
Lymphocytes (10^9/l)	**1.12**	1.3–4.1
Monocytes (10^9/l)	2.38	2.0–7.5
Eosinophils (10^9/l)	1	0–1.1
Basophils (10^9/l)	0	0–1.0
CHCM = cell haemoglobin concentration mean.		

BLOOD SMEAR EVALUATION

The erythrocyte morphology was unremarkable. A few neutrophils displayed toxic changes (diffuse cytoplasmic basophilia). Single or multiple, round, variable-sized, deeply basophilic morulae with irregular borders were frequently observed intracellularly within neutrophils (**Fig. 193.1**).

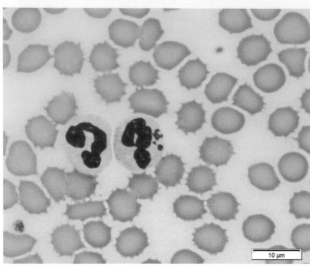

Analyte (units)	Result	Reference Interval
Glucose (mmol/l)	**7.27**	4.16–6.38
ALP (U/l)	**186**	20–120
ALT (U/l)	33	15–65
AST (U/l)	17	15–40
GGT (U/l)	4.2	2–8
Total bilirubin (μmol/l)	**5.3**	2.57–4.79
CK (U/l)	40	40–150
C-reactive protein (mg/l)	**768**	0–15
Urea (mmol/l)	8.93	6.43–16.13
Creatinine (μmol/l)	0.84	0.7–1.3
Sodium (mmol/l)	143	140–150
Chloride (mmol/l)	108	107–115
Potassium (mmol/l)	4.2	3.9–4.8

FIG. 193.1 Blood smear from the dog. Note the multiple, round, deeply basophilic morulae with irregular borders within a neutrophil. Modified Wright–Giemsa, ×100 (oil).

BIOCHEMISTRY

Analyte (units)	Result	Reference Interval
Total protein (g/l)	63.0	57–74
Albumin (g/l)	34.0	26–40
Globulins (g/l)	29.0	26–40

QUESTIONS

1 What is your assessment of these results?
2 What are the bases for the aetiology and pathogenesis for the present case?
3 What additional tests would be needed to confirm the likely diagnosis in this case?

CASE 194

An 8-week-old male Tibetan Mastiff showed an acute swelling on the head after playing with litter mates. Initially, it was small and flat, 1 × 0.5 cm (0.4 × 0.2 in) but was now 6 × 6 cm (2.4 × 2.4 in). A fine needle aspiration by the referring veterinarian revealed blood. The swelling was emptied with a syringe (2 ml) but it kept enlarging.

EXAMINATION FINDINGS

Pale mucous membranes were noted and the dog was slightly depressed.

COAGULATION PROFILE

Analyte (units)	Result	Reference Interval
aPTT (seconds)	**139**	71–102
PT (seconds)	13	12–17
Platelet count (10⁹/l)	250	200–500
BMBT	Not done	
D-dimer	**Negative**	1–4
PCV (%)	20	Not available for this age

QUESTIONS

1 What is your interpretation of these findings? Can you localise the bleeding problem to a specific part of the coagulation cascade?
2 What additional haemostatic tests are indicated?

CASE 195
A veterinary practitioner wants to assess the status of a cattle herd for a client.

QUESTIONS

1 Which acute-phase proteins (APPs) would you examine
to assess the health status of the cattle?
2 What actions does ceruloplasmin perform?

CASE 196
Foal number 1: 48 hours old. Presented with history of depression, possible blindness and seizures.
The serum Na^+ is 115 mmol/l (reference interval, 132–150). Foal number 2: 4 days old. Presented
with history of depression and had one seizure observed by groom. The serum Ca^{2+} is 2.0 mmol/l
(reference interval, 2.5–3.4). Foal number 3: 3 months old. Presented with history of diarrhoea for
the last 3 days and development within the last 24 hours of circling and head pressing and seizures.
Blood ammonia is 95 μmol/l (reference interval, <55).

QUESTIONS

1 For foal number 1, what are your main differential
diagnoses? What other tests may be helpful for
differentiating these diagnoses?
2 For foal number 2, is the slightly low calcium likely to be
the cause of the clinical signs? Why or why not?

3 For foal number 3, what are your differential diagnoses?
What other laboratory findings would provide support
for these diagnoses?

CASE 197
A 6-month-old male neutered Beagle was admitted with deep depression. The dog had been
adopted by the owner a few weeks ago.

EXAMINATION FINDINGS

Weakness, fever (39.6°C [103.3°F]); pale mucous membranes.

HAEMATOLOGY

Measurand (units)	Result	Reference Interval
RBC count (10^{12}/l)	**2.64**	5.70–8.56
Haemoglobin (g/l)	**60**	141–212
Haematocrit (l/l)	**0.18**	0.39–0.59
MCV (fl)	70	63.1–72.6
MCH (pg)	22.8	21.8–25.4
MCHC (g/l)	**326**	333–368
RDW (%)	**16.5**	11.6–14.7

Measurand (units)	Result	Reference Interval
Platelet count (10^9/l)	**85**	176–479
WBC count (10^9/l)	5.7	5.45–12.98
Neutrophils (10^9/l)	3.6	3.5–9.3
Lymphocytes (10^9/l)	1.7	1.1–3.8
Monocytes (10^9/l)	0.2	0.1–0.7
Eosinophils (10^9/l)	0.1	0–0.1

BLOOD SMEAR EVALUATION

The most relevant morphological changes are shown
(**Fig. 197.1**).

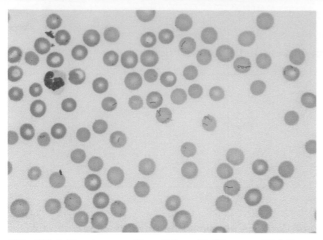

FIG. 197.1 Blood smear. May–Grünwald–Giemsa, ×50 (oil).

QUESTIONS

1 What are the most important morphological features of the blood smear?
2 What is the most probable pathogenesis of the disease diagnosed in this dog?
3 How can the diagnosis be confirmed?

CASE 198

An 18-month-old Jersey bull was kept on a dry lot with standard feeding and was current on vaccinations. He was scoop dehorned approximately 4 months ago. Sponges were inserted into the head, but it is uncertain if they were removed. He had been anorexic for the past 4 days.

EXAMINATION FINDINGS

There was a right-sided head tilt, swelling of the head, ventrolateral strabismus, exophthalmus, circling to the left and falling to the left (**Fig. 198.1**).

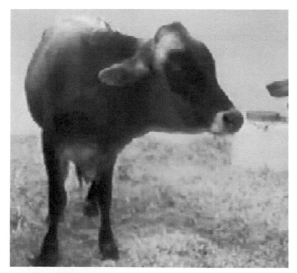

FIG. 198.1 Jersey bull showing depressed demeanour and circling to the left.

HAEMATOLOGY

Unremarkable except for fibrinogen of 0.8 g/l (reference interval, 0.2–0.4) and refractometer total protein of 84 g/l (reference interval, 55–80).

BIOCHEMISTRY

Analyte (units)	Result	Reference Interval
Albumin (g/l)	36	31–41
Glucose (mmol/l)	3.0	2.5–3.8
CK (U/l)	**233**	17–60
ALP (U/l)	77	3–86
GGT (U/l)	26	0–40
SDH (U/l)	12	0–15
Urea (mmol/l)	**23.8**	2.1–13.6
Creatinine (µmol/l)	**150**	62–115
Phosphorus (mmol/l)	2.36	1.49–2.36
Calcium (mmol/l)	2.56	2.23–2.73
Chloride (mmol/l)	102	92–102
Sodium (mmol/l)	**145**	135–144
Potassium (mmol/l)	3.9	3.5–5.0
TCO_2 (mmol/l)	32	24–32
Anion gap	14.9	12–22

CEREBROSPINAL FLUID ANALYSIS

Item	Result	Reference Interval
Macroscopic appearance	**Cloudy, white**	Clear, transparent
Erythrocytes (cells/µl)	7	<500
Leucocytes (cells/µl)	**4,100**	<10
Differential cell counts		
Neutrophils (%)	**90**	<5
Small mononuclear cells (%)	7	30–50
Large mononuclear cells (%)	3	40–60
Sodium (mmol/l)	145	<160
Glucose (mmol/l)	**0.5**	0.88–1.75

QUESTIONS

1 What is your assessment of these findings?
2 What are the most likely clinical diagnoses/differential diagnoses?

CASE 199

A 3-year-old male Drahthaar (hunting dog) presented because of haematuria and depression. The dog had spent some weeks in eastern Europe during the hunting season.

EXAMINATION FINDINGS

Weakness, fever (39.1°C [102.4°F]); slightly pale mucous membranes.

HAEMATOLOGY

Measurand (units)	Results	Reference Interval
RBC count (10^{12}/l)	5.88	5.70–8.56
Haemoglobin (g/l)	**135**	141–212
Haematocrit (l/l)	**0.38**	0.39–0.59
MCV (fl)	66.1	63.1–72.6
MCH (pg)	23	21.8–25.4
MCHC (g/l)	350	333–368
RDW (%)	12.9	11.6–14.7
Platelet count (10^9/l)	**135**	176–479
WBC count (10^9/l)	6.4	5.45–12.98
Neutrophils (10^9/l)	4.9	3.5–9.3
Lymphocytes (10^9/l)	**0.57**	1.1–3.8
Monocytes (10^9/l)	**0.9**	0.1–0.7
Eosinophils (10^9/l)	0	0–0.1

BLOOD SMEAR EVALUATION

The most relevant morphological changes are shown (**Fig. 199.1**).

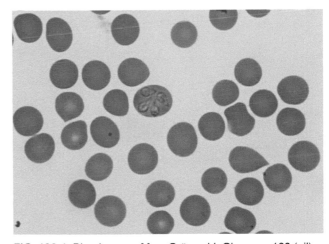

FIG. 199.1 Blood smear. May–Grünwald–Giemsa, ×100 (oil).

QUESTIONS

1 What are the structures in the cytoplasm of the erythrocytes?
2 What is the most probable pathogenesis of the disease diagnosed in this dog?
3 What other examination can be useful in the management of this disease?

CASE 200

A 9-month-old Hereford-cross steer weighing 400+ kg (880+ lb) was at pasture with 100 other steers of approximately equal weight and size, all intended for meat production. They were dewormed a month ago with ivermectin. Vaccinations are current. This steer was found depressed and not interested in eating and was rushed to the clinic.

EXAMINATION FINDINGS

Elevated RR and temperature.

HAEMATOLOGY

Measurand (units)	Result	Reference Interval
RBC count (10^{12}/l)	**8.45**	5.0–7.2
Haemoglobin (g/l)	114	87–124
Haematocrit (l/l)	**0.35**	0.25–0.33
MCV (fl)	41.5	38–51
MCH (pg)	14.5	14–19
MCHC (g/l)	**325**	340–380
Platelet count (10^9/l)	514	252–724
WBC count (10^9/l)	**21.3**	5.9–14.0
Neutrophils (10^{9}L)	**15.1**	1.80–7.20

Measurand (units)	Result	Reference Interval
Band neutrophils (10^9/l)	**0.52**	<0.30
Lymphocytes (10^9/l)	4.89	1.7–7.5
Monocytes (10^9/l)	0.784	0.0–0.9
Eosinophils (10^9/l)	0	0.0–1.3
Basophils (10^9/l)	0	0.0–0.3
Fibrinogen (g/l) (heat precipitation method)	**6**	2.0–5.0
Plasma protein (g/l) (refractometer)	76	55–80

QUESTIONS

1 What is your assessment of these findings?
2 What is/are your diagnosis/differential diagnoses?

Answers

CASE 1

1 What is your analysis of these results?

The most impressive findings in this case are the marked increase in CK and AST, supporting severe myopathy. Myopathy may involve skeletal and cardiac muscle, contributing to the collapse and death of this foal.

The severe myopathy is the most likely cause for the discoloured urine. The positive blood, protein and bilirubin reactions on dipstick are suspect because of the possibility of false-positive reactions due to the discolouration of the urine sample. With few erythrocytes in the sediment and a high CK and AST, the discoloured urine is likely due to myoglobin. Myoglobinuric nephrosis is supported by the red–brown granular casts (indicative of tubular damage) and marked increase in urea and creatinine. Differential diagnosis would be pre-renal damage, as the USG indicates concentrated urine. However, the presence of casts makes a solely pre-renal abnormality highly unlikely.

Additional abnormalities in GGT, GLDH and bile acids support hepatic dysfunction. The low albumin may be due to malnutrition related to poor ability to nurse associated with possible myopathy, but could also be due to decreased hepatic production. There may be some urinary protein loss, but this requires confirmation by other methods since the discoloured urine may interfere with the dipstick assessment.

The increase in phosphorus exceeds the age-related reference interval for foals, as expected with continued bone growth, and likely reflects renal injury/myoglobinuric nephrosis.

The hyponatraemia, hypokalaemia, hypocholaemia and hypocalcaemia likely reflect reduced intake. Increased renal loss may also contribute.

2 What are your differential diagnoses?

Toxicity (coffee weed ingestion or monensin toxicity), neurological disease (viral, developmental), equine rhabdomyolysis syndrome, botulism, rabies or trauma should all be considered, but in a foal between birth and 9 months of age with sudden collapse, nutritional myopathy should be a primary concern.

3 What additional testing would you recommend?

Additional history and examination of the pasture should be pursued to help rule out toxin exposure, possible exposure to rabid animals, botulism or trauma. Additional testing for vitamin E and glutathione peroxidase may help determine if vitamin E/selenium deficiency-associated nutritional myopathy is present.

Electrophoresis of the urine may provide the most definitive differentiation of myoglobinuria from haemoglobinuria.

FOLLOW UP
Further tests

Analyte (units)	Result	Reference interval
Glutathione peroxidase (µ/ml RBCs)	**3.7**	40–1,000
Vitamin E (µmol/l)	9.9	3–20

Glutathione peroxidase activity of erythrocytes may be a better indicator of long-term selenium status than serum selenium levels, since selenium is incorporated into erythrocytes during erythropoiesis. However, glutathione peroxidase activity may plateau above a certain level of selenium intake. Some animals may have levels of glutathione peroxidase below the reference interval without clinical signs.

A single vitamin E level within the reference interval does not completely rule out vitamin E deficiency. It has been suggested that a minimum of three samples should be used to determine vitamin E status since there may be marked variability in values between animals and within the same animal. Normal vitamin E levels may occur in deficient foals if there has been recent ingestion of colostrum.

POSTMORTEM DIAGNOSIS AND HISTOLOGICAL FINDINGS

Nutritional myopathy with renal, hepatic and cardiac failure.

CASE 2

1 What is your evaluation of the laboratory data?

There is slight hypochromic-normocytic anaemia. The increased RDW, increased aggregate reticulocyte count and few NRBCs are consistent with a marrow response to the anaemia. In the absence of a low total protein and clinical signs of external haemorrhage, haemolysis or ongoing internal haemorrhage are the primary considerations. The negative Coombs test does not completely rule out an immune-mediated basis for the anaemia, but does not provide any support for it.

The slight leucocytosis with absolute neutrophilia and monocytosis without concurrent lymphopaenia or eosinopaenia is consistent with an inflammatory leucogram.

The slight increase in ALT is consistent with hepatocellular damage. The slight hyperglycaemia is suggestive of stress or excitement at the time of collection. The possibility of a recent meal or diabetes mellitus cannot be completely ruled out, but there is no glucosuria or other features that support diabetes mellitus. The slight increase in pre-prandial and post-prandial bile acids are suggestive of hepatic dysfunction, but other causes of slight elevations, such as pancreatic or gastrointestinal disease, cannot be ruled out.

The negative FeLV/FIV ELISA results and negative PCR for feline haemotrophic *Mycoplasma* spp. suggests that the anaemia and/or inflammation are not due to chronic viral or *Mycoplasma* infection. The positive FeCoV titre is unlikely to be of significance in the absence of other findings suggestive of FIP (effusion, neurological signs, hypergammaglobulinaemia, lymphopaenia). The coagulation profile is unremarkable.

The cytology image contains a few hepatocytes whose features are not remarkable. There is moderate magenta/pink amorphous material consistent with amyloid. The cytological finding of material compatible with amyloid (see below) suggests hepatic dysfunction in association with increased pre-prandial and post-prandial bile acids.

2 What is your diagnosis/interpretation for this case?

This cat has the following problems: anaemia; inflammation (inflammatory leucogram); hyperglycaemia, likely related to stress; hepatocellular enzyme leakage and decreased hepatic function, associated with hepatic amyloidosis.

3 What pathophysiology is likely underlying the findings in this case?

The interpretation of hepatic amyloidosis is consistent with hepatocellular damage because of decreased blood flow and/or perivascular accumulation of amyloid with increased ALT and compromised function resulting in the slight increase in pre-prandial and post-prandial bile acids. The amyloid may cause intrahepatic rupture with intra-abdominal haemorrhage, resulting in the anaemia. The intra-abdominal location explains an absence of detection of a site of external haemorrhage. The presence of intracavitary haemorrhage may explain the inflammatory leucogram since no other site of inflammation has been identified. The possibility of hepatic inflammation cannot be ruled out because hepatic aspiration is relatively insensitive to focal or multifocal inflammation in the liver.

4 What other tests would you recommend performing, and why?

Hepatic biopsy would be helpful to confirm the amyloidosis and evaluate the extent of involvement and any other features that may be present.

FOLLOW UP AND CASE DISCUSSION

Hepatic biopsy confirmed hepatic amyloidosis with focal haemorrhage and slight impairment in hepatic function.

Amyloidosis is an uncommon disease in cats. It can be secondary to a systemic disease such as chronic inflammatory, infectious or neoplastic disease or exist as a breed-associated condition in which the cause is not known. In affected cats the precursor protein amyloid A, an amino terminal fragment of the acute-phase protein serum amyloid A, deposits in different organs such as the liver and kidney. Some systemic disorders have been described linked to amyloidosis in humans and dogs (e.g. multiple myeloma, lymphoma, blastomycosis, systemic lupus erythematosus and cyclic neutropaenia) but only a few associative disorders have been described in cats (e.g. feline infectious peritonitis). It has been advocated that any chronic inflammation process could cause secondary amyloidosis in cats, but otherwise it has never been proved.

Most published reports refer to the familial form in which accumulation of amyloid A occurs in the kidney, causing a glomerulopathy and chronic renal failure mainly in Abyssinian cats. In Siamese, Oriental and DSH cats, the accumulation is principally in the liver, causing ruptures and haemorrhages.

The signalment, signs on presentation and cytology were highly suggestive of amyloidosis; the final diagnosis was made with histology. It has been suggested that cytology from an FNA can replace biopsy for the diagnosis of liver amyloidosis; however, other authors have reported disagreement between cytology and histology.

No proven treatment is available for feline amyloidosis. Colchicine has been described for human cases (e.g. Mediterranean fever) and in dogs with amyloidosis. Treatment with this drug was offered but was declined by the owner in this case.

CASE 3

1 What is your evaluation of the laboratory data?

The erythrocytosis noted here could be relative or absolute. Relative erythrocytosis is likely in this dehydrated dog and further assessment after correction of the fluid deficits would allow confirmation. The azotaemia with hypercalcaemia, hyperkalaemia and hyponatraemia are highly supportive for hypoadrenocorticism, especially

	N	N (%) above RI	N (%) below RI
Urea	225	199 (88%)	0
Creatinine	225	147 (65%)	0
Sodium	298	1 (<1%)	243 (82%)
Potassium	298	277 (93%)	0
Na:K ratio (>27:1)	298	-	272 (91%)
Chloride	287	9 (3%)	138 (48%)
Calcium (total)	225	69 (31%)	21 (9%)
Calcium (ionised)	72	13 (18%)	18 (25%)
Glucose	295	41 (14%)	44 (15%)
N = number of dogs tested; RI = reference interval			

FIG. 3.1 Biochemical abnormalities reported in dogs with confirmed hypoadrenocorticism. Data extracted from Peterson *et al.* (1996) and Adler *et al.* (2007).

given the clinical presentation. The diagnosis is confirmed on the basis of the low cortisol concentrations before and after IV administration of tetracosactide.

In this case, the clinical presentation and laboratory abnormalities on initial screening tests are strongly supportive of hypoadrenocorticism. However, these profile changes are not always present and the absence of electrolyte changes (hyperkalaemia, hyponatraemia or Na:K ratio <27:1) does not exclude the diagnosis (**Fig. 3.1**). The sensitivity and specificity for a Na:K ratio of 27:1 have been reported as 89% and 97%, respectively. Results from the same study suggest that for a Na:K ratio <24:1, there is a high probability that the patient has hypoadrenocorticism.

Although both hyperglycaemia and hypoglycaemia are reported in confirmed cases, some patients present with weakness and seizures secondary to hypoglycaemia and hypoadrenocorticism should be considered in the causes of low blood glucose. Peterson *et al.* (1996) reported that 99 of 172 dogs (57.6%) with hypoadrenocorticism had a USG <1.030 despite the presence of azotaemia. This feature highlights the need for careful consideration of other differentials before diagnosing renal failure per se.

2 How might prior therapy affect confirmation of the diagnosis?

Recent therapy with prednisolone, prednisone and hydrocortisone may cause a false increase in cortisol concentration as a consequence of cross-reactivity of the drugs in cortisol assays. These drugs should be withdrawn 24 hours prior to performing an ACTH stimulation test. The results below are from a patient with suspected hypoadrenocorticism who was given prednisolone on the morning of the first ACTH stimulation test. A second test confirmed the diagnosis.

	Basal cortisol (nmol/l)	Cortisol post ACTH* (nmol/l)
Day 1: prednisolone given	106	111
Day 3: no therapy within 24 hours	<28	<28
* Sample collected 60 minutes after an IV injection of 250 µg of tetracosactide.		

Dexamethasone does not cross-react in laboratory assays for cortisol but may cause suppression of endogenous cortisol production from approximately 4–6 hours after administration. Where there is concern that prior steroid therapy could interfere with the interpretation of the dynamic test, measurement of aldosterone before and after administration of tetracosactide is recommended.

3 Briefly outline the pathophysiology underlying these laboratory abnormalities.

Cortisol and aldosterone are synthesised from cholesterol, via a pathway of intermediary steroids, in the adrenal cortex. Aldosterone plays a critical role in the homeostatic regulation of body water and it acts on the distal renal tubule, inducing sodium and chloride retention and excretion of potassium (and hydrogen).

Aldosterone secretion is stimulated by the renin–angiotensin system, the direct effect of hyperkalaemia on the zona glomerulosa, ACTH and hyponatraemia (**Fig. 3.2**).

Hypoadrenocorticism is a deficiency of glucocorticoids and, in most cases, mineralocorticoid hormone activity. Primary hypoadrenocorticism is caused by destruction of the adrenal gland by an immune-mediated process or, occasionally, by infiltrative disease or drug therapy. Primary hypoadrenocorticism commonly results in deficiencies of both glucocorticoid and mineralocorticoid activity, but a small percentage of affected dogs have normal electrolyte concentrations on initial presentation. These individuals may subsequently develop clinically significant electrolyte abnormalities.

A selective deficiency of glucocorticoid hormones is recognised in dogs with reduced pituitary–hypothalamic activity secondary to exogenous steroid administration or destructive lesions of the CNS (secondary hypoadrenocorticism). Mineralocorticoid hormone activity is spared in these patients. Measurement of endogenous ACTH may allow differentiation between primary disease, which is associated with high plasma ACTH concentrations, and secondary hypoadrenocorticism, in which the ACTH concentration is low. However, strict sample handling guidelines should be followed, including transporting the sample to the laboratory in a frozen state. In addition, ACTH rapidly decreases after exogenous steroid treatment and therefore the sample must be collected prior to therapy.

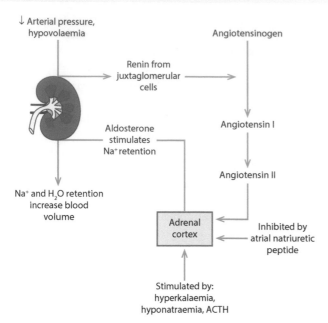

FIG. 3.2 Schematic representation of the mechanisms of control of aldosterone secretion from the adrenal cortex.

FOLLOW UP

For primary hypoadrenocorticism, mineralocorticoid therapy is required for the remainder of the patient's life. Approximately 50% of dogs also require long-term glucocorticoid supplementation. Medical therapy was introduced in this case and a follow-up electrolyte screen was performed 2 weeks later:

Analyte (units)	Result	Reference interval
Urea (mmol/l)	**10**	3.5–7.0
Chloride (mmol/l)	106	95–117
Sodium (mmol/l)	142	135–150
Potassium (mmol/l)	5.03	3.5–5.6
Sodium:potassium ratio	27:1	>27:1

REFERENCES AND FURTHER READING

Adler JA, Drobatz KJ, Hess RS (2007) Abnormalities of serum electrolyte concentrations in dogs with hypoadrenocorticism. *J Vet Intern Med* **21**:1168–1173.

Church DB (2004) Canine hypoadrenocorticism. In: *BSAVA Manual of Canine and Feline Endocrinology*, 3rd edn. (eds. CT Mooney, ME Peterson) British Small Animal Veterinary Association, Gloucester, p. 172.

Dunn KJ, Herrtage ME (1998) Hypocortisolaemia in a Labrador retriever. *J Small Anim Pract* **39**:90–93.

Peterson ME, Kintzer PP, Kass PH (1996) Pretreatment clinical and laboratory findings in dogs with hypoadrenocorticism: 225 cases (1979–1993). *J Am Vet Med Assoc* **208**:85–91.

Syme HM, Scott-Moncrieff JC (1998) Chronic hypoglycaemia in a hunting dog due to secondary hypoadrenocorticism. *J Small Anim Pract* **39**:348–351.

CASE 4

1 What is the anion gap (AG) in this case?
The AG = $(Na^+ + K^+) - (Cl^- + HCO_3^-)$ = $(145 + 6.5) - (124 + 10)$ = $151.5 - 134 = 17.5$. This is within the reference interval.

2 What is your assessment of the arterial pH?
The arterial pH is decreased, therefore this is an acidaemia.

3 What is your assessment of the likely underlying aetiology?
The bicarbonate is decreased, so the acidaemia is due to metabolic acidosis.

4 Is there appropriate compensation for this condition?
The $PaCO_2$ is decreased, as expected for compensation for a metabolic acidosis. The formula for compensation is:

$$PaCO_2 = 1.54 (HCO_3^-) + 8.4 \pm 1.1$$
$$PaCO_2 = 1.54 (10) + 8.4 \pm 1.1 = 15.4 + 8.4 \pm 1.1$$
$$= 23.8 \pm 1.1 = 22.7 \text{ to } 24.9$$

In this case, the measured $PaCO_2 = 24$. This is within the expected range for an adequate compensatory response.

5 Why is the K^+ increased in this case?
The K^+ is increased due to the buffering mechanism by which H^+ shifts from the extracellular fluid into the intracellular fluid in exchange for K^+.

6 Why is the Cl^- increased in this case?
The Cl^- is increased due to normal compensatory mechanisms based on the need to maintain electroneutrality. Since HCO_3^- has decreased, another anion must take its place. This suggests adequate Cl^- intake and absence of excessive loss from the kidney due to aldosterone influence.

7 What is a likely underlying aetiological mechanism for metabolic acidosis?
This is a secretional (hyperchloraemic or normal AG) acidosis resulting from loss of HCO_3^- in gastrointestinal fluids. In this case diarrhoea is the cause of the abnormalities. Administration of large amounts of sodium chloride (dilutional acidosis) can also cause hyperchloraemic metabolic acidosis that is not of secretional origin. However, these iatrogenic metabolic acidoses should be easily recognised because of the treatment history.

FURTHER READING

Dibartola SP (2012) *Fluid, Electrolyte and Acid-Base Disorders in Small Animal Practice*, 4th edn. Elsevier Saunders, St Louis.

CASE 5

1 Describe and discuss the significant biochemistry findings, and give the most likely cause of the icterus.

There is a severe hyperbilirubinaemia, which may be pre-hepatic, hepatic or post-hepatic in origin. In the face of normal haematology, pre-hepatic icterus is very unlikely. Severe hyperbilirubinaemia in combination with hypercholesterolaemia and increased ALP enzyme activity suggests cholestasis due to obstruction of bile ducts. Cholestasis is the most likely aetiology given the presence of mud-coloured faeces suggesting the absence of bile pigment. ALP, ALT and GLDH enzyme activities are severely increased. ALT is located intracytoplasmatically in hepatocytes and GLDH in mitochondria of hepatocytes. Thus, a severe increase of ALT and GLDH enzyme activity is indicative of severe hepatocellular damage. Mild hyponatraemia and hypochloraemia are also present, which are most likely due to loss of hypertonic fluid due to the vomiting and subsequent intake of pure water. The overall picture is suggestive of obstructive cholestasis as a cause for the icterus in this patient.

2 What further examinations are recommended to determine the aetiology of the disease in this dog?

Obstructive cholestasis is caused by pathological conditions impairing the bile flow through bile canaliculi or bile ducts. Probable aetiology includes stones (extremely rare in dogs), neoplasia and hepatitis/pancreatitis. The latter conditions may cause an obstruction of the bile ducts due to cellular swelling. Thus, the first step is an abdominal ultrasound to determine the probable underlying aetiology. Depending on the findings, laparotomy and/or biopsy of liver, pancreas and intestine are required. Infectious diseases such as leptospirosis should be considered as a cause for hepatitis.

FOLLOW UP
Abdominal ultrasound

During sonography, a severely dilated gallbladder and 2–3 markedly dilated bile ducts were visible. Only parts of the pancreas were detected, which was unremarkable at the time of examination.

Because of the severe obstructive cholestasis, laparotomy was performed, which revealed a small hepatic mass of 3 cm in diameter located near the gallbladder. The cystic duct was severely dilated. In the area of the papilla

magna, pancreas and mesenteric fat tissue were firm and nodular. The gallbladder was emptied and cholecysto-duodenostomy performed. Biopsies were taken from the hepatic mass near the gallbladder and from the firm nodules in the mesenteric fat tissue.

Histopathological examination

Biopsies from the hepatic mass were consistent with severely increased glycogen storage. Specimens of the mesenteric fat tissue were consistent with focal necrosis, haemorrhage and groups of lymphocytes. Based on these findings, a chronic pancreatitis with subsequent necrosis of the fat tissue was considered to be the most likely aetiology.

Leptospira serology

A serological survey of eight *Leptospira* serovars turned out negative.

Two days post operation, the dog was vomiting again. Amylase and lipase were assessed to evaluate the pancreas.

Analyte (units)	Result	Reference Interval
Amylase (U/l)	5,618	<1,157
Lipase (U/l)	2,726	<300

Clinical chemical analysis revealed severely increased amylase and lipase (more than 3 times the upper limit of the reference interval) suggestive of acute pancreatic necrosis.

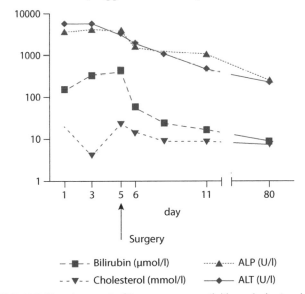

FIG. 5.2 Development of liver enzyme activities, cholesterol and bilirubin plasma concentrations prior to surgery and after cholecystoduodenostomy. Eighty days after surgery, the cholesterol plasma concentration is within the reference interval (3.3–8.6 mmol/l), whereas bilirubin plasma concentration as well as ALP and ALT enzyme activities are still mildly elevated, exceeding the reference intervals of <3.6 µmol/l, <131 U/l and <85 U/l, respectively.

Treatment included broad-spectrum antibiotics, anti-emetics, sucralphate, buprenorphine, continuous infusions of isotonic fluids, heparin and a plasma transfusion. The dog improved clinically and follow-up examinations demonstrated a gradual decrease of bilirubin, ALP, cholesterol and ALT (**Fig. 5.2**).

CASE 6

1 Does the anaemia appear regenerative?

The increased polychromasia, reticulocytosis and red cell indices (macrocytic [increased MCV], hypochromic [decreased MCHC] anaemia) indicate a regenerative anaemia. In addition, there are some NRBCs.

2 What is the significance of the blood smear picture?

The blood smear supports a regenerative response to the anaemia and the presence of small, dark-staining, dot- to rod-shaped organisms on the RBC indicates *Mycoplasma* spp. Organisms to consider are *Mycoplasma haemofelis* or *Candidatus Mycoplasma haemominutum*. The latter is usually smaller than *M. haemofelis*.

Usually, predisposing factors making the patient susceptible for the infection are needed. These could be FeLV or FIV infection, which can be ruled out in this cat. However, other systemic illnesses, trauma, neoplasia or other infections may lead to decreased immunocompetence of the patient and favour infection with *Mycoplasma* spp. Whether or not the described cardiomyopathy may be such a predisposing factor in this cat remains to be determined.

Mycoplasma infects erythrocytes and elicits a strong immune response, with antibodies either binding to parasite antigens on the erythrocyte surface or to altered RBC antigens. Finally, the spleen clears these RBCs from the circulation. A progressive regenerative haemolytic anaemia is the final result.

CASE 7

1 Name the abnormality visible in the blood smear.

Poikilocytic erythrocytes (abnormal shape) are visible. There are also moderate numbers of eccentrocytes (also known as bite cells, cross-bonded cells, or hemighosts).

2 List possible reasons for this finding for dogs, cats and horses. What is the reason in this case?

Eccentrocytes result from oxidative damage of erythro-cytes. In general possible causes include: inherited disorders (horse) (e.g. glucose–6–phosphate dehydrogenase deficiency, flavin adenine dinucleotide deficiency); ingestion of onions (horses, dogs, cats); ingestion of garlic (horses, dogs); red maple toxicity (*Acer rubrum*) (horse); vitamin K administration (dogs); acetaminophen treatment (dogs, cats); IV hydrogen peroxidase administration (cattle); various illnesses (e.g. diabetes mellitus, T-cell lymphoma, severe infections).

Lymphoma is described as resulting in eccentrocytes in cats. This is therefore the most likely cause of the abnormal RBC shape in this cat.

3 Describe the underlying pathological mechanism leading to this finding.

The above conditions lead to oxidative injury to erythrocytes. RBC membranes are altered, resulting in adherence of opposing areas of the cytoplasmic face of the RBC membrane. Therefore, haemoglobin is dislocated eccentrically, which leads to the typical appearance of the eccentrocytes. Collapsing of the cell membrane may lead to pyknocytes.

FURTHER READING

Stockham SL, Scott MA (2008) *Fundamentals of Veterinary Clinical Pathology*, 2nd edn. Blackwell Publishing, Oxford.

Weiss J, Wardrop KJ (2010) (eds) *Schalm's Veterinary Hematology*, 6th edn. Blackwell Publishing, Ames.

CASE 8

1 What is the most likely explanation for the laboratory abnormalities?

The haematology result shows a slight neutrophilia in the face of a normal leucocyte count. In general, causes may be acute or chronic inflammatory neutrophilia, steroid neutrophilia or physiological (epinephrine effect) neutrophilia. Rare Döhle bodies have been observed on the blood smear. Döhle bodies are cytoplasmic aggregates of rough endoplasmic reticulum. They contain RNA and are part of the signs of toxicity. These are consistent with a maturation defect due to accelerated myelopoiesis. However, Döhle bodies occur physiologically in small numbers in cats. As other signs of toxicity (e.g. basophilic cytoplasm, foamy cytoplasm) as well as band neutrophils are missing, inflammatory neutrophilia is unlikely. Lymphocyte and monocyte counts, as well as the number of eosinophils, are normal, which makes a steroid effect also unlikely. As cats are prone to fear and excitement, especially in the situation of seeing the veterinarian and blood sampling, an epinephrine effect should be considered. Catecholamines (e.g. epinephrine) lead to a dislocation of the marginated neutrophils in the blood vessel into the blood stream. As only the neutrophils in the central blood stream are sampled, this may be the cause of the present neutrophilia.

The erythron displays several abnormalities. While decreased RBC numbers and the haematocrit point to an anaemia, the increased haemoglobin concentration does not match with this finding. Very striking are the increased MCH and MCHC. In the face of haemolysis, leakage of haemoglobin out of RBCs and destruction of RBCs takes place. Therefore, increased haemoglobin associated with a decreased RBC number will be detected. The measured haemoglobin will not only contain the measured intraerythrocytic haemoglobin but also the free haemoglobin in the plasma. The haematocrit, MCH and MCHC are calculated by the haematology analyser according to the formulas:

$$Htc = \frac{MCV \times [RBC]}{1000} \quad MCH = \frac{[Hgb]}{[RBC]} \quad MCHC = \frac{[Hgb]}{Htc}$$

As the RBC number is altered by the haemolysis, the calculated Hct is also wrong (falsely decreased). An easy way to check if the haematocrit and haemoglobin concentration match and are detected accurately is the 'Rule of 3'. Using conventional units, the haemoglobin concentration is simply multiplied by three and results in the haematocrit ± 3. If SI units are used, the calculation is:

$$Hgb \times 0.003 = Htc \pm 3$$

Using this easy formula, the mismatch will be rapidly noticed and the problem detected. As the measured Hgb concentration and RBC number, as well as the calculated Hct, are altered, MCHC and MCH are also falsely increased, as seen in the formula above. Therefore, haemolysis is the most likely cause for the abnormalities in the erythrogram. Further evaluations will be needed to determine if this is iatrogenic haemolysis or is due to pathological intravascular haemolysis.

2 State and explain the causes for an increased MCHC.

The MCHC is the cellular haemoglobin concentration per average erythrocyte. This is one of the Wintrobe's erythrocyte indices and is used to characterise the erythrocytes in the peripheral blood. In the case of a normal MCHC the RBCs are described as normochromic, while a decreased MCHC presents as hypochromic RBCs. In theory, an RBC with an increased MCHC would be hyperchromic. However, a mature RBC's dry matter consists of about 95% haemoglobin. More than 95% haemoglobin in an erythrocyte is thereby not possible. An increased MCHC is therefore almost always related to some kind of artefact. Possible causes for an increased MCHC and MCH include:

- Haemolysis (see above), either intravascular haemolysis or *in-vitro* haemolysis.
- Spectral interferences: haemoglobin is detected via spectrophotometry. If the sample is highly lipaemic, is grossly icteric, displays a severe leucocytosis, or the patient's RBCs contain Heinz bodies, there may be interference with the haemoglobin assay.
- There will be an interference with light transmission in the spectrophotometer and a falsely increased MCHC.
- Eccentrocytes are RBCs with an abnormal shape due to oxidative damage of the erythrocyte (such as onion ingestion, some NSAIDs, other drugs). Because of the oxidative change, part of the RBC membranes fuse and the haemoglobin is condensed, leading to a proportional loss of cell volume and a potentially increased MCHC. This condition, however, is rare.

3 How do you explain the biochemistry changes in light of the abnormalities discussed in the first two questions?

The biochemical changes can be explained by looking at the methodology of sodium, phosphate and glucose measurement. Many analyzers use spectrophotometry for their detection. As indicated above, haemoglobin interferes with spectrophotometric assays.

Spectrophotometry (simplified scheme: Fig. 8.1):
The analyte in the sample absorbs light of a specific wavelength. The detector measures how much light

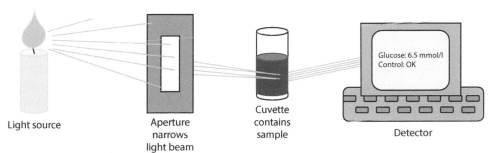

FIG. 8.1 Simplified spectrophotometry schematic. A light source projects a beam of a selected wavelength, which is focused (narrowed) by an aperature, and light that is transmitted through the sample is measured by a detector. The concentration of a substance in the sample is calculated based on the amount of light transmitted through the sample.

has been absorbed and calculates the concentration of the analyte. As haemoglobin interferes with the light transmission, it may lead to falsely increased/decreased results. In this case, false hyperphosphataemia and hyperglycaemia may be present. Because of this possible interference, it is always important to know which interferences influence which analyte and in what way. This information should be available in the user's manual for the biochemistry instrument.

FURTHER READING

Stockham SL, Scott MA (2008) *Fundamentals of Veterinary Clinical Pathology*, 2nd edn. Blackwell Publishing, Oxford.

CASE 9

1 Is this azotaemia likely to be pre-renal, renal or post-renal? Why?

The increase in urea and creatinine indicates a moderate azotaemia. Azotaemia may be pre-renal (hypovolaemia due to dehydration, decreased cardiac output due to cardiac insufficiency or shock), renal (kidney dysfunction) or post-renal (urinary obstruction). There are several elements that suggest this is a pre-renal azotaemia, likely secondary to the polyuria (which is driving polydipsia):

- There is a slight increase in total protein and albumin, which is likely due to haemoconcentration secondary to dehydration.
- There is an asynchronous increase in urea compared to creatinine (urea is 1.5 times the upper reference limit and creatinine is just slightly over the reference interval). This is likely due to dehydration because in this condition, urea is resorbed by the renal tubules, increasing the levels in the peripheral blood. The possibility of digestion of blood associated with high intestinal or gastric bleeding should also be considered when urea is disproportionately increased compared with creatinine.
- There is no evidence of chronic renal failure because the dog is in good body condition, there is no evidence of anaemia and the PU/PD had a sudden onset. Urinalysis is often helpful in distinguishing between pre-renal and renal azotaemia, although in this case it is not helpful because of the hypercalcaemia, which interferes and lowers the USG.

2 How would you explain the low USG?

The USG is low (<1.007) and is hyposthenuric. There is no hypersthenuria, as would be expected considering the evidence of a pre-renal azotaemia. The cause of this is the hypercalcaemia, which has caused a nephrogenic diabetes insipidus, a group of renal and extrarenal diseases in which ADH is present but the renal tubules are not responsive to it. Increased ionised calcium inhibits ADH activity via dysregulation of aquaporins, a group of proteins of the cell membrane that regulate the flow of water. In addition, the presence of increased calcium reduces tubular resorption of sodium and chloride in the ascending limb of the loop of Henle, which reduces the osmotic gradient needed for water resorption in the distal nephron.

3 Explain the possible cause of the reported hypercalcaemia.

There is a moderate increase in total calcium, which may be due to several conditions. High total calcium is observed with: increased calcium mobilisation from bone or absorption in intestine; increased vitamin D activity; decreased urinary excretion of calcium; increased protein-bound calcium; and idiopathic cases (cats).

Increased calcium mobilisation from bone or absorption from intestine may be due to primary hyperparathyroidism, which is characterised by an increase in secretion of parathyroid hormone (PTH), which also causes hypophosphataemia because of its phosphaturic action. Therefore, in this case PTH may be measured to assess primary hyperparathyroidism, although this is considered unlikely because hypercalcaemia is not associated with hypophosphataemia. Another possible differential is humoral hypercalcaemia of malignancy, which is due to the production of a specific hypercalcaemic agent (PTHrP) by neoplastic cells. Increased vitamin D is another cause of increased total calcium and concurrent hyperphosphataemia because it promotes intestinal absorption of calcium and phosphate. Vitamin D can be measured and in this case could be a possible cause of the hypercalcaemia considering the concurrent hyperphosphataemia. Hypercalcaemia can also be caused by decreased urinary excretion of calcium because of renal failure. However, dogs with renal failure may have increased total calcium because of an increased concentration of calcium bound to ions that have not been excreted by the kidney, but have a decrease in free calcium that is lost by the kidneys. Measurement of ionised calcium when hypercalcaemia is present may be helpful to exclude a possible renal cause of the hypercalcaemia. In this case the azotaemia is likely to be pre-renal, but an underlying renal disease caused by the hypercalcaemia cannot completely be excluded. Occasionally, idiopathic conditions can cause hypercalcaemia, especially in the cat.

For these reasons PTH, PTHrP and vitamin D were measured. Low-normal PTH excludes hyperparathyroidism, low PTHrP excludes hypercalcaemia of malignancy. High vitamin D, hypercalcaemia and hyperphosphataemia reflects hypervitaminosis D.

Analyte (units)	Result	Reference interval
PTH (pg/ml)	**18.5**	20–65
PTHrP (pmol/l)	<0.1	0–0.5
Vitamin D (ng/ml) 25(OH)D3	**64.6**	19.3–43.6

4 What is your diagnosis?

Hypervitaminosis D. The psoriasis cream ingested by the dog contained high levels of vitamin D and is likely to be the cause. There is a concurrent nephrogenic diabetes insipidus, which is likely secondary to hypercalcaemia and is the cause of the PU/PD and the consequent dehydration.

FURTHER READING

Stockham SL, Scott MA (2008) *Fundamentals of Veterinary Clinical Pathology*, 2nd edn. Blackwell Publishing, Oxford.

Villiers E (2005) Disorders of erythrocytes. In: *BSAVA Manual of Canine and Feline Clinical Pathology*, 2nd edn. (eds. E Villiers, L Blackwood) British Small Animal Veterinary Association, Gloucester, pp. 33–37.

CASE 10

1 Are all these aspects demonstrated in the clinical history and laboratory tests to confirm suspicion of DIC?

DIC can be caused by severe systemic inflammation, which is evidently present in the present case. The clinical signs of systemic inflammatory response syndrome (increased HR and RR and increased temperature) along with a clear inflammatory leucogram (neutrophilia and increased concentration of band neutrophils) and finally a markedly increased C-reactive protein (major acute-phase protein) confirms that the pancreatitis is affecting the patient systemically. The clinical development of pancreatitis is usually thought to happen over days, which should allow fibrinogen to also increase as an acute-phase protein. The low normal fibrinogen at admission could thus indicate an increased fibrinogen consumption, as the inflammatory process will induce increased production by the liver. The slight anaemia is most likely due to a prolonged inflammatory response of the bone marrow. Despite the treatment, the systemic inflammatory activity seems to persist, as evidenced by persisting clinical signs and lack of decrease in the concentration of C-reactive protein. Therefore, an obvious clinical cause for DIC is present.

Activation of coagulation is demonstrated by prolonged aPTT, prolonged PT and decreased platelet concentration. A decreasing trend of platelet concentration over time, as seen, is usually viewed as a very strong marker of consumption due to activated coagulation. Increased

fibrinolytic activity is evidenced by the increased concentration of D-dimer, a specific fibrin degradation product from cross-linked fibrin.

However, the panel of laboratory tests presented does not include a marker of inhibitor consumption. Abnormally low activities of inhibitors are necessary to demonstrate that the increased activity is uncontrolled/uncompensated. Protein C, protein S and antithrombin activities are examples of markers of inhibitor activity.

FURTHER READING

Bick RL, Arun B, Frenkel EP (1999) Disseminated intravascular coagulation. Clinical and pathophysiological mechanisms and manifestations. *Haemostasis* **29**:111–134.

Kjelgaard-Hansen M, Jacobsen S (2011) Assay validation and diagnostic applications of major acute phase protein testing in companion animals. *Clin Lab Med* **31**:51–70.

Wiinberg B, Jensen AL, Johansson PI *et al.* (2010) Development of a model-based scoring system for diagnosis of canine disseminated intravascular coagulation with independent assessment of sensitivity and specificity. *Vet J* **185**:292–298.

CASE 11

1 What crystals can be seen on the picture?

The picture shows a less common modification of struvite crystals in cat urine.

2 What is the most important differential diagnosis?

The most important differential is cystinuria. However, cystinuria is a rare inherited disorder of renal tubular transport.

3 How can you differentiate between these two types of crystals?

The struvite crystals are eight-sided; usually, some more or less 'normal' looking struvite crystals are found. They dissolve in 10% acetic acid. Cystine crystals are typically more or less regularly six-sided.

4 What do the crystals shown indicate?

These struvite crystals have the same meaning as other modifications. They may or may not be an indication of struvite urolithiasis. They may or may not be of clinical significance.

FURTHER READING

Nelson RW, Couto CG (2009) *Small Animal Internal Medicine*, 2nd edn. Mosby Elsevier, St. Louis, p. 643.

Osborne CA, Stevens JB (1999) *Urinalysis: A Clinical Guide to Compassionate Patient Care*. Bayer Corporation, Shawnee Mission.

CASE 12

1 Describe and discuss the laboratory abnormalities. What is the most likely diagnosis?

There is a moderate leucocytosis associated with a moderate neutrophilia with regenerative left shift and a moderate lymphocytosis. These findings are consistent with chronic active inflammation, with acute need for neutrophils and deceased bone marrow storage pool for segmented neutrophils. Mild eosinophilia may occur in the face of parasitic or allergic disease or in the face of chronic inflammatory neutrophilia. Eosinophilia may be the result of irritation/inflammation involving mucous membranes, such as the urinary bladder.

The decreased RBC count, haematocrit and haemoglobin concentration are consistent with slight normocytic-normochromic anaemia. If a response to the anaemia does not become apparent in the peripheral blood over the next 3–7 days, a chronic non-regenerative anaemia is confirmed. Causes for non-regenerative anaemia include anaemia of inflammatory disease, reduced erythropoiesis due to decreased erythropoietin concentration and bone marrow disorder. In the face of severe renal disease (isosthenuric USG, increased urea and creatinine), inadequate erythropoietin production by the kidneys is likely. Further mechanisms leading to non-regenerative anaemia associated with chronic renal disease include decreased RBC life span, an inadequate bone marrow response to erythropoietin as well as the possibility of intestinal blood loss due to uraemic ulcers.

There is a mild to moderate azotaemia consistent with a decreased GFR due to pre-renal, renal or post-renal disease. As the urine is isosthenuric, renal concentration ability is impaired, supporting renal insufficiency. Decreased GFR further leads to decreased phosphate excretion via the kidneys and hyperphosphataemia.

There is a marked proteinuria, which may be pre-renal, renal or post-renal. As no lower urinary tract infection is present and the urine protein:creatinine ratio is markedly increased, renal proteinuria (e.g. due to glomerular or tubular damage) is most likely. Therefore, protein-losing nephropathy (PLN) is present. Slight hypoproteinaemia is associated with a slight to moderate hypoalbuminaemia. The hypoalbuminaemia in this case is most likely due to loss via the kidneys. Other conditions leading to hypoalbuminaemia include decreased protein intake, defective intestinal protein absorption, increased loss via intestines (protein-losing enteropathy [PLE]), blood loss or decreased albumin synthesis in the liver. Mild hypercholesterolaemia is most likely caused by secondary hyperlipoproteinaemia due to increased hepatic production of VLDLs and defective lipolysis in face of nephrotic syndrome/PLN. Hypercholesterolaemia is further observed in a variety of other diseases (cholestasis, acute pancreatitis, diabetes mellitus, hypothyroidism, hyperadrenocorticism) or after a high dietary fat intake. However, in the absence of laboratory support for and clinical hints towards these diseases, they seem highly unlikely.

Diagnosis: chronic inflammatory disease with chronic renal insufficiency; PLN and nephrotic syndrome. The chronic renal insufficiency has further led to non-regenerative anaemia.

2 How is this diagnosis defined?

Nephrotic syndrome is characterised by the presence of hypoalbuminaemia, proteinuria, hypercholesterolaemia and oedema. In some cases, oedema, secondary to hypoalbuminaemia and diminished oncotic pressure, is not present (incomplete nephrotic syndrome). Several diseases display a nephrotic syndrome, including amyloidosis, membranous nephropathy and hereditary nephritis.

FURTHER READING

Closterman ES, Pressler BM (2011) Nephrotic syndrome in dogs: clinical features and evidence-based treatment considerations. *Top Companion Anim Med* **26**:135–142.

CASE 13

1 What is your interpretation of the agarose gel serum protein electrophoresis?

The interpretation is that of a likely biclonal gammopathy. Two peaks are not clearly defined in the densitometry tracing, but are suggested by the tall relatively narrow spike (slightly exceeds the width of the albumin peak) with a 'shoulder' in the gamma globulin region. Two distinct bands are apparent in the gel, providing further support for two populations of gammaglobulin.

2 What are the differential diagnoses in this case?

Differential diagnoses should include lymphoproliferative disease (lymphoma, myeloma, lymphoid leukaemia), but some infections (leishmaniosis, babesiosis, other infections) may occasionally present with this type of pattern.

3 What other type of serum protein electrophoresis may be helpful in confirming the finding suggested by the agarose gel electrophoresis?

Capillary zone electrophoresis may be of benefit since it may more clearly demonstrate biclonal peaks within the gammaglobulin region. The capillary zone serum protein electrophoresis pattern in this patient is shown (**Fig. 13.3**). The albumin peak is located at the far left. Note that the biclonal nature of the gammaglobulin peaks is clearly demonstrated.

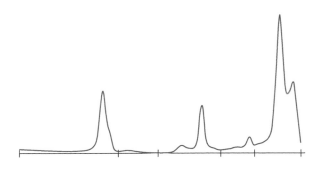

FIG. 13.3 Capillary zone electrophoretogram of a dog with biclonal gammopathy.

FURTHER READING

Facchini RV, Bertazzolo W, Zuliani D *et al.* (2010) Case report: detection of biclonal gammopathy by capillary zone electrophoresis in a cat and a dog with plasma cell neoplasia. *J Vet Clin Pathol* **39**:440–446.

CASE 14

1 What is the most likely explanation for the laboratory abnormalities? Describe the pathomechanism.

The most striking finding in this case is the markedly increased feline pancreatic lipase (fPLI) concentration, which is consistent with pancreatitis and matches the non-specific clinical signs in this cat. There is a mild hyperbilirubinaemia and a slight increase in ALP and ALT enzyme activities. Hyperbilirubinaemia may occur in the face of pre-hepatic (e.g. haemolysis), hepatic or post-hepatic disease. As no haemolysis has been reported and anaemia is not present, pre-hepatic causes can be excluded. Pancreatic inflammation may lead to impaired bile flow through the common bile duct, thereby leading to post-hepatic hyperbilirubinaemia. Patients with pancreatitis frequently have concurrent disease, such as hepatic lipidosis, hepatitis, intestinal inflammation or intestinal neoplasia. Increased enzyme activity of ALP may also point to cholestasis due to impaired bile flow. In cats, increased ALP is also reported with hepatic lipidosis, another possible cause for hepatic bilirubinaemia. Hepatic lipidosis may also be the reason for hepatocellular damage as exemplified by the increased ALT enzyme activity. Extension of the pancreatic inflammation to the liver may further contribute to increased ALT enzyme activity.

There is a mild azotaemia characterised by a mild increase in urea and creatinine concentrations as well as a mild hyperphosphataemia. This is consistent with a decreased GFR and may be pre-renal, renal or post-renal in origin. As the patient shows a decreased appetite, diminished fluid intake leading to dehydration as a pre-renal cause for the azotaemia should be considered. In the face of severe pancreatitis, vascular leakage may also contribute to pre-renal azotaemia as extravasation of fluid in the third space takes place. However, definitive exclusion of renal or post-renal disease is only possible by urinalysis. Special consideration should be given to the USG as well as signs of lower urinary tract disease.

Mild hypoproteinaemia based on a mild hypoalbuminaemia may occur in the face of vascular leakage, malnutrition, impaired intestinal absorption of protein and/or diminished hepatic albumin synthesis. The exact reason for the hypoalbuminaemia cannot be determined based on the present results. Finally, mild hyperglycaemia is present and may be stress induced in a chronically ill cat. In addition, the inflamed pancreas may release glucagon in higher concentrations than insulin. Glucagon leads to increased gluconeogenesis and glycogenolysis, thus augmenting glucose serum concentration. Diabetes mellitus is another risk factor for pancreatitis and, of course, should also be considered, although the hyperglycaemia is only slight.

2 What further analyses would you recommend, and why?

Urinalysis is recommended to determine if there is a renal cause for the azotaemia. Repeated glucose monitoring is further warranted to include/exclude diabetes mellitus. Although hepatic enzyme activities are only slightly increased, fine needle aspiration of the liver may be informative to rule in/out hepatic lipidosis. This may occur in overweight cats with anorexia or decreased appetite, as reported in the history.

Morphological diagnosis of pancreatitis can only be done by histological examination of biopsy specimens. Therefore, consideration must be given to the fact that lesions may occur multifocally in the organ and results of the histology may be falsely negative.

Feline trypsin-like immunoreactivity (fTLI) may be assessed in a cat with pancreatitis, but sensitivity and specificity are not as good as fPLI and negative results do not rule out pancreatitis. fTLI may further be increased in the face of intestinal disease, which is a common risk factor for pancreatitis.

FURTHER READING

Kaneko JJ, Harvey JW, Bruss ML (2008) *Clinical Biochemistry of Domestic Animals*, 6th edn. Elsevier, San Diego.
Stockham SL, Scott MA (2008) *Fundamentals of Veterinary Clinical Pathology*, 2nd edn. Blackwell Publishing, Oxford.

CASE 15

1 What is your analysis of these results?

There is slight normocytic-normochromic anaemia. The moderate leucocytosis with moderate neutrophilia and slight monocytosis and the absence of lymphopaenia supports inflammation. The slight increase in lymphocytes may be due to immune stimulation or neoplasia. The features of the atypical lymphoid cells in the peripheral blood smear support the presence of lymphoproliferative disease, of which chronic lymphocytic leukaemia (CLL) or lymphoma are the primary considerations. By definition, CLL is defined by the presence of increased lymphocytes morphologically indistinguishable from normally differentiated lymphocytes. The atypia of these lymphocytes and the presence of multiple enlarged lymph nodes more strongly support lymphoma rather than CLL. The typical age of horses at the time of diagnosis of lymphoma is 5–10 years, but lymphoma has been reported in horses from birth to >20 years of age. Neoplastic lymphocytes in the peripheral blood are estimated to occur in 30–50% of horses with lymphoma.

The low platelet estimate is typical of these conditions and may be due to a combination of decreased platelet production associated with bone marrow involvement or platelet consumption, sequestration or destruction secondary to the presence of neoplasia. The anaemia may be due to paraneoplastic immune-mediated destruction and/or bone marrow involvement.

There is a moderate increase in total protein with a slight increase in globulins. The increase in globulins may be due to increased acute-phase reactant proteins associated with inflammation, as suggested by the leucogram, but increased gammaglobulins associated with monoclonal or polyclonal gammopathy of lymphoma is considered likely.

There is unlikely to be any significance associated with a low CK concentration, but low levels due to decreased muscle mass associated with muscle wasting/catabolism cannot be ruled out.

Liver enzymes AST, GLDH and GGT are within normal limits, which excludes hepatocellular damage. Increase in total bilirubin is therefore likely to be due to anorexia and/or haemolysis. These findings suggest that significant hepatic neoplastic infiltration is not present.

The hypercalcaemia is likely due to neoplastic production of increased PTHrP resulting in pseudohyperparathyroidism. Metastatic mineralisation of the kidney is considered unlikely because of the absence of elevation in urea and creatinine.

2 What are your differential diagnoses?

The interpretation is that of generalised lymphoma. Intestinal, mediastinal or cutaneous lymphoma (the other forms of lymphoma reported in the horse) are not supported by the clinical and laboratory findings. The morphological features support lymphoid origin, but in some cases with marked variation in cell morphology, a differential diagnosis may be myeloid leukaemia.

3 What additional testing would you recommend?

Additional testing that may be helpful includes:

● Bone marrow aspiration and lymph node aspirates as part of clinical staging.
● Serum protein electrophoresis to characterise the elevation in globulins.
● Coombs test to determine if the anaemia may have an immune-mediated basis.
● Urinalysis and urine culture to provide baseline data for continued monitoring.
● Evaluation of clonality and flow cytometry may be of interest for further confirmation of neoplasia and lymphoid cell type of origin, respectively, although these findings are unlikely to alter the prognosis or treatment. However, these types of testing are not routinely available for horses.

CASE 16

1 What is your diagnosis?

Mild non-regenerative anaemia, hypercholesterolaemia, low thyroxine (T4) and increased canine thyrotropin (thyroid stimulating hormone; cTSH) provide support for hypothyroidism. Positive thyroglobulin autoantibodies (TgAAs) indicate underlying lymphocytic thyroiditis.

2 Explain how the profile abnormalities relate to the diagnosis.

A mild non-regenerative anaemia, secondary to a reduced metabolic rate and tissue oxygen requirement, is reported in approximately 40–50% of dogs with hypothyroidism.

Hypercholesterolaemia, identified in approximately 75% of hypothyroid dogs, is characterised by an increased concentration of LDL cholesterol. In man, it has been demonstrated that hypothyroidism (via a deficiency in triiodothyronine) causes downregulation of the hepatic LDL receptor, resulting in impaired clearance of this lipoprotein class from the circulation.

Hypertriglyceridaemia is also noted in some hypothyroid dogs. A decreased activity of lipoprotein lipase, the enzyme responsible for the hydrolysis of triglycerides in triglyceride-rich lipoproteins, is believed to be responsible.

Low T4 is expected in most hypothyroid dogs. However, the test has a specificity of approximately 70–75% and a low T4 concentration does not confirm the diagnosis. In one study of 223 dogs with non-thyroidal illness (Kantrowitz et al., 2001), 31% of dogs had a low T4 concentration. When classified according to the severity of disease, 7% of dogs with mild illness (treated as outpatients), 28% with moderate illness and 60% of dogs with severe illness (requiring intensive care) had serum

T4 concentrations below the reference range. The non-thyroidal diseases included hyperadrenocorticism, diabetes mellitus, hepatic disease, renal failure, cardiac disease and neoplasia.

In addition, drug therapies, especially glucocorticoids, phenobarbitone (phenobarbital) and sulphonamides, are reported to decrease canine T4 concentrations (Daminet & Ferguson, 2003). The effects of drugs and non-thyroidal illness on thyroid hormones may be the consequence of reduced protein binding, the influence of circulating cytokines and increased hepatic metabolism.

cTSH is a useful adjunct to the diagnosis of hypothyroidism. The concentration is reported to be less affected by non-thyroidal illness than total T4 (Kantrowitz et al., 2001) but increases are noted in 8–18% of euthyroid dogs with non-thyroidal illness (Dixon & Mooney, 1999; Peterson et al., 1997). If a diagnosis of hypothyroidism is to be established in a dog with pre-existing disease, then free T4 measured by equilibrium dialysis (FT4D) is a useful inclusion since Kantrowitz et al. (2001) identified only 4 of 223 (1.8%) dogs with non-thyroidal illness to have low T4 and FT4D and high cTSH.

TgAAs are produced in dogs with lymphocytic thyroiditis, although antibody production appears to wane in older animals. They are identified in approximately one half of hypothyroid dogs but there is considerable breed variation and the English Setter, Golden Retriever and Boxer are reported to be among the breeds with a higher prevalence of TgAA-positive hypothyroidism (Graham et al., 2007). The presence of antibodies does not provide information regarding thyroid function or confirm clinical hypothyroidism, but approximately 5% of euthyroid dogs with circulating TgAAs go on to develop hypothyroidism within 12 months. A small number of hypothyroid dogs have antibody production against T4 and T3, which interferes with routine assays for these hormones. Most of the dogs with anti-T4 antibodies also have circulating TgAAs, which can be used as an indicator of whether antibody production might have falsely increased the T4 concentration.

FOLLOW UP
In this case, the clinical presentation, absence of other identifiable disease and the laboratory abnormalities support hypothyroidism secondary to lymphocytic thyroiditis. The dog responded well to thyroid supplementation.

REFERENCES AND FURTHER READING
Daminet S, Ferguson DC (2003) Influence of drugs on thyroid function in dogs. *J Vet Intern Med* **17**:463–472.

Dixon RM (2004) Canine hypothyroidism. In: *BSAVA Manual of Canine and Feline Endocrinology*, 3rd edn. (eds CT Mooney, ME Peterson) British Small Animal Veterinary Association, Gloucester, pp. 172–181.

Dixon RM, Mooney CT (1999) Evaluation of serum free thyroxine and thyrotropin concentrations in the diagnosis of canine hypothyroidism. *J Small Anim Pract* **40**:72–78.

Graham PA, Lunquist RB, Refsal KR et al. (2001) 12-month prospective study of 234 thyroglobulin antibody-positive dogs which had no laboratory evidence of thyroid dysfunction (abstract). *J Vet Intern Med* **14**:298.

Graham PA, Refsal KR, Nachreiner RF (2007) Etiopathologic findings of canine hypothyroidism. *Vet Clin North Am Small Anim Pract* **37**:617–631.

Kantrowitz LB, Peterson ME, Melián C et al. (2001) Serum total thyroxine, total triiodothyronine, free thyroxine and thyrotropin concentrations in dogs with nonthyroidal illness. *J Am Vet Med Assoc* **219**:765–769.

Peterson ME, Melián C, Nichols R (1997) Measurement of serum total thyroxine, triiodothyronine, free thyroxine and thyrotropin concentrations for diagnosis of hypothyroidism in dogs. *J Am Vet Med Assoc* **211**:1396–1402.

CASE 17

1 What is your assessment of the arterial pH?
The arterial pH is decreased, therefore this is an acidaemia.

2 What is your assessment of the likely underlying aetiology?
The bicarbonate is decreased, so the acidaemia is due to metabolic acidosis.

3 What is the anion gap (AG) in this case?
$AG = (Na^+ + K^+) - (Cl^- + HCO_3^-) = (146 + 5.9) - (108 + 12) = 151.9 - 120 = 31.9$. The AG is increased, which indicates titrational metabolic acidosis regardless of the blood pH, the PCO_2 or the bicarbonate concentration.

4 Is there appropriate compensation for this condition?
The $PaCO_2$ is decreased, as expected for compensation for a metabolic acidosis. The formula for compensation is:

$$PaCO_2 = 1.54\,(HCO_3^-) + 8.4 \pm 1.1$$
$$PaCO_2 = 1.54\,(12) + 8.4 \pm 1.1 = 18.48 + 8.4 \pm 1.1$$
$$= 26.9 \pm 1.1 = 25.8 \text{ to } 28$$

In this case, the measured $PaCO_2 = 25$. This is nearly within the expected range for an adequate compensatory response. With this degree of deviation, this is likely to be an adequate compensatory response.

5 What is a likely underlying aetiological mechanism for this condition?
This is a titrational metabolic acidosis (hypochloraemic acidosis or increased AG acidosis). The underlying

pathophysiology involves buffering (titrating) of a large amount of acids in the blood stream by bicarbonate. Bicarbonate is thereby utilised and decreased in concentration. Various endogeneous or exogeneous sources of acid may lead to titrational metabolic acidosis. Based on the history and clinical signs in this cow, grain overload is the underlying cause.

Grain consists of easily fermentable carbohydrates. If the animal is not used to carbohydrates and/or the amount of ingested carbohydrates is too high, the number of gram-positive bacteria in the rumen increases markedly. Bacteria, especially *Streptococcus bovis*, start producing lactic acid, which accumulates rapidly. The ruminal pH changes into an acidotic environment and impairs growth of other organisms, further favouring growth of lactic acid-producing bacteria. Lactate can be measured in serum and leads to metabolic acidosis.

FURTHER READING

Stockham SL, Scott MA (2008) *Fundamentals of Veterinary Clinical Pathology*, 2nd edn. Blackwell Publishing, Oxford.

CASE 18

1 Describe and discuss the abnormalities of the haemogram, clinical biochemistry profile and blood gas analysis as well as the findings of the urinalysis. Calculate the AG (i.e. the difference between routinely measured cations and routinely measured anions) using the formula:

$$AG = ([Na^+] + [Ca^{2+}]) - ([Cl^-] + [HCO_3^-])$$
(reference interval <20 mmol/l)

What anion is most likely responsible for the abnormal AG in this cat?

There is a severe leucopaenia characterised by a severe neutropaenia, a moderate lymphopaenia and a slight monocytosis. Lymphopaenia and monocytosis suggest endogenous glucocorticoid effect due to stress and/or inflammation. Given the history, neutropaenia is most likely due to a peracute inflammation with a demand for neutrophils exceeding the actual storage pool and capacity of regeneration of the bone marrow.

The most striking finding in the biochemistry is a severe hyperphosphataemia. Possible causes include a decreased urinary phosphate excretion, mainly due to reduced GFR or bladder rupture, increased phosphate absorption from the intestine, and a shift of phosphate from the intracellular fluid to the extracellular fluid caused by cellular necrosis (e.g. tumour lysis, myopathies). A slight azotaemia may indicate reduced GFR due to pre-renal,

renal or post-renal causes. However, it is not considered the main aetiology for hyperphosphataemia, as the severity of elevation in phosphate plasma levels tends to parallel the magnitude of azotaemia.

There is a marked hypocalcaemia and hypomagnesaemia. In the face of severe, acute hyperphosphataemia, hypocalcaemia may be caused by three processes:

- High phosphate plasma concentrations result in formation of $CaHPO_4$ complexes with ionised calcium.
- The high $Ca^{2+} \times PO_4^{2-}$ product may cause metastatic calcification of tissues and thus subsequent hypocalcaemia.
- The increased renal phosphate excretion may be accompanied by the excretion of cations including Ca^{2+}. Hypomagnesaemia is most likely caused by the same processes as hypocalcaemia.

There is a moderate to marked hypernatraemia. Given the history and the other laboratory findings, an increased intestinal sodium uptake due to a sodium phosphate-containing enema is most likely. An enema-induced loss of pure water in the intestine due to osmosis may further contribute to hypernatraemia. Moderate hypernatraemia is associated with borderline hyperchloraemia. Generally, changes in chloride parallel changes in plasma sodium concentration to maintain electrical neutrality. A non-parallel increase in sodium and chloride concentration suggests the presence of an increased AG (with an increased concentration of an anion other than bicarbonate or chloride) because electrical neutrality must be maintained. Serum is always electrically neutral (i.e. total positive charges equal total negative charges). However, some anions, such as proteins, organic anions, SO_4 and PO_4, cannot be routinely measured so there is always a difference between routinely measured cations and routinely measured anions, called the AG.

The major purpose of calculating the AG is to identify significantly increased concentrations of unmeasured anions such as ketones, ethylene glycol and methaldehyde. The AG in this patient, using the formula shown in the question, is:

$$([164 \text{ mmol/l}] + [0.5 \text{ mmol/l}]) - ([111 \text{ mmol/l}] + [9.1 \text{ mmol/l}]) = 44.4 \text{ mmol/l (normal: <20 mmol/l)}$$

Editors' note: An alternative formula for AG is used commonly: $([Na^+] + [K^+]) - ([Cl^-] + [HCO_3^-])$.

In this cat, the increased AG of 44.4 mmol/l is caused by the significant hyperphosphataemia.

Moderate hyperglycaemia is most likely glucocorticoid mediated given the haemotological findings suggestive of stress. Diabetes mellitus, however, cannot entirely be ruled out. Therefore, the determination of plasma fructosamine concentration is recommended if the finding is persistent. There is a slight increase in ALT activity suggesting slight hepatocellular damage.

Blood gas analysis shows a severe acidaemia, a severely decreased concentration of HCO_3^- and normal pCO_2, which is consistent with metabolic acidosis. A probable aetiology is the excess generation of H^+ or a loss of HCO_3^- via the intestine or kidneys. In this patient, the severe increase of phosphate acting as an acid is most likely responsible for the metabolic acidosis.

In the face of hypertonic dehydration, normosthenuria with a USG of 1.025 is considered to be too low and suggests renal failure. There is a proteinuria, which falsely elevates SG so that the renal ability to concentrate the urine might be even lower. Microhaematuria and subsequent proteinuria are most likely caused by sampling (cystocentesis).

2 What is the most likely aetiology of the abnormalities in this cat?

Given the history and the magnitude of the hyperphosphataemia, administration of an enema containing sodium phosphate is the most likely aetiology of the observed abnormalities.

3 What is the prognosis in this patient?

The most striking laboratory abnormalities reported in the literature after experimental or accidental treatment of cats and small dogs with a sodium phosphate-containing enema included hypernatraemia, hypocalcaemia and hyperphosphataemia. These severe electrolyte abnormalities were fatal in several cases, so that phosphate-containing enemas should not be applied to cats and small dogs, especially if the patients are dehydrated or have concurrent colonic diseases.

FOLLOW UP

The cat was treated at the intensive care unit of the hospital for 16 days and extensive monitoring of electrolytes was performed. Treatment included application of IV crystalloid fluids, broad-spectrum antibiotics and substitution of potassium chloride if necessary. Constipation was treated with lactulose and paraffin given orally and a phosphate-free enema. The cat improved significantly and was discharged with normal electrolytes apart from a slight hyponatraemia.

FURTHER READING

Atkins CE, Tyler R, Greenlee P (1985) Clinical, biochemical, acid-base, and electrolyte abnormalities in cats after hypertonic sodium phosphate enema administration. *Am J Vet Res* **46**:980–988.

Jorgensen LS, Center SA, Randolph JF *et al.* (1985) Electrolyte abnormalities induced by hypertonic phosphate enemas in two cats. *J Am Vet Med Assoc* **187**:1367–1368.

Tomsa K, Steffen F, Glaus T (2001) Life-threatening metabolic disorders after application of a sodium phosphate containing enema in the dog and cat. *Schweiz Arch Tierheilkd* **143**:257–261.

CASE 19

1 Describe and discuss the laboratory abnormalities present.

There is a mild to moderate leucocytosis based on the moderate neutrophilia and mild lymphopaenia. Possible causes are acute inflammatory disease or corticosteroid effect (stress response). Differentiation of the two conditions could be enhanced by examination of a blood smear (exclusion of toxic and band neutrophils, which would support inflammatory disease) or assessment of acute-phase proteins (APPs). The latter would be increased in cases of systemic inflammation.

2 Which analytes would you examine to assess the acute-phase response (APR) in this patient?

The APR is part of the innate immune system of the patient. After a wide variety of different insults (e.g. trauma, infectious diseases, neoplasia, drugs, toxins) local inflammatory cells are stimulated. These then synthesise various cytokines, most importantly IL-6 and IL-1, as well as TNF-α and interferon-γ. These cytokines are crucial for initiation of hepatic synthesis of many APPs. Assessment of APR involves evaluation of a panel of APPs. Major APPs are characterised by an immediate (within the first 24–48 hours after the insult) 100–1,000-fold rise in concentration. In health, major APPs are predominantly present in very low concentrations, often <1 mg/l. In contrast therefore, moderate APPs display a lower rise, often 5–10-fold, which peaks later in the course of disease (e.g. after 2–3 days). Finally, negative APPs do not show a rise but a decline in the face of an APR.

In canines, a panel of APPs should include either CRP or serum amyloid A (SAA) as major APPs. Currently, only limited tests are available to measure SAA in dogs. On the other hand, a species-specific CRP test can be performed. Moderate APPs include haptoglobin or alpha-1-acid glycoprotein. Albumin is the most important negative APP.

3 What actions does C-reactive protein perform in the body?

C-reactive protein (CRP) functions as an opsinin. It scavenges bacteria and leads to complement activation and subsequent uptake of bacteria by macrophages. In addition, it leads to the induction of cytokines, further amplifying the APR. A third action involves the action of neutrophils. It inhibits chemotaxis and modulates the action of neutrophils.

FOLLOW UP

Analyte (units)	Result	Reference Interval
CRP (mg/l)	**140**	0–10

CRP concentration was markedly increased consistent with systemic inflammation and justifying further diagnostics. Ultrasonography of the abdomen revealed thickened intestinal walls and subsequent full-thickness biopsy was consistent with lymphoma.

FURTHER READING

Cerón JJ, Eckersall PD, Martínez-Subiela S (2005) Acute phase proteins in dogs and cats: current knowledge and future perspectives. *J Vet Clin Pathol* **34**:85–99.

Eckersall PD, Bell R (2010) Acute phase proteins: biomarkers of infection and inflammation in veterinary medicine. *Vet J* **185**:23–27.

CASE 20

1 What is the parasite in the thyroid aspirate and the blood smear?

It is a microfilaria (L1) of *Dirofilaria immitis*, which must be distinguished from *Dipetalonema reconditum* (may sometimes be difficult) because the presence of the *D. reconditum* does not require expensive and potentially harmful arsenical therapy, as does *D. immitis*. *Dirofilaria repens* is another possible differential.

Characteristics of *Dipetalonema reconditum* and *Dirofilaria immitis*

	Number in blood	Shape	Length (microns)
D. reconditum	Few	Curved body and blunt head	250–288
D. immitis	Many	Straight body and tail. Tapered head	295–325

2 What haematological and serum abnormalities might you expect related to this parasitic infection?

Haematological and serum abnormalities may be useful in providing support of this disease. Low-grade non-regenerative anaemia, neutrophila, eosinophilia and basophilia may be observed. Thrombocytopaenia and DIC may be present after adulticidal therapy. In a small proportion of animals with severe infection, an increase in liver enzymes and a pre-renal azotaemia may be observed as a consequence of heart failure. If there is concurrent glomerulonephritis, albuminuria and serum hypoproteinaemia may also be noted.

FURTHER READING

Ettinger SJ, Feldman ED (2005) *Textbook of Veterinary Internal Medicine*, 6th edn. Elsevier Saunders, St. Louis.

CASE 21

1 Name the type of poikilocytosis of erythrocytes present in the blood smear.

The erythrocytes are present as codocytes, also known as target cells or 'Mexican hat cells'.

2 Describe the mechanism that leads to the presence of this type of abnormal RBC shape.

In codocytes the erythrocyte membrane is increased in comparison to the haemoglobin content of the cell. In particular, the cholesterol and phospholipid concentrations of the RBC membrane are increased, leading to the typical shape of the target cell.

3 In which diseases does this type of poikilocytosis occur? What is the most likely cause in this patient?

Diseases in which codocytes frequently can be observed include the following: hepatic disease, especially cholestatic liver disease; iron deficiency; renal disease; post splenectomy; in association with regenerative anaemia

In this cat, the biochemistry shows increased GGT, ALP and ALT enzyme activity. While an increase in ALT is consistent with hepatocellular damage, GGT and ALP increases in cats are typical for hepatic lipidosis. Given the history, this is likely. Fine needle aspiration of the liver would lead to a definitive diagnosis.

FURTHER READING

Stockham SL, Scott MA (2008) *Fundamentals of Veterinary Clinical Pathology*, 2nd edn. Blackwell Publishing, Oxford.

Weiss J, Wardrop KJ (2010) (eds) *Schalm's Veterinary Hematology*, 6th edn. Blackwell Publishing, Ames.

CASE 22

1 Briefly discuss the factors that can lead to variation in laboratory test results. Define the index of individuality (IoI) and how it is calculated.

If serial results of an analyte are generated in the laboratory, several sources of variation have to be considered:

(1) Pre-analytical variation, which includes varying sampling sites, varying tube filling levels, time of occlusion of the blood vessel and different people sampling. (2) The machine itself does not always perform in the same way. Intra- and inter-assay precision is therefore an integral part of method validation studies. This part is typically known as analytical variance or analytical coefficient of variation (CV_A). Post-analytically, errors in reporting the results may occur, although this is less likely because of the increasing use of electronic data transfer and is mostly neglected in studies of biological variation. (3) Every analyte has inherent biological changes known as biological variation. This variation may be within individuals (intra-individually [CV_I]) or between individuals (inter-individually [CV_G]) and includes hormonal influences, seasonal variation, metabolic variations and age-related changes.

The IoI is a value describing the amount of variation of an analyte in a particular species of interest. The formulae below fully include the CV_A, CV_I and CV_G. Basically, two variants to calculate the IoI exist and both are used in the literature, leading to confusion in the interpretation of results if the reader is not aware of the type of formula used:

$$(1)\ \mathrm{IoI} = (CV_I^2 + CV_A^2)^{1/2}/CV_G \quad \text{or}$$
$$(2)\ \mathrm{IoI} = CV_G/(CV_I^2 + CV_A^2)^{1/2}$$

The IoI can be used to judge whether population-based reference intervals are appropriate for interpretation of results or if it is preferable to use subject-based reference intervals (also called the critical difference or reference change value).

When using the first formula, a low (<0.6) IoI (CV_G >CV_I) means that high individuality exists and that subject-based reference intervals should be favoured over population-based reference intervals. The second formula is more intuitive; a low (<0.6) IoI (CV_I >CV_G) indicates low individuality and population-based reference intervals are appropriate for use.

The authors prefer the second formula, as it is intuitively easier to understand (low IoI = low individuality). When the second formula returns a high result (>1.6), there is high individuality for an analyte and use of the subject-based reference intervals (the critical difference or reference change value or significance change value) is likely to provide the best interpretation of changes in serial results.

2 Why is it important to know the degree of biological variation in a patient?

Every analyte always shows variation around a fixed haemostatic setting point. The degree of biological variation, therefore, may be small or large for an analyte, as the red and lilac bars, respectively, show (**Fig. 22.1**).

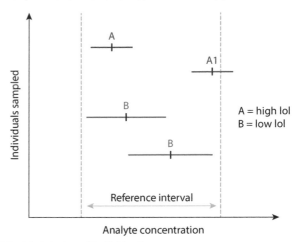

FIG. 22.1 Index of individuality.

Analyte A shows a high individuality (high IoI, second formula) and analyte B shows a low individuality (low IoI, second formula).

Usually, population-based reference intervals are generated to include 95% of the 'normal' individual results obtained from reference individuals. Every reference individual is sampled once. Imagine patient A1 in the graph showing high individuality of the analyte. If this patient had an increased concentration of the analyte with a narrow range, an increase in the value of the analyte would be abnormal for the individual patient, but still be within the population-based reference range, and no concern would be raised when interpretation is based on the 95% population-based reference interval. In this case, subject-based reference intervals would be preferable to correctly identify pathological changes of the analyte.

Information about biological variation can therefore be used to judge the applicability of population-based reference intervals or subject-based reference intervals. There are calculations that can be done to determine desirable bias, CV and total allowable error based on biological variation, and these may be helpful in defining performance criteria for a machine when selecting a machine and method for analyte determination. (See also Appendix 2, p. 264.)

FURTHER READING

Carney PC, Ruaux CG, Suchodolski JS *et al.* (2011) Biological variability of C-reactive protein and specific canine pancreatic lipase immunoreactivity in apparently healthy dogs. *J Vet Intern Med* **25**:825–830.

Carney PC, Ruaux CG, Suchodolski JS *et al.* (2012) Letter to the editor. *J Vet Intern Med* **26**, 2.

Pagitz M, Frommlet F, Schwendenwein I (2007) Evaluation of biological variance of cystatin C in comparison with other endogenous markers of glomerular filtration rate in healthy dogs. *J Vet Intern Med* **21**:936–942.

Walton RM (2012) Subject-based reference values: biological variation, individuality, and reference change values. *J Vet Clin Pathol* **41**:175–181.

Walton RM (2012) Letter to the editor. *J Vet Intern Med* **26**, 1.

CASE 23

1 What is your evaluation of the laboratory data?
Normal laboratory values for llamas are not well established, especially for haematology. Serum chemistry values tend to follow those of other species such as goats. The most remarkable finding as far as laboratory data is concerned is the lack of severe abnormalities in an animal that is slowly dying. In this clinician's experience it is common to have thin llamas and alpacas that waste away without having laboratory work that is definitive for any given disease.

The only condition that may point to severe underlying disease is the presence and increasing number of band neutrophils. While the total leucocyte count is within normal limits, the increasing number of of band neutrophils suggests a degenerative left shift. This condition resembles diminished bone marrow storage capacities of segmented neutrophils.

There is, however, a consistently low albumin and a mild anaemia. Hypoalbuminaemia may occur in the face of loss via kidneys, intestine or skin or in association with an acute-phase response, as albumin is a negative acute-phase protein. Anaemia is mild and appears non-regenerative. Anaemia of chronic inflammatory disease is the most likely cause, considering the hypoalbuminaemia, band neutrophils and clinical changes. Apart from the low numbers of eggs on faecal examination and the difficulty passing a nasogastric tube at the last examination, these laboratory results could be compatible with chronic parasitism. However, while the parasites certainly did

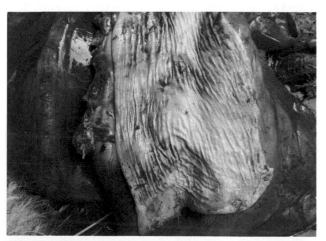

FIG. 23.1 Photo of the necropsy of the llama. Note the width of the oesophagus compared with the lung.

not help, necropsy demonstrated the real reason for the 'starvation in the midst of plenty'.

FOLLOW UP AND CASE DISCUSSION
The necropsy results demonstrated oesophageal dilation (twice normal size) from near the thoracic inlet to the entrance of C1. The rest of the organs appeared grossly normal (**Fig. 23.1**).

Editors' Note: This case illustrates well the fact that llamas can be suffering from serious illness, eventually resulting in death, with few laboratory abnormalities. In this case the continued decline in albumin is a poor prognostic indicator.

CASE 24

1 What are the principal causes of hypercalcaemia?
The main causes of hypercalcaemia are summarised in the HARDION acronym: **H**yperparathyroidism; **A**ddison's disease; **R**enal disease; vitamin **D** toxicosis; **I**diopathic (in cats), **I**nflammatory disease (granulomatous disease); **O**steolysis; **N**eoplasia (lymphoma, anal sac adenocarcinoma, other), **N**utritional.

In this case, the clinical suspicion of hypercalcaemia associated with malignancy is high, as a perianal mass was detected on clinical examination. Hypercalcaemia develops through secretion of parathyroid hormone-related protein (PTHrP) by the neoplastic cells, leading to a suppression of PTH secretion by the parathyroid glands.

2 What are the principal causes of thrombocytopaenia?
A decrease in the number of circulating platelets can be secondary to splenic sequestration, increased consumption, primary or secondary immune-mediated destruction or decreased production. Several pathogens (*Ehrlichia* spp., *Leishmania, Babesia, Leptospira* spp., parvovirus) can cause thrombocytopaenia. Toxic causes have also to be considered, as many drugs are known to have antiplatelet effects (chloramphenicol, penicillin, sulphonamides, azathioprine, cyclophosphamide, doxorubicin, oestrogen). Primary or secondary immune-mediated diseases are typically associated with a severe thrombocytopaenia (i.e. $<50 \times 10^9$/l).

3 What further tests are required?
Fine needle aspiration of the perianal mass is necessary to eliminate or confirm the presence of neoplasia.

FOLLOW UP
A diagnosis of anal sac adenocarcinoma was made cytologically. Staging of the tumour is the next step to

take, as anal sac adenocarcinomas have a high metastatic potential (sublumbar lymph nodes), with surgical excision of the mass and pathohistological examination.

FURTHER READING

Stockham SL, Scott MA (2008) *Fundamentals of Veterinary Clinical Pathology*, 2nd edn. Blackwell Publishing, Oxford.

CASE 25

1 What abnormality do you detect in the cell on the cytological slide?

The fine needle aspirate shows a macrophage containing several *Leishmania* amastigotes.

2 Describe the laboratory abnormalities present and discuss their association with the underlying cause of disease.

Slight normocytic-normochromic anaemia is present. Increased numbers of polychromatophils are not detected on the blood smear, so the anaemia is non-regenerative. As a chronic disease, leishmaniasis leads to an iron distribution disorder, making iron less available for erythropoiesis and resulting in chronic inflammatory/infectious anaemia, which is non-regenerative. Differential diagnoses for this type of anaemia are recent blood loss or bone marrow disease.

Biochemistry reveals slight to moderate hyperproteinaemia with hypoalbuminaemia and hyperglobulinaemia most likely due to polyclonal gammopathy. Like many other infectious diseases, *Leishmania* organisms lead to stimulation of the immune system and production of immunoglobulins. In fine needle aspirates from lymph nodes, liver, spleen or bone marrow, lymphoplasmacytic inflammation may also be visible. Dogs with clinical leishmaniasis often show high serological titres for the disease. Hypoalbuminaemia may develop due to various pathological mechanisms. As albumin is a negative acute-phase protein, it decreases in the face of an acute-phase response. Renal proteinuria (see below) may contribute to hypoalbuminaemia because of loss of albumin. Cases with severe hyperglobulinaemia may show a hyperviscosity syndrome, leading to further impaired renal function and coagulation disorders. Thrombocytopathy, thrombocytopaenia, impaired secondary haemostasis and/or fibrinolysis may be observed.

Mild azotaemia with hyperphosphataemia is present owing to a decreased GFR due to pre-renal, renal or post-renal disease. Infected dogs develop immune complexes that lead to glomerulonephritis and tubulointerstitial nephritis. Therefore, a renal cause is most likely. Most dogs with clinical leishmaniasis die because of renal failure.

In summary, leishmaniasis is a systemic disease affecting several different organ systems. Therefore, a wide variety of laboratory changes can be expected, which are all non-specific. No pathognomonic biochemical abnormalities are present. Several differential diagnoses must be taken into account when evaluating the laboratory data.

3 How is the disease transmitted?

Leishmania spp. are parasites transmitted by sand flies of the genera *Phlebotomus* (in the Mediterranean region and Africa) and *Lutzomyia* (in Central and South America).

FURTHER READING

Solano-Gallego l, Koutinas A, Miró G *et al.* (2009) Review: directions for the diagnosis, clinical staging, treatment and prevention of canine leishmaniasis. *Vet Parasitol* **165**:1–18.

CASE 26

1 What is your interpretation of these findings?

The clinical signs, biochemistry findings and results of the ACTH stimulation test are consistent with hyperadrenocorticism (HAC).

2 What is the pathophysiology associated with these findings?

85–90% of cases of canine HAC are caused by a tumour of the pars intermedia and pars distalis of the pituitary gland, resulting in hypersecretion of ACTH. The remaining 10–15% of cases are due to an adrenal tumour or iatrogenic HAC.

In pituitary-dependent HAC, increased ACTH results in stimulation of the adrenal glands and excessive production of cortisol. In adrenal tumours, ACTH is not increased and increased cortisol is produced by the neoplastic cells. Iatrogenic HAC is caused by administration of exogenous steroids.

PU/PD occurs in 85–95% of dogs with HAC. Glucocorticoids are thought to interfere with antidiuretic hormone (ADH) release and activity, resulting in polyuria, with compensatory polydipsia. The slight decrease in creatinine in this case may be due to renal medullary washout associated with polyuria. The slight decrease in potassium may also be due to renal loss, although decreased intake should also be considered.

The pendulous abdomen is due to redistribution of fat to the abdomen, wasting of abdominal muscles and hepatomegaly (associated with accumulation of glycogen). Muscle wasting is due to corticosteroid-induced protein catabolism.

A thin skin and bilaterally symmetrical truncal alopecia (with sparing of the head and extremities) are common findings, with atrophy of the hair follicles, epidermis and sebaceous glands. The increase in ALP and ALT are due to steroid induction of these enzymes and may be contributed to by hepatocellular compromise.

3 What other tests for hyperadrenocorticism are routinely available, and how does their sensitivity and specificity compare with those of the ACTH stimulation test?

Tests used in diagnosis of HAC include:

Test	Use	Sensitivity	Specificity	Miscellaneous
Urine cortisol: creatinine ratio	Best collected at home (reduced stress). Careful selection of animals in which this test is used will help reduce false-positive results	High sensitivity in detection of increased cortisol secretion.	Poor specificity – may be increased in non-adrenal illness with stress	A positive test in an animal with clinical signs and supportive findings of HAC justifies further testing by ACTH stimulation test and/or LDDST
ACTH stimulation test	Diagnosis of HAC (pituitary-dependent or adrenal tumour) and iatrogenic HAC. Diagnosis of hypoadrenocorticism.	80–85% sensitivity (false negatives may occur in 15–20% of dogs with HAC)	Good specificity (85%)	More expensive test than LDDST because of cost of synthetic ACTH. Does not help distinguish between pituitary-dependent HAC and adrenal tumour
LDDST	Diagnosis of HAC. May help differentiate pituitary-dependent HAC from adrenal tumour	High sensitivity (95%)	Moderate specificity (44–73%)	More likely than ACTH stimulation test to give false-positive result in animals with non-adrenal illness
HDDST	Differentiate pituitary-dependent HAC from adrenal tumour	N/A – requires prior diagnosis of HAC	N/A – requires prior diagnosis of HAC	None
Endogenous ACTH	Differentiation of pituitary-dependent HAC from adrenal tumour	High sensitivity	High specificity	Handling of specimen is critical. Requires rapid separation of plasma, freezing and submission of frozen specimen. Deviation from protocol may result in deterioration of ACTH and failure to detect its presence, or misinterpretation as a low result indicative of adrenal tumour

FURTHER READING

Peterson ME (2007) Diagnosis of hyperadrenocorticism in dogs. *Clin Tech Small Anim Pract* **22**:2–11.

Zerbe CA (2000) Differentiating tests to evaluate hyperadrenocorticism in dogs and cats. *Comp Cont Ed Pract Vet* **22**:149–157.

CASE 27

1 Describe the abnormalities that are present and indicate the most likely diagnosis based on the present findings.

There is a moderate anaemia with an abnormally high MCV, which could indicate regeneration with macrocytic erythrocytes. Evaluation of a reticulocyte count and blood film (looking for polychromasia) is needed to determine if this is a regenerative anaemia. Additionally, the RBCs are 'hyperchromic' (increased MCHC), which is an artefact due to the present haemolysis. Further possible causes include lipaemia or Heinz bodies.

Causes for haemolytic anaemia include immune-mediated diseases, infectious disease, mechanical damage to erythrocytes (e.g. intravascular coagulation or vasculitis) or other conditions affecting the metabolism of erythrocytes.

The latter include oxidative damage to erythrocytes or defects in the production of ATP, the major energy source of erythrocytes. In addition to hypophosphataemic haemolysis, these defects include hereditary diseases such as phosphofructokinase (PFK) deficiency and pyruvate kinase (PK) deficiency. As PFK deficiency is described in English Springer Spaniels and the history, physical examination and erythrogram match with this condition, it is most likely that this dog is suffering from this disease. There is a genetic test to identify individuals who are affected with PFK deficiency or are carriers or clear of the disease (http://www.vetgen.com/canine-pfk.html [Accessed 16th December 2013]).

2 Describe the underlying pathophysiology of the disease. How do the haemolytic crises develop?

PFK deficiency is an autosomal recessive hereditary disease affecting the anaerobic glycolysis, also known as the Embden–Meyerhof pathway. To really understand the pathophysiology, a little more detail is required.

Anaerobic glycolysis is the biochemical pathway to generate four moles of ATP by converting glucose over various steps to pyruvate and finally to lactate. The enzyme PFK is the rate-limiting step in this pathway and converts fructose-6-phosphate to fructose-1,6-diphosphate. PFK consists of three subunits: M- (muscle), L- (liver), and P- (platelet). The muscle subunit dominates with 86% in PFK in erythrocytes. In PFK-deficient patients, the gene coding for the M-subunit is mutated, leading to a loss of 40 amino acids in the enzyme. This morphological change in the enzyme makes it prone to degradation, and possibly also result in the loss of the enzyme.

As PFK concentration is reduced in affected dogs, anaerobic glycolysis cannot generate ATP and lactate any more, leading to decreased concentrations of these substances in the patient. Another important effect includes reduced 2,3-diphosphoglycerate (DPG) concentration. DPG is generated in a branch in addition to anaerobic glycolysis, the diphosphoglycerate shunt or the Rapaport–Luebering cycle. It is a major anion in RBCs with a dominant function of decreasing the affinity of haemoglobin for oxygen and thereby facilitating oxygen delivery to tissues.

How do haemolytic crises develop in PFK-deficient patients? As concentrations of the major erythrocyte anion DPG are markedly reduced in affected dogs, chloride anions move into RBCs, leading to an increased pH in the RBCs. Unfortunately, RBCs become extremely fragile at an alkaline pH making changes in pH (e.g. due to respiratory changes) highly dangerous. Every situation in which the patients start hyperventilating, thus releasing CO_2 and increasing the pH, have to be considered. These may include panting, barking, episodes of exercise or a high environmental temperature. All these situations may lead to an acute haemolytic crisis in the PFK-deficient patient.

Despite the haemolysis, why do the patients show such a high RBC regeneration? As mentioned above, DPG leads to a reduced haemoglobin affinity for oxygen. In the face of decreased DPG concentrations, the affinity of haemoglobin for oxygen is increased, making it more difficult to release oxygen into tissues. Therefore, a relative tissue hypoxia may develop, further stimulating erythropoietin production and erythropoiesis.

PFK deficiency is described in English Springer Spaniels, American Cocker Spaniels, Whippets and mixed-breed dogs.

3 What further diagnostics would you perform to support your diagnosis?

Suspicion of PFK deficiency can be ascertained by PCR. Patients have a normal life expectancy if life-threatening hyperventilation is avoided.

FURTHER READING

Kaneko JJ, Harvey JW, Bruss ML (2008) *Clinical Biochemistry of Domestic Animals*, 6th edn. Elsevier, London.

Stockham SL, Scott MA (2008) *Fundamentals of Veterinary Clinical Pathology*, 2nd edn. Blackwell Publishing, Oxford.

CASE 28

1 What is your evaluation of the laboratory data?

There is slight anaemia. The small increase in MCV may reflect some degree of bone marrow response. The absence of polychromasia is expected since reticulocytes are not released into the peripheral blood of horses, donkeys or mules. The anaemia is likely associated with chronic disease (see discussion of biochemistry below). There is slight leucocytosis and neutrophilia without lymphopaenia, which is suggestive of inflammation.

The persistent increase in ALP and GGT supports cholestasis or hepatocholangitis, although there is no current indication of an increase in total bilirubin. The increases in urea, creatinine and calcium are consistent with decreased glomerular filtration rate. In combination with the isosthenuric USG, these findings are consistent with renal failure. Hypercalcaemia is a relatively common finding in equids since there is very efficient intestinal absorption of calcium and urinary excretion of calcium is the primary means of calcium elimination.

The moderate persistent increase in CK likely reflects muscle damage associated with increased 'down' time due to the laminitis. It is less likely to be due to muscle catabolism since this donkey continued to eat until day 14. The slight increase in AST may reflect ongoing muscle damage, but may also be contributed to by hepatocellular damage.

In the absence of hyperglycaemia likely exceeding the renal threshold for glucose, the glucose in the urine suggests renal tubular damage. The slight increase in bilirubin may also reflect decreased renal function. The USG is in the isosthenuric range and, in conjunction with the biochemistry findings, supports renal failure. The slight increase in protein may reflect glomerular damage.

2 What is your diagnosis/interpretation of this case?

The present findings suggest renal failure, ongoing muscle damage and possible hepatobiliary disease.

3 What other tests could be performed and why?

The following may be of benefit:

- Bile acids assay to further assess liver function.
- Ultrasound of liver and kidneys to determine if abnormalities suggestive of certain conditions are present.
- Liver biopsy to determine the type and extent of liver disease.
- Renal biopsy to determine the type and extent of renal disease.

FOLLOW UP

The donkey was euthanised 2 days later primarily because of an inability to control its pain. A necropsy was performed. Severe icterus, small kidneys and a fibrotic liver were noted (**Figs. 28.1, 28.2**). It is surprising that the total bilirubin levels were low on the final serum chemistry panel run only 2 days prior to euthanasia. Clinically, the donkey was not icteric until the very end.

Histological evaluation of tissues collected at post-mortem examination had diagnoses of:

● Severe, diffuse, chronic bridging hepatic fibrosis with bile duct proliferation, oval cell hyperplasia and minimal lymphoplasmacytic portal hepatitis.
● Multifocal to locally extensive, subacute to chronic, lymphoplasmacytic interstitial nephritis with multifocal glomerular sclerosis, segmental glomerular amyloid and subacute tubular necrosis and regeneration with multifocal interstitial fibrosis and focal eosinophilic and neutrophilic interstitial and intratubular nephritis.

The pathologist's comment suggested toxic injury, particularly mycotoxin, as a possible cause for the severe hepatic injury. The pattern of injury and fibrosis of the kidneys was suggestive of multifocal infarction and/or pyelonephritis.

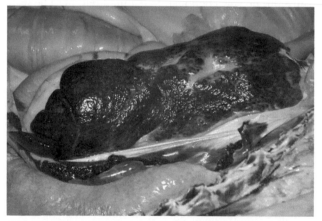

FIG. 28.1 Liver. Nodular appearance with depressed areas.

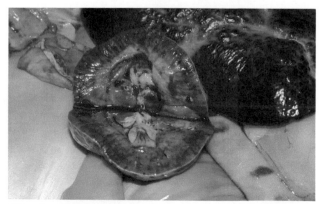

FIG. 28.2 Kidney. Note the multiple white cortical foci and the dilated renal pelvis.

The presence of intratubular inflammation suggests pyelonephritis is most likely in this case.

On further discussion of these findings with the owners, one of the caretakers remembered a bag of feed that was apparently mouldy and had been thrown out about 1 month before any illness in either the donkey or the pony. Because multiple people are known to feed at this location, this mouldy feed may have been inadvertently fed. The histology findings are compatible with a chronic long-term problem, and knowing for certain the exact cause is not possible.

CASE 29

1 What organisms are apparent in the lymph node aspirate smear?

Leishmania amastigotes. These are extracellular, but are often also seen intracellularly.

2 What is your interpretation of the haematologic findings?

A non-regenerative anaemia, most likely caused by chronic inflammation. The marked neutrophilia and the mild monocytosis could also indicate ongoing inflammation.

3 What other biochemistry analyte would be good to look at in this case?

Albumin. The globulins could then be calculated; moreover, albumin is a negative acute-phase protein (i.e. inflammation causes a mild decrease in albumin). Albumin was not analysed in this case.

4 How would you describe the crystals present in the urine sediment?

Small globular yellow–brown crystals occurring together in clumps. The crystals vary in size from about 2–10 μm in diameter and small protrusions are present on some of them.

5 What are the most important differentials?

The crystals are consistent with xanthine or ammonium urate. These cannot be distinguished by appearance alone; infrared spectroscopy identified these crystals as xanthine.

6 Which medication can cause these crystals?

Allopurinol was used in this case to treat leishmaniasis: the *Leishmania* organism falsely incorporates allopurinol into its RNA instead of hypoxanthine, which leads to impaired protein synthesis and a decreased ability to reproduce.

7 What is the mechanism of formation?

Allopurinol is a structural isomer of hypoxanthine and competitively inhibits the enzyme xanthine oxidase, thus causing a decreased production of uric acid and an increase in the levels of xanthine and hypoxanthine. Xanthine is poorly soluble and a higher dose of allopurinol may result in crystalluria or xanthine urolithiasis.

Note: This case has been modified from a presentation on crystalluria in the dog given by E. Hooijberg, J. Leidinger and E. Leidinger at the ESVCP meeting in Toulouse, France, in 2010.

FURTHER READING
Osborne CA, Lulich JP, Swanson LL *et al.* (2009) Drug-induced urolithiasis. *Vet Clin North Am Small Anim Pract* **39**:55–64.

van Zuilen CD, Nickel RF, van Dijk TH *et al.* (1997) Xanthinuria in a family of Cavalier King Charles spaniels. *Vet Q* **19**: 172–174.

CASE 30

1 What is your assessment of the arterial pH?
The arterial pH is decreased, therefore this is an acidaemia.

2 What is your assessment of the underlying aetiology?
The bicarbonate is decreased, so the acidaemia is due to metabolic acidosis.

3 What is the anion gap (AG) in this case?
AG = $(Na^+ + K^+) - (Cl^- + HCO_3^-) = (145 + 6.5) - (107 + 10) = 151.5 - 117 = 34.5$. The AG is increased, which indicates titrational metabolic acidosis regardless of the blood pH, the $PaCO_2$ or the bicarbonate concentration.

4 Why is the K+ increased in this case?
The K^+ is increased because of the buffering mechanism by which H^+ shifts from the extracellular fluid into the intracellular fluid in exchange for K^+.

5 What is a likely underlying aetological mechanism for the condition in this dog?
This is a titrational metabolic acidosis. This condition occurs as a result of bicarbonate consumption by titration (buffering) of excessive amounts of acids entering the blood. An acid is an anion that is weakly associated with a hydrogen proton. When an acid enters the blood, the sodium from sodium bicarbonate associates with the anion and the bicarbonate associates with the hydrogen proton. This results in the sodium concentration remaining stable, but an increase of one mEq of unmeasured anion (hence, an increase of one in the anion gap) for every mEq of bicarbonate utilised in buffering the acid. Titrational metabolic acidoses increase the anion gap, but usually do not change the plasma chloride concentration. As a result, titrational metabolic acidoses are sometimes called 'euchloraemic' or 'normochloraemic metabolic acidoses' and 'increased anion gap metabolic acidoses'. The term 'titrational metabolic acidosis' more accurately reflects the pathophysiological process that is occurring.

History, clinical signs and time of the year as well as the titrational metabolic acidosis suggest that ethylene glycol (EG) intoxication should be considered. EG is metabolised into glycoaldehyde and further on to glycolic acid, one of the metabolites responsible for the development of the acidosis. Further processing of glycolic acid results in formic acid, oxalate and other substances aggravating metabolic acidosis.

Differential diagnoses for titrational metabolic acidosis are endogenous sources of acids due to shock (lactic acid, pyruvic acid and others), extreme anaerobic metabolism (lactic acid, pyruvic acid and others), ketoacidotic stage of diabetes mellitus (keto acids), starvation (keto acids) and late renal failure (phosphates, sulphates and others).

6 What further test may strengthen your diagnosis?
It is possible to measure EG levels in blood, but this test may not always be available. A combination of history and other laboratory findings is often used for a presumptive diagnosis. There is development of azotaemia due to nephrotoxic potential of glycolic acid and cytotoxicity of oxalates. As EG is osmotically active, increased serum osmolality as well as an osmolal gap are present. Calculation of the osmolal gap can be performed using the following formula:

$$\text{Osmolal gap} = 1.86 \, [Na^+ + K^+] + [\text{urea}] + [\text{glucose}]$$

(**Note:** If analytes are not measured in SI units, they should be converted to SI units before applying the formula.)

Urinalysis may be of benefit as oxalate combines with calcium to form calcium oxalate crystals. Calcium oxalate monohydrate crystals are typically predominant and when present in moderate to large numbers they are highly supportive of EG toxicity.

FURTHER READING
Dibartola SP (2012) *Fluid, Electrolyte and Acid-Base Disorders in Small Animal Practice*, 4th edn. Elsevier Saunders, St. Louis.

CASE 31

1 How would you describe this azotaemia, and what does this indicate?
There is evidence of a moderate azotaemia, which has become severe in 72 hours. The presence of isosthenuric urine indicates a primary renal azotaemia due to kidney dysfunction. Clinical history is important to differentiate AKI from chronic renal failure. The acute onset of symptoms and

the oliguria indicate AKI, which is caused by a renal disease or an insult that markedly decreases the GFR.

2 How would you explain the high anion gap?

Anion gap is a calculated measure that is representative of the unmeasured ions in plasma or serum. The high anion gap in this case may be due to increased phosphate, which cannot be excreted by the kidney. Renal failure may also cause high anion gap acidosis by decreased acid excretion and decreased bicarbonate reabsorption. Blood gas analysis is recommended in order to confirm this (evaluation of pH, HCO_3^-).

3 What is the crystal indicated by the arrow?

It is a sulphonamide crystal, which frequently occurs with sulphonamide administration. It may cause AKI by intratubular crystal precipitation.

4 What is the main differential diagnosis for this case?

The clinical history and the laboratory results are indicative of AKI, likely caused by an idiosyncratic trimethoprim-sulphadiazine (TMPS) drug reaction. When the owner was questioned further based on the crystals found, it was discovered that this patient had been prescribed TMPS by another veterinarian. This dog received aggressive fluid therapy and urea and creatinine returned to normal levels after 2 weeks.

CASE 32

1 Describe and discuss the significant biochemistry and urinalysis findings.

There is a marked hyperglycaemia, which is consistent with diabetes mellitus (DM). In theory, a differential diagnosis is stress-induced hyperglycaemia but the magnitude as well as the species makes this differential unlikely.

Urea concentration is slightly decreased. In this case glucosuria is present, which may have led to decreased tubular urea absorption. Decreased urea synthesis because of hepatic disease may contribute.

The plasma is severely lipaemic, which leads to interference with spectrophotometric assays. Therefore, moderate hyperphosphataemia, total protein concentration and globulin concentration are most likely falsely increased. Slight hyperalbuminaemia is consistent with hypovolaemia. Clinically, signs of dehydration should be evaluated. Moderate hypertriglyceridaemia and mild hypercholesterolaemia are frequently observed in patients suffering from DM due to accelerated synthesis of the lipids. An important differential is HAC.

Liver enzyme activities are slightly to moderately elevated, which is indicative of hepatocellular damage,

most likely due to a metabolic disorder such as lipidosis, which is frequently associated with DM. Moderately increased ALP enzyme activity points to intra- or post-hepatic cholestasis with induction of the liver-specific ALP isoenzyme. Cholestasis may result from metabolic disease (e.g. DM), lipidosis or HAC.

There is a marked glucosuria in the face of hyperglycaemia, which indicates that the reabsorption capacity of the renal proximal tubules for glucose is exceeded. Slight proteinuria may be physiological in males.

In summary, this dog is suffering from DM with subsequent hepatocellular disease, most likely hepatic lipidosis.

2 What further tests would you recommend, and why?

Further recommended tests include:

- Abdominal ultrasonography as well as assessment of canine pancreatic lipase to rule in/out pancreatitis as a probable cause of DM. Potential hepatic lipidosis should also be evaluated.
- Fine needle aspiration of the liver to confirm hepatic lipidosis and cholestasis.
- Urine culture, as diabetic patients frequently develop urinary tract infections due to glucosuria. This may occur in the absence of pyuria.
- Phosphate and protein concentrations should be repeated in a non-lipaemic sample. Ultracentrifugation may be used to clear a lipaemic sample, if available. There are some chemical methods that may also be used to clear lipaemic samples. Sometimes sufficient clearing may be obtained by putting the sample in the freezer where rapid cooling will result in separation of lipid in a 'cream' layer at the top of the tube and clear (or less lipaemic) serum below this layer.
- If the DM is difficult to stabilise, HAC may be contributing. An ACTH stimulation test may be performed.

CASE 33

1 What is your interpretation of these findings?

These findings are consistent with a mild selective glomerular proteinuria (albumin >40%, gamma globulin <5%, mild increases in alpha-1 and beta globulins). This is typical of increased glomerular filtration of albumin in early or mild glomerular disease.

2 What other categories of renal proteinuria can be determined by agarose gel urine protein electrophoresis?

Based on the electrophoretic trace, renal proteinuria can often be further categorised into:

- Mild selective glomerular proteinuria.
- Severe selective glomerular proteinuria. More pronounced increases in albumin, alpha-1 and beta globulins with a relative absence of higher molecular proteins (α2 macroglobulin and immunoglobulins).
- Non-selective glomerular proteinuria. Increased glomerular permeability leads to higher concentrations of higher molecular weight proteins (alpha-2 and beta-2 globulins).
- Tubular proteinuria. Urine protein:creatinine ratio <2.0. Diminished tubular resorptive capacity results in an increase in urinary excretion of globulins, typically demonstrated by increased alpha-2 and beta globulins.
- Mixed glomerular and tubular proteinuria.
- Overflow proteinuria. High plasma protein concentrations of low molecular weight proteins are filtered through the glomeruli in increased amounts and exceed the resorptive capacity of the renal tubules, typically associated with paraproteinaemias.

3 What are the indications for agarose gel urine protein electrophoresis and the pitfalls in the use of agarose gel urine protein electrophoresis?
Agarose gel urine protein electrophoresis is indicated for differentiation of glomerular and tubular proteinuria, assessment of protein selectivity in renal glomerular disease and investigation of monoclonal gammopathies (identification of Bence-Jones proteinuria).

Pitfalls include: (1) a concentration step is required prior to protein electrophoresis to achieve reliable densitometry results; (2) interpretation is subjective; (3) there is poor sensitivity for the detection of Bence-Jones proteins (BJP) (optimal sample would be a 24-hour urine collection; a BJP peak may be masked by an overspill proteinuria; (4) poor access to immunoelectrophoresis means that individual globulins and paraproteins cannot be characterised further.

CASE 34

1 What is your assessment of the significant profile changes, and what are the possible causes?
Azotaemia exemplified by increased urea and creatinine concentrations, as well as hyperphosphataemia, generally may occur in pre-renal, renal or post-renal disease. Given the hyperproteinaemia, dehydration could contribute to increased renal parameters, although the magnitude of increase would be unusual. Renal failure (acute or chronic), urinary tract obstruction or urinary tract

trauma are further pathologies to consider. Urinalysis is highly recommended to rule in/out renal or post-renal disease.

Hyperkalaemia is noted in the oliguric or anuric phases of renal failure and especially in AKI. It is generally not expected with chronic polyuric renal failure. This electrolyte disturbance is also commonly noted with urinary tract obstruction and trauma.

FOLLOW UP
Given the history in this case, urinary tract trauma was considered a possibility. A conservative approach was elected and the patient treated with fluid therapy. Imaging or abdominocentesis in an attempt to identify uroperitoneum was not attempted. Acute uroabdomen is characterised by the presence of a transudate or modified transudate (protein concentration <30 g/l), with concentrations of creatinine and potassium higher than those in serum.

The renal parameters in this cat improved considerably within a short period of time and the azotaemia had resolved by day 14.

Analyte (units)	Result (day 6)	Result (day 14)	Reference Interval
Total protein (g/l)	67	63	55–78
Albumin (g/l)	36	35	26–40
Globulins (g/l)	31	28	19–48
Urea (mmol/l)	**22.1**	7.8	3.5–8.0
Creatinine (μmol/l)	**251**	165	40–180
Calcium (mmol/l)	2.46	2.63	2.0–2.8
Phosphorus (mmol/l)	**2.3**	**1.7**	0.81–1.61
Sodium (mmol/l)	145	145	141–155
Potassium (mmol/l)	4.2	4.4	3.5–5.5

FURTHER READING
Stockham SL, Scott MA (2008) *Fundamentals of Veterinary Clinical Pathology*, 2nd edn. Blackwell Publishing, Oxford.

CASE 35

1 What is your interpretation of these findings?
The test results enable classification of the possible haemostatic deficiency. PT and aPTT are markers of various aspects of a secondary haemostasis, with PT reflecting the function of the extrinsic and common pathway, while aPTT reflects the function of the intrinsic and common pathway, both mainly reflecting the activity of the soluble factors involved in fibrin formation. BMBT evaluates the function of a primary haemostasis (i.e. formation of a functional platelet plug) and the platelet concentration is a measure of the presence of sufficient numbers of platelets.

The results in this case indicate that the haemostatic defect is in primary haemostasis owing to the thrombocytopaenia with or without concurrent platelet dysfunction.

CASE 36

1 What is your evaluation of the laboratory data?

There is slight anaemia. Because of a concurrent moderate decrease in total protein with proportionate decreases in albumin and globulins suggestive of loss of serum, haemorrhage should be a primary consideration and loss of blood into the gastrointestinal tract in association with diarrhoea is one consideration. Haemolysis or decreased marrow production cannot be ruled out. The possibility of anaemia of chronic disease or associated with poor nutrition should be considered due to the very thin body condition.

The slight leucocytosis with slight neutrophilia and monocytosis is supportive of inflammation.

There is a moderate decrease in total protein with slightly to moderately decreased albumin and a borderline to slight decrease in globulins. This may be due to haemorrhage, but this pattern is highly suggestive of protein-losing enteropathy. The deworming history suggests parasitism is not likely to be the underlying cause. The hypoproteinaemia/hypoalbuminaemia is the likely cause for the oedema noted clinically.

The slight increase in total bilirubin may be due to decreased hepatic blood flow associated with anorexia and/or cholestasis.

The decreases in Na^+, Cl^- and Ca^{2+} may be due to intestinal loss with diarrhoea and/or decreased consumption. The decrease in calcium may also be attributable to the decreased albumin (decreased protein binding). The increase in K^+ may reflect acidosis associated with intestinal bicarbonate loss with diarrhoea or may be associated with haemolysis or delay in removal of serum from the clot in the collection tube.

The slight increases in ALP and phosphorus are attributable to continued bone growth in this age foal.

2 What is your diagnosis/interpretation?

The primary consideration is *Lawsonia intracellularis* infection resulting in proliferative enteritis. Differential diagnoses include infectious enteritis, sand impaction, parasitism, gastroduodenal ulcers and intoxication with plants and chemicals including pharmacological agents such as NSAIDs. Infectious agents that may be implicated in weanling diarrhoea are numerous and include *Salmonella* spp., *Rhodococcus equi*, *Clostridium* spp., *Ehrlichia risticii*, *Campylobacter jejuni*, rotavirus and adenovirus. However, these conditions are unlikely to cause outbreaks of disease characterised by weight loss, diarrhoea, colic and hypoproteinaemia in foals of this age group.

3 What pathophysiology is likely underlying the findings in this case?

L. intracellularis is an obligate intracellular organism. The method of infection and transmission of the disease in the horse is unknown, although the faecal–oral route is most likely. Oedema occurs in the serosal layer of the intestine, resulting in necrosis and mucosal thickening. Crypt cells expand and elongate, and the bacteria may be seen in the apical cytoplasm of these cells. Mitotic cells are abundant, resulting in proliferative enteropathy, while inflammatory cells and goblet cells are reduced or absent. Immature animals around weaning age are most often affected. Affected older animals are more likely to have proliferative enteritis with intestinal haemorrhage. In these cases, the mucosal thickening is not as apparent, congestion of the mucosal blood vessels occurs and inflammatory cells are consistently present in the lamina propria. These changes lead to poor intestinal absorption resulting in protein-losing enteropathy and diarrhoea, with potential for altered intestinal motility and colic.

4 What other tests would you recommend performing?

There is a serological test for *L. intracellularis* conducted on serum and PCR tests available for detection of this organism in faeces (University of Minnesota). Diagnosis is based on a positive silver staining demonstrating organisms in small intestinal tissue sections. It is not possible to culture the organism using routine methods.

FURTHER READING

Frank N. Fishman CE, Gebhart CJ *et al.* (1998) *Lawsonia intracellularis* proliferative enteropathy in a weanling foal. *Equine Vet J* **30**:549–552.

Lavoie JP, Drolet R, Parsons D *et al.* (2000) Equine proliferative enteropathy: a cause of weight loss, colic, diarrhea and hypoproteinemia in foals on three breeding farms. *Equine Vet J* **32**:418–425.

Lawson GH, Gebhart CJ (2000) Proliferative enteropathy. *J Comp Pathol* **122**:77–100.

CASE 37

1 Discuss the significant haematological and biochemistry findings.

There is a borderline leucocytosis based on a slight mature neutrophilia, suggesting stress (epinephrine or glucocorticoid effect). A moderate normocytic-normochromic anaemia is present, which is non-regenerative at the time of the sample because of the absence of polychromasia, hypochromasia and macrocytosis of erythrocytes.

In the face of haemorrhagic thoracic effusion, hypoproteinaemia and markedly prolonged coagulation times, anaemia due to acute to subacute haemorrhage prior to onset of regeneration (<3 days) is most likely.

The slight increase in urea concentration in the face of normal creatinine concentration suggests gastrointestinal haemorrhage, although a decreased GFR or diet effect should also be considered. Moderate hyponatraemia, slight to moderate hypochloraemia as well as slight hypokalaemia and hypocalcaemia are consistent with third-space fluid losses due to thoracic effusion. This results in hypovolaemia and therefore subsequent secretion of ADH and a thirst response. Uptake of pure water causes a dilution of extracellular fluid.

There is a slight hypoproteinaemia based on a slight hypoalbuminaemia and low normal globulins, which is most likely due to haemorrhage. Slight to moderate hyperglycaemia suggests stress-induced glucocorticoid effect. Diabetes mellitus or iatrogenic infusion of glucose are probable differential diagnoses, but less likely given the history and further findings in this dog. The borderline increase in triglyceride concentration is clinically not significant.

2 Describe and discuss the coagulation profile. What is the most likely aetiology of the disease?

There is a severely prolonged aPTT and a moderately prolonged PT, suggesting a disorder of secondary haemostasis affecting the extrinsic and intrinsic or common pathway. The magnitude of PT prolongation is greater than the prolongation of aPTT. This pattern is highly suggestive of acute coumarin (rodenticide) intoxication, as factor VII has the shortest half-life and is affected first in the absence of vitamin K.

Differential diagnosis includes DIC; however, the first variable affected in DIC tends to be aPTT rather than PT. Moreover, in the case of DIC, thrombocytopaenia and decreased fibrinogen would be expected. Measurement of D-dimers is helpful to rule in/out DIC, but it should be considered that haemorrhage in body cavities may also result in increased D-dimers.

3 What are the prognosis, treatment and monitoring of this disease?

The prognosis is good to guarded depending on the severity of clinical signs, the location of the haemorrhage (e.g. CNS would be an unfavourable location) and how early treatment is initiated. Treatment should be performed with vitamin K_1 (4–5 mg [up to 10 mg]/kg body weight q12h diluted in a saline infusion). After 2–3 days, vitamin K_1 can be given orally and the dosage can be reduced to 1–2 mg/kg q12h. In the case of first-generation coumarin

derivatives (e.g. warfarin), treatment should be continued for at least 7 days, whereas second-generation coumarin derivatives (e.g. diphacinon) require therapy of at least 3 weeks duration. If confirmation of rodenticide toxicity is desired, normalisation of the coagulation profile while on vitamin K therapy would provide good support for coumarin intoxication. Two to five days after discontinuation of treatment, PT should be measured. If PT is still prolonged, therapy should be continued for a further 2 weeks.

FOLLOW UP

This dog received a blood transfusion and vitamin K_1 and the coagulation profile was unremarkable 24 hours after initiation of treatment.

FURTHER READING

Sheafor SE, Couto CG (1999) Anticoagulant rodenticide toxicity in 21 dogs. *J Am Anim Hosp Assoc* **35**:38–46.

CASE 38

1 What is your diagnosis?

Low T4 and free T4 measured by FT4D and the presence of TgAAs are consistent with hypothyroidism secondary to lymphocytic thyroiditis.

2 Comment on the profile abnormalities, the underlying pathophysiology and the degree of confidence each result contributes to the diagnosis.

T4 is decreased in hypothyroid dogs and in association with non-thyroidal illness and drug therapy. In one study (Gaskill *et al.*, 2000) 32% of epileptic dogs had T4 concentrations below the reference range at 6 and 12 months after starting phenobarbitone therapy. Given the potential difficulty of confirming hypothyroidism in a dog receiving long-term anticonvulsant therapy, a more comprehensive thyroid panel was requested for this patient, rather than the commonly used screening combination of T4 and cTSH.

FT4D is less affected by nonthyroidal illness and drug therapy than total T4 (Peterson *et al.*, 1997). Although the low FT4D result in this patient increases the probability of hypothyroidism, a definitive diagnosis is still not possible since decreased FT4D has been reported in dogs receiving phenobarbitone therapy (Daminet *et al.*, 2003).

Most hypothyroid dogs have increased cTSH concentrations, but several studies report a number of hypothyroid dogs with cTSH concentrations within the reference interval (13–38% of hypothyroid dogs; Dixon & Mooney, 1999; Peterson *et al.*, 1997; Scott-Moncrieff *et al.*, 1998). Phenobarbitone is reported to have the potential to increase the cTSH concentration (Gaskill *et al.*, 1999), although studies in this area are not in universal agreement (Daminet & Ferguson, 2003).

Veterinary Clinical Pathology

The presence of TgAAs provides no information regarding thyroid function but indicates the presence of lymphocytic thyroiditis. Antibody production peaks at 4–8 years and older dogs are less likely to have positive results (Graham *et al.*, 2007).

FOLLOW UP

This patient poses a diagnostic dilemma. The finding of low T4, FT4D and normal cTSH may be noted in both hypothyroid dogs and euthyroid dogs with non-thyroidal illness. At the time of presentation, the seizures were well controlled and there was no evidence of additional disease, including cardiac disease. A presumptive diagnosis of hypothyroidism was made based on the clinical presentation, thyroid hormone results and the demonstration of lymphocytic thyroiditis. A more confident diagnosis would have been possible if the cTSH concentration had also been increased, since Kantrowitz *et al.* (2001) found only 4 of 223 (1.8%) dogs with non-thyroidal illness to have low TT4 and FT4D and high cTSH.

This patient was treated with thyroid supplementation and responded well.

REFERENCES AND FURTHER READING

Daminet S, Ferguson DC (2003) Influence of drugs on thyroid function in dogs. *J Vet Intern Med* **17**:463–472.

Dixon RM, Mooney CT (1999) Evaluation of serum free thyroxine and thyrotropin concentrations in the diagnosis of canine hypothyroidism. *J Small Anim Pract* **40**:72–78.

Gaskill CL, Burton SA, Gelens HC *et al.* (1999) Effects of phenobarbital treatment on serum thyroxine and thyroid-stimulating hormone concentrations in epileptic dogs. *J Am Vet Med Assoc* **215**:489–496.

Gaskill CL, Burton SA, Gelens HC *et al.* (2000) Changes in serum thyroxine and thyroid-stimulating hormone concentrations in epileptic dogs receiving phenobarbital for one year. *J Vet Pharmacol Ther* 4:243–249.

Graham PA, Refsal KR, Nachreiner RF (2007) Etiopathologic findings of canine hypothyroidism. *Vet Clin North Am Small Anim Pract* **37**:617–631.

Kantrowitz LB, Peterson ME, Melián C *et al.* (2001) Serum total thyroxine, total triiodothyronine, free thyroxine and thyrotropin concentrations in dogs with nonthyroidal illness. *Journal of the American Veterinary Medical Association* **219**:765–769.

Peterson ME, Melián C, Nichols R (1997) Measurement of serum total thyroxine, triiodothyronine, free thyroxine and thyrotropin concentrations for diagnosis of hypothyroidism in dogs. *J Am Vet Med Assoc* **211**:1396–1402.

Scott-Moncrieff JCR, Nelson RW, Bruner JM *et al.* (1998) Comparison of serum concentrations of thyroid-stimulating hormone in healthy dogs, hypothyroid dogs, and euthyroid dogs with concurrent disease. *J Am Vet Med Assoc* **212**: 387–391.

CASE 39

1 How do you interpret the clinical chemistry data?

Serum amyloid A (SAA) is the major APP in cats. Haptoglobin is one of the moderate APPs in cats. In the literature, there is no indication of a rise in CRP in cats in the face of an acute-phase response (APR). In this patient, SAA is showing a 12-fold increase and haptoglobin a more than 5-fold increase consistent with an APR and systemic inflammation. There is slight hypoalbuminaemia. In addition to decreased protein intake, decreased albumin synthesis and loss of albumin via the kidneys or intestines, the APR may be the cause for the decrease in albumin. In the face of an APR, albumin acts as a negative APP in the majority of species and declines in the course of disease. Usually the decrease is slight.

In summary, these parameters support an APR and systemic inflammation. It is important to remember that this is a non-specific reaction, which may occur in a wide variety of diseases. A specific aetiologic diagnosis cannot be made based on these parameters. However, as the changes are marked, further diagnostics including blood work, radiography and ultrasonography are warranted to determine the cause of the inflammation.

2 What actions does haptoglobin perform in the body?

Most importantly, haptoglobin is a haemoglobin scavenger. Free haemoglobin in the plasma, possibly resulting from haemolysis, is toxic and induces a pro-inflammatory response. Therefore, haptoglobin protects the body from the negative effects of free haemoglobin. Consideration should be given to the fact that in the face of haemolysis, haptoglobin may be low in concentration, as the haptoglobin–haemoglobin complex is cleared by the reticuloendothelial system. Furthermore, binding of haemoglobin is a bactericidal process, as haemoglobin-iron is thus unavailable for bacterial growth. In addition, haptoglobin inhibits the chemotaxis and phagocytosis of granulocytes. This further affects the inflammatory response.

FURTHER READING

Cerón JJ, Eckersall PD, Martínez-Subiela S (2005) Acute phase proteins in dogs and cats: current knowledge and future perspectives. *J Vet Clin Pathol* **34**:85–99.

Eckersall PD, Bell R (2010) Acute phase proteins: biomarkers of infection and inflammation in veterinary medicine. *Vet J* **185**:23–27.

Ulutas B, Bayramli G, Ulutas PA *et al.* (2005) Serum concentration of some acute phase proteins in naturally occurring canine babesiosis: a preliminary study. *J Vet Clin Pathol* **34**:144–147.

CASE 40

1 Does the anaemia appear regenerative?

The lack of polychromasia and reticulocytosis in the face of a severe anaemia indicates a non-regenerative anaemia. High numbers of NRBCs as a sole finding do not indicate bone marrow regeneration. NRBC numbers increase with many regenerative anaemias, but increases may also be seen with many non-regenerative anaemias.

NRBCs cannot be adequately determined and enumerated by current haematology analysers. In contrast, as nucleated cells they may be counted as WBCs by a haematology analyser, leading to a falsely increased WBC count. If more than 10 NRBCs are encountered on a blood smear, a correction of the total WBC count has to be performed after counting the number of NRBCs per 100 WBCs. The formula to correct the measured WBC count is:

$$\text{Corrected WBC count} = (\text{uncorrected WBC count} \times 100)/(100 + \text{NRBCs per 100 WBCs})$$

The corrected WBC count in this patient is:

$$(20 \times 100)/(100 + 32) = 2,000/132 = 15.15\ (10^9/l)$$

2 What is the significance of the blood smear pictures?

Blast cells (immature cells with visible nucleoli) are an abnormal finding in peripheral blood smears of cats. These cells appear to be rubriblasts and that, along with the non-regenerative anaemia and high number of NRBCs, suggests erythroleukaemia (AMl-M6).

In cats, FeLV infection is most commonly associated with erythroleukaemia. In this cat the ELISA for FeLV is negative. ELISA tests detect the nucleocapsid protein p27. This test may be positive in the face of infection. However, false-negative results may occur in the face of viraemia in about 10% of FeLV infected cats. A further test to definitively rule in/out FeLV infection in this case would be PCR for provirus detection.

FOLLOW UP

A bone marrow examination revealed marked erythropoiesis with a maturation arrest typical of erythroleukaemia. An FeLV provirus PCR done on the bone marrow was positive. Therefore, FeLV-induced erythroleukaemia is present in this case.

FURTHER READING

Lutz H, Addie D, Belák S *et al.* (2009) Feline leukaemia, ABCD guidelines on prevention and management. *J Feline Med Surg* **11**:565–574.

Weiss DJ, Wardrop KJ (2010) Acute myeloid leukemia. In: *Schalm's Veterinary Hematology*, 6th edn. Wiley Blackwell, Ames, p. 481.

CASE 41

1 How would you interpret this anaemia?

There is a moderate microcytic-hypochromic anaemia with mild evidence of regeneration, confirmed by the presence of small numbers of polychromatophils on the blood smear. Microcytosis and hypochromasia are due to defective haemoglobin synthesis caused by iron deficiency. Iron deficiency is commonly observed in chronic external blood loss, which may result from blood loss into the gastrointestinal, urogenital or respiratory tracts or from the skin surface.

2 What is the significance of the codocytes?

Codocytes or target cells have a central area of haemoglobin surrounded by a pale rim with haemoglobin at the periphery of the cell. They also have increased amounts of cholesterol resulting in an increase in the surface area of the erythrocyte membrane. Codocytosis is frequently observed in hypochromic states (e.g. iron deficiency).

3 What is the significance of the eosinophilia?

There is a mild eosinophilia, which is commonly observed in hypersensitivity conditions and parasitic infection. Eosinophilia may also be paraneoplastic and is frequently associated with mast cell tumours, because of chemoattractants released from mast cells, and with other neoplasms (lymphoma, carcinoma) caused by the release of eosinophilia-inducing factors, mainly IL-5. There are also several idiopathic eosinophilic conditions that have been described in cats and, less frequently, in dogs (eosinophilic granuloma complex and hypereosinophilic syndrome in cats, eosinophilic myositis, gastroenteritis and pneumonia in dogs).

4 How would you explain the high urea?

High urea with normal creatinine may reflect decreased urinary excretion due to pre-renal conditions such as hypovolaemia (dehydration) or decreased cardiac output (cardiac insufficiency, shock). Gastrointestinal haemorrhage may also cause increased urea because the marked haemoglobin degradation increases ammonia (NH_4) delivery to hepatocytes, which convert this into urea.

5 Give a possible explanation to this case. What further investigations would you suggest?

There is evidence of an iron deficiency anaemia, which is likely due to external blood loss. A positive faecal occult blood test confirmed the suspicion of gastrointestinal blood loss. This condition may be due to ulceration, parasitism, neoplasia or inflammatory bowel disease. Faecal examination was performed and was positive for *Strongyloides* spp., a nematode that lives in the adult stage in the mucosa of the small intestine and may cause haemorrhagic enteritis.

FURTHER READING

Stockham SL, Scott MA (2008) *Fundamentals of Veterinary Clinical Pathology*, 2nd edn. Blackwell Publishing, Oxford.

CASE 42

1 Discuss the laboratory findings and their significance.

There is a slight anaemia, which is marginally microcytic and hypochromic. This is consistent with anaemia of inflammatory disease (AID) with sequestration of iron (AID can also be normocytic-normochromic) or iron deficiency anaemia (chronic blood loss usually). The possibility of chronic blood loss is supported by the positive faecal occult blood and may be due to gastrointestinal ulceration.

AID results from decreased iron availability (increased uptake of iron by macrophages, local binding of iron by apolactoferrin released by neutrophils, decreased iron absorption from the gut) and can occasionally lead on to the microcytic, hypochromic anaemia expected in iron deficiency. Iron sequestration has an antibacterial effect. Erythrocyte survival is also decreased in AID (premature removal by macrophages due to erythrocyte surface alterations), as is erythropoiesis (cytokines [e.g. IL-1, TNF-α] decreased erythropoietin production).

Decreased serum TIBC and increased serum ferritin can be used, if necessary, to distinguish AID from iron deficiency anaemia, where TIBC is high and serum ferritin low. The latter is a good indicator of total body iron stores.

The moderate neutrophilia, slight left shift and monocytosis suggest inflammation with necrosis. The hypoproteinaemia, which is due to low albumin and marginally increased globulins, suggests protein-losing enteropathy. ALP is increased but, with a normal GGT of this horse and GLDH, it is likely to be due to the young age (2 years) of this horse and continued bone growth. The increased CK and AST suggest mild muscle damage, possibly as a result of the colic behaviour.

The oral glucose absorption test shows a flatter than normal curve, with an increase of 80% over baseline. This suggests partial malabsorption (15–85% absorption) but such values can be seen in some normal horses.

The peritoneal fluid analysis supports an inflammatory condition. Faecal occult blood should be interpreted with caution, but in this case it might be significant as the haematology indicated blood loss as a possibility.

2 What is your interpretation of these findings and what are your recommendations?

From the history and results, a relatively mild protein-losing enteropathy with the presence of inflammation is likely, and previous parasitic damage is high on the list (granulomatous enteritis). Although rectal biopsy might help further characterisation in this case, oral prednisolone was started without further diagnostic investigation and the problem resolved completely.

CASE 43

1 What is your evaluation of the urinalysis findings?

The abnormal colour (red–brown) with an absence of erythrocytes in the urine sediment is suggestive of haemoglobin or myoglobin in the urine. Correlation with the serum appearance is recommended; red discolouration of serum due to haemolysis is suspected in the presence of haemoglobinuria, while spillover of myglobin into the urine will occur in the absence of serum discolouration. The positive dipstick protein and bilirubin may be due the presence of these elements, but are suspect due to the fact that discoloured urine may make evaluation of colour changes on dipstick pads difficult or impossible. The positive haemoglobin/blood may be due to discolouration interfering with pad colour and/or the presence of haemoglobin, since no increase in erythrocytes is present in the urine sediment. The slight decrease in USG may not be of clinical significance, but continued monitoring is recommended to determine if a pattern of abnormality can be detected.

These findings are highly suggestive of haemoglobinuria associated with intravascular haemolysis. Evaluation of an FBC and peripheral blood film morphology is needed to help determine if anaemia is present or if there are features or parasites that may explain the haemolysis.

2 What is your evaluation of the haematological findings and the photomicrograph of the peripheral blood film?

The haematological findings do not indicate anaemia, although there is a borderline decrease in the RBC count. However, developing anaemia may not yet be evident since the presenting complaint is of acute development. No abnormalities are identified in the other automated haematological data.

The peripheral blood film indicates the presence of numerous eccentrocytes (haemoglobin concentrated eccentrically at one pole of the erythrocyte with a clear area surrounded by the erythrocyte membrane at the opposite pole of the erythrocyte). This is likely causing haemolysis and causing haemoglobinuria.

3 What conditions/differential diagnoses do you suspect, and what is the pathophysiological basis for this condition?

Eccentrocytosis in dogs has been associated with drug administration, onion or garlic and/or chive toxicity, vitamin K antagonist toxicity, ketoacidotic or compensated diabetes mellitus, T-lymphoid lymphoma, severe infections and occasionally with other conditions.

The mechanism for eccentrocyte formation is oxidative damage to haemoglobin.

FOLLOW UP

On further questioning, the owners revealed that the dog had consumed two orders of battered onion rings the evening prior to presentation. The take-away delivery had been left unguarded on the counter and he had helped himself. With supportive treatment and fluid therapy to help prevent haemoglobinuric nephrosis, the dog recovered without complications.

FURTHER READING

Caldin M, Carli E, Furlanello T *et al.* (2005) A retrospective study of 60 cases of eccentrocytosis in the dog. *J Vet Clin Pathol* **34**:224–231.

CASE 44

1 What cells can be seen in Fig. 44.1?

Leucocytes (segmented neutrophils) and RBCs.

2 What do they indicate in urine?

The leucocytes indicate inflammation in the urogenital tract. Infection can only be suspected if bacteria are found microscopically or by urine culture. This is difficult to tell from the picture shown here. More than 10^4 rods or $>10^5$ cocci/μl are required to detect bacteria in urine sediment. Sensitivity of detection of bacteria can be improved by staining an air-dried sediment smear.

3 Does the ratio of these cells indicate inflammation or bleeding?

The ratio of leucocytes to RBCs indicates inflammation, likely with diapedesis bleeding. With bleeding the ratio to be expected would be 1 leucocyte in approximately 500 RBCs. However, the use of ratios may not always be reliable, particularly in samples that are not examined within 30 minutes of collection (since cell degeneration or lysis may occur) or in which samples are split into aliquots

for other types of testing (may result in uneven distribution of cells in the various aliquots).

4 Is the +++ positive leucocyte esterase test on the dipstick an indication of pyuria?

A positive leucocyte esterase test on the dipstick is NOT an indication for the presence of leucocytes in sediment. False-positive reactions occur frequently in different dipstick systems. The reason for this is not clear, but it has been demonstrated that the leucocyte esterase test for leucocytes in feline urine is positive in many samples that do not contain leucocytes and so microscopic sediment evaluation is the preferred method for detection of leucocytes in feline urine. In cats, the leucocyte esterase dipstick test has moderate sensitivity (77%) but low specificity (34%) compared with microscopic sediment evaluation. In dogs, the leucocyte esterase test has low sensitivity (34%) but high specificity (93.2%) for evaluation of pyuria in urine specimens. Therefore, when a leucocyte esterase test is positive in dog urine, it is highly likely that pyuria is present. However, a negative test does not rule out the possibility of pyuria.

5 Is the nitrite test available on some dipsticks suitable for use in dogs and cats?

Nitrate, originating from the diet, is a normal constituent of urine. The reduced form, nitrite, is not normally found in urine but is produced by some bacteria. A positive result suggests significant bacteriuria. Osborne and Stevens (1999) indicated that clinical evaluations of urine dipstick nitrite are not consistent in the detection of significant bacteriuria in dogs and cats and, therefore, are not suitable for use in these species.

REFERENCE AND FURTHER READING

Holan KM, Kruger JM, Gibbons SN *et al.* (1997) Clinical evaluation of a leukocyte esterase test strip for detection of feline pyuria. *J Vet Clin Pathol* **26**:126–131.

Osborne CA, Stevens JB (1999) *Urinalysis: A Clinical Guide to Compassionate Patient Care.* Bayer Corporation, Shawnee Mission.

Swenson CL, Boisvert AM, Gibbons-Burgener SN *et al.* (2011) Evaluation of modified Wright staining of dried urinary sediment as a method for accurate detection of bacteriuria in cats. *J Vet Clin Pathol* **40**:256–264.

CASE 45

1 What is your assessment of these findings and the physiological bases for them?

The 'ping' noted on auscultation with percussion and abdominal distension is consistent with abomasal displacement resulting in partial anorexia and decreased milk production. The increase in RBCs, haemoglobin, haematocrit, total protein and albumin all support the presence of dehydration. Dehydration is suggested by partial anorexia and removal of the abomasal reflux. The neutrophilia and increased fibrinogen support the presence of inflammation. The increased creatinine may be due to pre-renal (dehydration), renal or post-renal conditions. Urinalysis and measurement of USG is recommended to help determine if conditions other than dehydration may be contributing.

The hypokalaemia may be due to decreased intracellular potassium because of partial anorexia, loss of K^+-rich fluid in the abomasal reflux and/or metabolic alkalosis (see below). The hypochloraemia is likely due to chloride sequestration in the abomasum and loss of chloride with removal of the reflux fluid. It is likely to be further compounded by an alkalosis.

The increased TCO_2 is consistent with metabolic alkalosis. The abomasum normally secretes large amounts of HCl for digestion and this is neutralised by bicarbonate secretion in the duodenum stimulated by passage of a food bolus from the abomasum into the duodenum. With abomasal displacement, the abomasum is functionally obstructed, resulting in sequestration of H^+, Cl^- and K^+-containing fluids. K^+ is further depleted by decreased food intake. Without ingesta passing into the intestine, bicarbonate is retained and metabolic alkalosis results.

2 What is your diagnosis?
Displaced abomasum with resulting metabolic alkalosis, hypokalaemia and hypochloraemia.

3 What might you expect to find in the urine, and why?
A paradoxical aciduria is expected in the urine. In response to dehydration, increased aldosterone secretion will stimulate Na^+ resorption and retention of water in the kidney. Usually Cl^- is absorbed with Na^+, but with concurrent hypochloraemia, HCO_3^- is absorbed to maintain electroneutrality and the urine becomes more acidic. Na^+ can also be absorbed in exchange with K^+ or H^+. With hypokalaemia, H^+ is exchanged for Na^+, further contributing to the acidic urine.

Urine chloride concentration is expected to be low (<10 mmol/l) owing to the hypochloraemia.

4 What treatment is needed?
Treatment is aimed at correction of the abomasal displacement and abomasopexy. Correction of serum Cl^- and K^+ levels with fluid therapy is needed to help resolve the dehydration, metabolic alkalosis and paradoxical aciduria.

CASE 46

1 Describe and discuss the haematological abnormalities.
There is a moderate to marked leucocytosis based on a moderate eosinophilia, a slight to moderate neutrophilia with slight left shift, a moderate lymphocytosis, moderate monocytosis and slight basophilia.

Causes for the eosinophilia and basophilia include hypersensitivity reactions, idiopathic disease, parasitic infections, fungal disease, neoplasia or hypoadrenocorticism. Allergic disorders are frequently associated with eosinophilia, mostly involving flea-bite dermatitis, but allergic respiratory disease is also a common cause. Idiopathic eosinophilia (hypereosinophilic synodrome) shows extensive infiltration of tissues with eosinophils. Lungs, muscle tissue, the gastrointestinal tract or bones (eosinophilic panosteitis) may be affected in idiopathic eosinophilia. A wide variety of parasites may lead to increased numbers of eosinophils. Besides ectoparasites, heartworms (*Dirofilaria* spp.), *Angiostrongylus* spp., *Strongyloides* spp. or *Trichuris* spp. should be considered. Larvae that may result in pulmonary disease include *A. vasorum, Crenosoma vulpis, Oslerus osleri* and *Oslerus (Filaroides) hirthi*. Eosinophilia may be involved in primary neoplasia (e.g. rare eosinophilic leukaemia) or as a paraneoplastic syndrome. Although the latter is mostly described in mast cell tumours, paraneoplastic eosinophilia has also been reported in other benign and malignant neoplasms such as T-cell lymphoma. The underlying mechanism may involve cytokines such as IL-2 or IL-5.

Neutrophilia with left shift, lymphocytosis and monocytosis further indicates chronic inflammation. The normocytic-normochromic, non-regenerative anaemia may be anaemia of chronic disease. Confirmation by repeated analysis to determine if this is a persistent finding is recommended. A further differential in theory includes bone marrow disease. Although this is highly unlikely in the presence of increased leucocytes, this could be excluded by bone marrow examination (e.g. via cytological and/or histological examination).

In summary, as this dog clinically shows signs of respiratory disease, eosinophilic bronchopneumonia or lung worms should be considered. Further recommended analyses include bronchioalveolar lavage with cytological examination as well as faecal parasite analysis. If no cause for the laboratory abnormalities can be detected, the other differentials must be ruled out. There is an ELISA test for *A. vasorum*. A Baermann procedure may be successful in obtaining larvae from faeces that have been coughed up and swallowed.

2 What preformed proteins are released from the eosinophilic-specific granules and what actions do they perform?

The eosinophilic-specific granule proteins are listed below:

Major Preformed Protein	Function
Major basic protein	• Cytotoxic to parasites, protozoa, bacteria and cells • Leads to mediator release from mast cells • Platelet activation • Bronchospasmic complement activation
Eosinophil peroxidase	• Generation of toxic oxygen radicals • Induces release of histamine from mast cells • Inactivation of leucotrienes
Eosinophil cationic protein	• Toxic to microorganisms and tracheal epithelium • Neurotoxic • Promotes mast cell degranulation • Heparin neutralisation
Eosinophil-derived neurotoxin	• Toxic to myelinated nerve fibres • Antiviral activity

FURTHER READING

Stockham SL, Scott MA (2008) *Fundamentals of Veterinary Clinical Pathology*, 2nd edn. Blackwell Publishing, Oxford.

Weiss DJ, Wardrop KJ (2010) (eds) *Schalm's Veterinary Hematology*, 6th edn. Blackwell Publishing, Ames.

CASE 47

1 There is no clear cause of the polydipsia, but what is your interpretation of the abnormalities present?

Hyperkalaemia at this level is spurious. Reported causes of pseudohyperkalaemia include leakage of potassium from platelets and leukaemic cells. Haemolysis may cause serum increases in cattle, horses and some breeds of dog (e.g. Akita) but is not reported in the cat. In this case the combination of non-detectable calcium and pseudohyperkalaemia suggests contamination of the sample with the anticoagulant K_3-EDTA. The EDTA binds calcium, rendering it unavailable for assay, while the potassium in the anticoagulant is measured as serum potassium. Other assays that require divalent cations as cofactors (e.g. ALP requires free ionised magnesium) are also affected.

FURTHER READING

Stockham SL, Scott MA (2008) *Fundamentals of Veterinary Clinical Pathology*, 2nd edn. Blackwell Publishing, Oxford.

CASE 48

1 What is your interpretation of this electrophoresis?

The narrow tall spike in the gamma globulin region is consistent with a monoclonal gammopathy. The width of the spike is no wider than that of the albumin peak. Remember that this is judged without the post-albumin shoulder, which is poorly defined in this case.

2 What is the most likely clinical diagnosis?

The most likely clinical diagnosis is lymphoproliferative disease (lymphoma or myeloma). Occasionally, non-neoplastic conditions will result in monoclonal gammopathy, but this is rare. A few transient monoclonal gammopathies of unknown origin have been reported in the horse.

FURTHER READING

Geelen SMJ, Bernadina WE, Grinwis GCM *et al.* (1997) Monoclonal gammopathy in a Dutch Warmblood mare. *Vet Quart* **19**:20–32.

CASE 49

1 What is the most likely diagnosis based on the haematological abnormalities, breed, age and clinical signs? What test could you perform to confirm your diagnosis?

The present findings are highly suspicious for canine leucocyte adhesion deficiency (CLAD), which is a homozygous autosomal recessive disease in Irish Setters. As in this case, puppies of a few weeks of age suffer from various inflammatory conditions associated with a pronounced leucocytosis based on a neutrophilia. Definitive diagnosis is by PCR testing in specialised laboratories.

2 Describe the underlying clinicopathological abnormality.

Affected dogs with the homozygous form of the disease are missing the beta-2 integrin CD18, a surface glycoprotein of leucocytes essential for leucocyte adhesion to the endothelial surface and transmigration to the site of infection.

3 Summarise all the events and involved structures in the adhesion and transmigration of leucocytes from the vascular endothelium to a site of injury.

Injurious agents at the site of injury are engulfed by macrophages, which afterwards secrete cytokines, most importantly TNF and IL-1. These, as well as other mediators such as histamine, act on endothelial cells, inducing expression of adhesion molecules, E- and P-selectin, as well as the adhesion molecules of the immunoglobulin family, VCAM-1 and ICAM-1, on the cellular surface.

Leucocytes express sialylated Lewis X oligosaccharides, which, after binding to selectins on the endothelial cell surface, allow a low-affinity connection of leucocytes and endothelial cells. The blood flow disconnects this interaction, leading to a fast off-rate of leucocytes and initiating the process of rolling.

In the next step, rolling leucocytes are activated by chemokines bound to proteoglycans on endothelial cells. Activation leads to a conversion of leucocyte integrins (LFA-1 [beta-2 integrin, CD11a/CD18] and VLA-4 [beta-1 integrin]) from a low-affinity state to a high-affinity state, stopping rolling and initiating pavementing. Therefore, leucocyte integrins bind to adhesion molecules of the immunoglobulin family of endothelial cells.

Diapedesis of leucocytes through the interendothelial space is also initiated by chemokines. Structures important in this process are adhesion molecules that bind to each other, PECAM-1 and, again, members of the immunoglobulin superfamily. Collagenases are thought to facilitate the flow of leucocytes through the basement membrane.

Finally, beta-1 integrins of leucocytes make them adhere to the extracellular matrix, thus allowing them to function against the injurious agents.

FURTHER READING

Ettinger SJ, Feldman EC (2005) *Veterinary Internal Medicine*, 6th edn. Elsevier Saunders, St. Louis.

Kumar V, Fausto A, Abbas A (2004) *Robbins & Cotran Pathologic Basis of Disease*, 7th edn. Elsevier Saunders, St. Louis.

CASE 50

1 What is the anion gap (AG) in this case?
AG = $(Na^+ + K^+) - (HCO_3^- + Cl^-)$ = $(145 + 6.5) - (27 + 104)$ = $151.5 - 131 = 20.5$. The AG is within the reference interval.

2 What is your assessment of the arterial pH?
The arterial pH is decreased, therefore this is an acidaemia.

3 What is your assessment of the likely underlying aetiology for this arterial pH?
A decrease in HCO_3^-, which would be expected with metabolic acidosis, is not present. The $PaCO_2$ is significantly increased, so this is a respiratory acidosis. Anaesthesia has led in this cat to alveolar hypoventilation, which impairs excretion of CO_2 and accumulates H^+.

4 Is there appropriate compensation for this condition, and does it suggest an acute or a chronic condition?
Yes, there is appropriate compensation with an increase in HCO_3^- as expected to compensate for the increase in $PaCO_2$.

If this is an acute respiratory acidosis, it is expected that a 10 mmHg increase in $PaCO_2$ would cause an increase of 1.5 mmol/l HCO_3^-. If this is a chronic respiratory acidosis, it is expected that a 10 mmHg increase in $PaCO_2$ would cause an increase of 3.5 mmol/l HCO_3^-.

In this case, the $PaCO_2$ is increased by 30 mmHg from the middle of the reference interval for $PaCO_2$. This would be expected to result in an increase of 4.5 mmol/l of HCO_3^- in an acute condition and an increase of 10.5 mmol/l of HCO_3^- in a chronic condition.

The HCO_3^- is increased by 5 mmol/l from the middle of the reference interval for HCO_3^-. Therefore, as this is closest to an increase of 4.5 mmol/l of HCO_3^-, this cat has an acute respiratory acidosis. This is expected in this case, because no ongoing respiratory impairment is present in the kitten and anaesthesia is the cause of the respiratory acidosis.

FURTHER READING

Dibartola SP (2012) *Fluid, Electrolyte and Acid-Base Disorders in Small Animal Practice*, 4th edn. Elsevier Saunders, St. Louis.

CASE 51

1 How do you interpret the laboratory findings?
The most striking finding is the severely decreased cTLI concentration. The TLI assay gives information concerning the function of the exocrine pancreas, as it detects trypsinogen and trypsin as well as trypsin molecules bound to protein-ase inhibitors. Markedly decreased cTLI concentrations are consistent with exocrine pancreatic insufficiency (EPI), as the pancreas cannot maintain its secretion of zymogens and TLI concentration in serum will be decreased. The clinical signs in this patient are typical for this disease and occur if about 90% of the excretory function of the pancreas is lost. In addition, the age and breed of the patient match. Rough-coated Collies and German Shepherd Dogs are reported to commonly suffer from EPI. Caution is needed when interpreting TLI if a fasted sample has not been examined or if the patient shows impairment in GFR. A post-prandial increase in TLI has been reported. As TLI is excreted via the kidneys, renal insufficiency may also lead to an increase in TLI.

The slight increase in ALT enzyme activity points to hepatocellular damage. Causes may include increased intestinal permeability leading to increased exposure of the liver to hepatotoxic substances.

Hypocholesterolaemia and hypotriglyceridaemia are frequently observed in patients with EPI but are unlikely to be of clinical significance.

2 What further diagnostics are necessary in this patient, and why?
Pancreatic acinar atrophy, chronic pancreatitis or pancreatic neoplasia may be a cause of EPI. Diagnostic imaging

(radiography and ultrasound) may help detect pancreatic abnormalities/neoplasia. Further useful laboratory tests include assessment of cobalamin. In patients with EPI, the cobalamin concentration is frequently decreased due to two possible reasons: (1) malabsorption may lead to secondary intestinal bacterial overgrowth and increased consumption of cobalamin by bacteria; (2) the pancreas is secreting the intrinsic factor, which assembles with cobalamin in the intestine and is essential for cobalamin absorption in the ileum. In the face of EPI, concentrations of the intrinsic factor may be diminished, leading to impaired cobalamin absorption and hypocobalaminaemia.

FURTHER READING

Westermarck E, Wiberg M. (2003) Exocrine pancreatic insufficiency in dogs. *Vet Clin North Am Small Anim Pract* **33:**1165–1179.

CASE 52

1 What is your assessment of these findings?

There is slight responding anaemia as 2+ polychromatophils are present. The anaemia is likely the result of the haemorrhagic diarrhoea. The slight decrease in refractometer total protein, hypoalbuminaemia and hypophosphataemia may also be due to gastrointestinal loss and decreased absorption associated with haemorrhage and diarrhoea.

There is slight leucopaenia and neutropaenia, which may reflect increased loss of neutrophils, likely into the gastrointestinal tract in association with the diarrhoea. There may be loss of fibrinogen in the gastrointestinal tract since fibrinogen is not increased and the protein:fibrinogen ratio is <10%. Often, inflammation is associated with increased fibrinogen and a protein:fibrinogen ratio >10% as fibrinogen is an acute-phase protein.

The increased platelet count may reflect marrow stimulation due to the anaemia and leucopaenia. It could also be due to rebound if previous thrombocytopaenia has been present.

The slight increase in chloride may reflect dehydration. With dehydration, the degree of anaemia, hypoproteinaemia, hypoalbuminaemia and hypophosphataemia may be greater than reflected by these results. Often, secretional metabolic acidosis accompanies diarrhoea, although the TCO_2 is not decreased and, therefore, a mixed acid–base disorder with concurrent alkalosis should be investigated. The decreased anion gap is likely due to decreased negative charges (unmeasured anions) associated with hypoalbuminaemia.

2 What additional laboratory tests would you recommend?

Since diarrhoea is present, faecal parasitology is recommended. Arterial blood gas evaluation may be helpful in assessment of the acid–base status. Urinalysis

may also be of benefit in determining if ketosis is present due to negative energy balance.

FOLLOW UP

Faecal flotation showed 1,500 *Eimeria* spp. oocysts per gram of faeces. The clinical diagnosis is that of 'nervous coccidiosis'. This condition may be epidemic or sporadic in cattle in the wintertime in the United States of America and Canada. It is caused by *Eimeria* or *Isospora* spp. The neurological manifestation has high mortality (>80%). There is no known effective therapy for the neurological form. For the remainder of the cattle, treatment with a coccidiostat, reduction of crowding, efforts to clean the environment and minimisation of stress are recommended.

CASE 53

1 Describe and discuss the significant biochemistry findings.

There is a severe hypoproteinaemia based on a severe hypoalbuminaemia and a moderate hypoglobulinaemia. Probable causes include decreased protein uptake due to chronic anorexia and decreased albumin synthesis due to liver failure or protein loss via the intestine, kidneys, haemorrhage or severely exudative skin diseases. Given the dog's history, protein-losing enteropathy is most likely; however, renal loss and liver dysfunction should be ruled out. Renal protein loss should be considered especially in a Bernese Mountain Dog, but is generally associated with hypercholesterolaemia rather than a decreased cholesterol concentration. Hypocholesterolaemia may be associated with portosystemic shunts or protein-losing enteropathy because of decreased cholesterol production. In this dog, the latter is most likely.

There is a mild ionised hypocalcaemia, which may be caused by an inadequate absorption from the intestine. A slight increase of ALT activity is present, which is suggestive of mild hepatocellular insult.

2 What further tests are required to determine the aetiology of the significant abnormalities in this dog?

Urinalysis, including evaluation of a dipstick, sediment and UPCR, should be performed to rule out renal protein loss. Liver function testing (e.g. determination of pre- and post-prandial bile acid concentrations) is indicated to rule out hypoalbuminaemia due to hepatic dysfunction. Abdominal ultrasound is helpful to detect abnormalities of the gastrointestinal tract, liver and kidneys. If there is no evidence of severe liver failure or protein-losing nephropathy, enteral protein loss is most likely. Endoscopy and biopsy would be the last diagnostic steps to detect the underlying aetiology. The results in this patient are shown below:

- Urinalysis

Item	Result	Reference Interval
USG	**1.038**	>1.030
Dipstick Evaluation		
pH	7.5	Acidic
Bilirubin	**++**	Negative
Blood	Negative	Negative
Glucose	Negative	Negative
Protein	Negative	Negative to trace
UPCR	**0.1**	<0.2
Sediment Analysis		
Erythrocytes	<5	0–5/hpf
Leucocytes	<5	0–5/hpf
Epithelial cells	<5	0–5/hpf
Crystals	0	Variable
Casts	0	Variable/lpf
Bacteria	0	None
hpf: ×40 magnification		

There is no evidence of renal protein loss.

- **Bile acid stimulation test.** No evidence of liver dysfunction.
- **Abdominal ultrasound.** A moderately enlarged lymph node in the central abdomen was detected.
- **Endoscopy.** Endoscopic examination of the stomach revealed a slightly granular mucosa. Duodenal villi were oedematous and numerous white yellow–white stipples indicative of lymphangiectasia were observed. Biopsies were taken and submitted for histopathological examination.
- **Histopathological examination.** Biopsies of the stomach were consistent with a mild chronic lymphocytic–plasmacytic gastritis. Specimens of the duodenum demonstrated severe lymphangiectasia and mild lymphocytic–plasmacytic gastritis.

A diagnosis of protein-losing enteropathy due to lymphangiectasia of the duodenum was made.

Treatment of protein-losing enteropathy includes dietary management with a fat-restricted, calorie-dense and highly digestable diet. Glucocorticoids may be beneficial if a lymphocytic–plasmacytic infiltration of the lamina propria is present. Response to treatment is unpredictable; however, a remission of clinical signs may be achieved for months and even several years. Generally, the overall long-term prognosis is poor.

CASE 54

1 What is the most likely diagnosis based on the present findings?
Miniature and Toy Poodles who display macrocytic erythrocytes without anaemia and associated with giant or hypersegmented neutrophils are consistent with a diagnosis of Poodle marrow dyscrasia.

2 What further diagnostics would you perform to support your diagnosis?
Although the pathogenesis of the syndrome is unclear, a pronounced bone marrow dyserythropoiesis is observed in these cases. Therefore, cytological bone marrow examination is recommended. Features often visible in the sample include megaloblasts, bi- or multinucleation of erythroid precursors and an abnormal nuclear shape, with the most characteristic sign of the syndrome being nuclear bridging of rubricytes. Mitotic figures may be seen in higher frequency.

3 How do you interpret the condition for the well-being of the patient?
This syndrome is not reported to be associated with clinical problems. Nevertheless, it is a hereditary condition affecting both sexes, so breeding with affected individuals should be avoided.

FURTHER READING

Stockham SL, Scott MA (2008) *Fundamentals of Veterinary Clinical Pathology*, 2nd edn. Blackwell Publishing, Oxford.
Weiss DJ, Wardrop KJ (2010) (eds) *Schalm's Veterinary Hematology*, 6th edn. Blackwell Publishing, Ames.

CASE 55

1 What are the common clinicopathological findings in canine monocytic ehrlichiosis (*E. canis*)?
Common clinocipathological findings in canine cases of monocytic ehrlichiosis include thrombocytopaenia, pancytopaenia, lymphocytosis with presence of granular lymphocytes, hypoalbuminaemia, hyperglobulinaemia and increased serum activity of hepatic enzymes. Severe thrombocytopaenia was the only haematological abnormality in this case. This is thought to result from decreased production secondary to bone marrow hypoplasia, along with sequestration, consumption and secretion of platelet-inhibition factor by infected lymphocytes.

2 What does the serum protein electrophoretic tracing indicate?
The serum protein electrophoresis indicates moderate hypoalbuminaemia along with marked gammopathy.

As the gammaglobulin peak is narrower than the albumin peak, monoclonal gammopathy is present. A monoclonal spike is the result of the presence of a single clone producing one class of immunoglobulin. The differential diagnoses for monoclonal gammopathy are B-cell neoplasia (i.e. multiple myeloma, lymphoma) or infection (less common). In cases of canine monocytic ehrlichiosis, protein electrophoresis may also reveal the presence of a polyclonal gammopathy or monoclonal gammopathy (rarely). Hypoalbuminaemia could be related to decreased hepatic production in the face of an acute-phase reaction (negative acute-phase protein reaction) or increased renal loss.

FURTHER READING
Little S (2010) Ehrlichiosis and anaplasmosis in dogs and cats. *Vet Clin North Am Small Anim Pract* **40**:1121–1140.
Stockham SL, Scott MA (2008) *Fundamentals of Veterinary Clinical Pathology*, 2nd edn. Blackwell Publishing, Oxford.

CASE 56

1 What is your interpretation of these findings?
The clinical signs, electrolyte results and results of the ACTH stimulation test are consistent with hypoadrenocorticism.

2 What is the pathophysiology associated with these findings?
Hypoadrenocorticism is most often due to primary disease of the adrenal gland. This is due to immune-mediated destruction of the adrenal glands. Secondary hypoadrenocorticism is rare and may be due to trauma, a tumour or congenital defects of the pituitary gland resulting in decreased ACTH production, or it may be iatrogenic following abrupt withdrawal of prolonged corticosteroid therapy. Hypoadrenocorticism may be termed 'atypical' if there is only decreased glucocorticoids without concurrent decreased mineralocorticoids (no electrolyte abnormalities). The absence of destruction of adrenal medulla with adrenocortical destruction may explain such 'atypical' cases.

The altered electrolytes seen in most cases are due to mineralocorticoid deficiency with renal loss of Na^+, Cl^- and water, and retention of K^+ and H^- ions. Lack of sodium results in inadequate circulating blood volume, leading to decreased cardiac output and reduced perfusion of organs, especially the kidneys. Hypovolaemia, hypotension and hypoperfusion of tissue with reduced cardiac output underlies the development of neurological and gastrointestinal compromise, pre-renal uraemia, cardiac arrhythmias and shock.

FURTHER READING
Feldman EC, Nelson RW (1996) Hypoadrenocorticism. In: *Canine and Feline Endocrinology and Reproduction*, 2nd edn. (eds EC FGeldman, RW Nelson) Saunders, Philadelphia, pp. 55–77.
Greco DS (2000) Hypoadrenocorticism in dogs and cats. *Vet Med* **95**:468–476.

CASE 57

1 What is your interpretation of this finding?
The aPTT assay is used to evaluate the contact pathway of the coagulation cascade and is dependent on adequate activity of the following coagulation factors: I, II, V, VIII, IX, X, XI and XII. Prolonged aPTT times can be due to the presence of inhibitors or to true factor deficiency, and differentiating between them is done by mixing equal amounts of pooled normal canine plasma and plasma of the patient, which should normalise the aPTT if the prolongation is due to factor deficiencies. In the present case, the aPTT is not normalised and the presence of an inhibitor is thus confirmed. With no history of anticoagulant treatment, the most likely cause of the markedly prolonged aPTT is the presence of antiphospholipid antibodies (previously named 'lupus anticoagulants'). The presence of antiphospholipid antibodies will cause an *in-vitro* disturbance of the assay due to neutralisation of the activating factor of the assay (the phospholipids in the reagent) with no relation to an *in-vivo* coagulopathy. Additional tests (e.g. a modified aPTT or specialised tests such as the Russell's viper venom test) are necessary to confirm that a reduction of phospholipids is the likely cause.

2 Does the finding confirm that a coagulopathy is present in this dog?
The finding does not confirm that a coagulopathy is present. Based on the results and history, the prolonged aPTT is most likely an *in-vitro* phenomenon.

FURTHER READING
Lubas G, Caldin M, Wiinberg B *et al.* (2010) Laboratory testing of coagulation disorders. In: *Schalm's Veterinary Hematology*, 6th edn. (eds DJ Weiss, KJ Wardrop) Blackwell Publishing, Ames, pp. 1082–1100.

CASE 58

1 Discuss the laboratory findings and their significance.
The main finding is the high triglycerides, which is well into the range (>5.0 mmol/l) diagnostic for hyperlipaemia. Ponies, Shetland ponies in particular, and miniature horses

are predisposed to develop this condition. This diagnosis is also consistent with the clinical signs and clinical findings. The less markedly increased cholesterol compared with triglycerides is typical of hyperlipaemia. Increased non-esterified fatty acids released from adipose tissue during fasting (due to increased hormone-sensitive lipase activity – induced by glucagon, glucocorticoids, catecholamines and made worse by ponies [especially pregnant/lactating ponies] being relatively insulin resistant), results in triglyceride accumulation in the liver. The amount of triglyceride overwhelms the liver's capacity to convert it to VLDL-triglyceride, therefore triglycerides accumulate in the liver (and kidney) and VLDL accumulates in the blood. Hypoglycaemia is a common but not consistent finding.

The increase in GGT, GLDH and bile acids indicates significant cholestasis, hepatocellular damage and impaired hepatic function as a result of the fatty liver. Most bilirubin is free (unconjugated), as is usually the case in horses, regardless of the underlying cause.

The high urea and creatinine are probably partly due to dehydration but renal function may also be impaired. Urinalysis is warranted to gain further insights into the cause of the azotaemia.

The oedema is unlikely to be due to hypoalbuminaemia (not low enough). Subcutaneous vascular thrombosis secondary to lipaemia and fat embolism is the most common cause of dependent oedema in patients with hyperlipaemia. Vascular thrombosis may also be seen in the lungs, kidneys and brain. Azotaemia may further exacerbate hyperlipaemia because it prevents lipid removal from the blood by interfering with lipoprotein lipase.

Calcium is normal and phosphorus is insignificantly low. Calcium was measured to check for hypocalcaemia, an important differential diagnosis for depression in this pony before the triglyceride result was obtained.

2 What is your interpretation?

The findings are consistent with hyperlipaemia precipitated by the recent foaling and current lactation. There is concurrent hepatic and likely renal damage due to triglyceride accumulation and possible thrombosis.

3 What is the prognosis?

The prognosis for hyperlipaemia is poor. Mortality is estimated to occur in 60–100% of patients with this condition.

CASE 59

1 Give a short overview of the pathophysiology of NT-proBNP. Where does it come from, why does it increase and what actions does it perform?

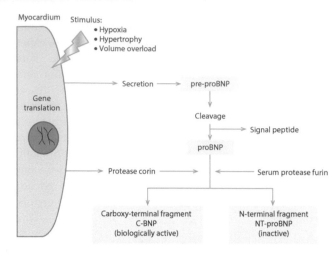

FIG. 59.1 Pathophysiology of the formation of NT-proBNP. Different stimuli lead to BNP gene translation in the myocardium, which subsequently secretes the hormone pre-proBNP. Further cleavage leads to the formation of proBNP. Either the myocardial protease corin or the ubiquitous protease furin split proBNP into the biologically active carboxy-terminal fragment C-BNP and the inactive form NT-proBNP.

B-type natriuretic peptide (BNP) is produced in the cardial myocytes together with the atrial natriuretic peptide (ANP) (Fig. 59.1).

The actions of C-BNP take place after binding to natriuretic peptide receptors in the kidneys, lungs, adrenal glands and vasculature. Specifically, C-BNP activates the renal A-type natriuretic peptide receptor (NPR-A), which leads to natriuresis by inhibition of tubular sodium transport in the inner medullary collecting duct of the kidneys. C-BNP therefore counteracts the actions of the renin–angiotensin–aldosterone system (RAAS), which leads to sodium retention. Natriuresis is accompanied by increased water retention in the tubules with production of diuresis. In the kidneys, C-BNP further inhibits the formation of renin. Aldosterone release is inhibited in the adrenal glands. The vasculature of the lungs is also affected by the actions of NPR-A. Relaxation of the systemic and pulmonary arterioles can be noted. The final outcome of C-BNP action is decreased systemic and pulmonary resistance. BNP therefore influences blood pressure, but in the opposite direction to the action of the RAAS. Other effects of BNP are antifibrotic and antihypertrophic.

NPR-C, the C-type natriuretic peptide receptor, mediates renal clearance of BNP. Selectivity of the receptor is greater for ANP than for BNP, possibly explaining the longer half-life of BNP in plasma. Clearance of NT-proBNP is slower than that of C-BNP, leading to an even longer half-life.

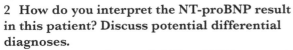
2 How do you interpret the NT-proBNP result in this patient? Discuss potential differential diagnoses.

As stated above, an increase in NT-proBNP is expected after hypoxia, hypertrophy or volume overload having an impact on the myocardium and leading to increased transcription of BNP. Therefore, congestive heart failure may be the cause of the increased NT-proBNP results. However, a more detailed look at how to interpret the NT-proBNP result is required.

NT-proBNP seems to be especially useful in the examination of patients with respiratory distress of unknown cause. While an experienced cardiologist may rely on clinical examination, the NT-proBNP value may give a first hint about the reason for the respiratory signs to a general practitioner, who is uncomfortable with cardiology or his/her ability with cardiac auscultation. NT-proBNP can help differentiate between congestive heart failure and respiratory disease as a potential cause of the respiratory signs. Sensitivity and specificity therefore depend on the cut-off used. A general guideline in the interpretation of the result is shown below:

NT-proBNP (pmol/l)	Interpretation
<900	Highly specific for respiratory disease
900–1,800	Intermediate result; further cardiological evaluation of the patient warranted
>1,800	Highly specific for congestive heart failure

Nevertheless, one should have in mind that the test is quite new and reference intervals, as well as recommended cut-off values, may change if more studies become available and/or the assay is refined. As indicated above, results at the lower and higher end of the scale will give a more specific answer than intermediate results, which require further diagnostics.

Despite cardiological or respiratory disease, renal disease may alter the NT-proBNP result, as the peptide is cleared by the kidneys. In patients with azotaemia, NT-proBNP results above the reference interval may be seen. Chronic renal disease may also lead to increased transcription of the BNP gene if the myocardium is stretched in the face of volume overload and diastolic dysfunction. Therefore, renal disease should always be excluded if an increased NT-proBNP result is observed.

Biological variation is another cause of potentially increased NT-proBNP results. Day-to-day variation, as well as profound weekly variations, have been observed in healthy dogs. Potential causes of these changes may be changes in the diet or water intake increased exercise or neurohormonal changes, all of which can affect the volume status of the dog.

Finally, systemic and pulmonary hypertension of any cause, drugs that alter the volume status of the patient (e.g. diuretics) as well as infectious disease may cause an increase in NT-proBNP.

3 What pre-analytical precautions do you need to consider?

NT-proBNP is quite unstable and time, as well as temperature, has an impact on the result. Therefore, EDTA samples should be spun immediately after venipuncture and plasma should be transferred to a special tube containing a protease inhibitor. These tubes are usually provided by the diagnostic laboratory. Unless the sample is taken to the laboratory on the day of collection, the sample at best is kept in the refrigerator. Some laboratories recommend using cold centrifugation and freezing the sample at −70°C until analysis.

FOLLOW UP

Therapy was instituted and radiography and ultrasound performed after the dog was stabilised. Congestive heart failure could therefore be verified.

FURTHER READING

Connolly DJ (2010) Natriuretic peptides: the feline experience. *Vet Clin North Am Small Anim Pract* **40**:559–570.
Oyama MA, Singletary GE (2010) The use of NT-proBNP assay in the management of canine patients with heart disease. *Vet Clin North Am Small Anim Pract* **40**:545–558.
Sisson DD (2004) Neuroendocrine evaluation of cardiac disease. *Vet Clin North Am Small Anim Pract* **34**:1105–1126.

CASE 60

1 Describe and discuss the significant haematological findings, as well as the coagulation profile.

Slight mature neutrophilia and monocytosis suggest corticosteroid effect ('stress' leucogram). There is a slightly regenerative anaemia, which is most likely due to subacute haemorrhage (>3 days) given the history and physical examination. A moderate thrombocytopaenia is present. Generally, thrombocytopaenia may be due to consumption, loss or decreased production of platelets. The latter, however, is unlikely as the presence of large and giant platelets indicates regeneration.

Both PT and aPTT are severely prolonged, exceeding the upper detection limit of the test, which is consistent with a disorder affecting both the intrinsic and extrinsic and/or common coagulation pathway. There is a severe hypofibrinogenaemia, a moderate decrease in antithrombin and a marked increase in D-dimer concentrations. Increased D-dimers in the blood plasma are indicative of an increased fibrinolysis of cross-linked fibrin and therefore an elevation in coagulation activity.

This combination of findings suggests hyperfibrinolysis following hypercoagulation and a subsequent consumption of platelets, coagulation factors, fibrinogen and inhibitors of coagulation such as antithrombin. The overall picture is compatible with a diagnosis of DIC. Given the physical examination findings in this dog, neoplasia (mammary tumour) is the most probable aetiology.

2 What is the most likely aetiology of the abnormalities, and what prognosis is associated with the diagnosis?

The overall picture is consistent with DIC, most likely due to a mammary tumour. Metastases may predispose to DIC, but other factors associated with malignancy may also predispose to DIC. The prognosis is poor as these cases are generally not responsive to treatment unless the tumour is removed. Surgery, however, cannot be recommended given the poor coagulation status.

ADDITIONAL COMMENTS

Mammary carcinomas have been demonstrated in the literature to tend to lead to DIC and hyperfibrinolysis. Generally, increased plasma levels of D-dimers are observed in dogs with thromboembolism, end-stage renal failure, DIC, neoplasia, immune-mediated anaemia and other diseases associated with hypercoagulability, as well as profound haemorrhage in body cavities.

The diagnosis of DIC can only be made if 3–4 variables out of eight (platelets, PT, aPTT, thrombin time, fibrinogen, antithrombin, D-dimers, presence of schistocytes in the blood film) are abnormal.

FURTHER READING

Abbrederis N (2005) *Validierung von laborparametern zur Diagnose einer DIC [validation of clinical pathological variables for diagnosis of DIC].* Tierärztliche Faktultät der ludwig-Maximilians-Universität München.

Carr AP, Panciera, Dl, Kidd L (2002) Prognostic factors for mortality and thromboembolism in canine immune-mediated hemolytic anemia: a retrospective study of 72 dogs. *J Vet Intern Med* **16**:504–509.

Griffin A, Callan MB, Shofer FS *et al.* (2003) Evaluation of a canine D-dimer point-of-care test kit for use in samples obtained from dogs with disseminated intravascular coagulation, thromboembolic disease, and hemorrhage. *Am J Vet Res* **64**:1562–1569.

Mischke R, Freund, M, Leinemann-Fink *et al.* (1998) Veränderungen der Hämostase bei Hunden mit akuter lymphoblastenleukämie [hemostatic changes in dogs with acute lymphoblastic leukemia]. *Berl Munch Tierarztl Wochenschr* **111**:53–59.

Mischke R, Wohlsein P, Busse L *et al.* (1998) Verbrauchskoagulopathie und Hyperfibrinolyse bei Hunden mit metastasiertem Mammakarzinom [disseminated intravascular coagulation and hyperfibrinolysis in dogs with metastatic mammary carcinoma]. *Schweiz Arch Tierheilkd* **140**:497–505.

Monreal L (2003) D-dimer as a new test for the diagnosis of DIC and thromboembolic disease. *J Vet Intern Med* **17**:757–759.

Nelson OL, Andreasen C (2003) The utility of plasma D-dimer to identify thromboembolic disease in dogs. *J Vet Intern Med* **17**:830–834.

Scott-Moncrieff, JC, Treadwell, NG, McCullough, SM *et al.* (2001) Hemostatic abnormalities in dogs with primary immune-mediated hemolytic anemia. *J Am Anim Hosp Assoc* **37**:220–227.

Stokol T (2003) Plasma D-dimer for the diagnosis of thromboembolic disorders in dogs. *Vet Clin North Am Small Anim Pract* **33**:1419–1435.

Stokol T, Brooks MB, Erb HN *et al.* (2000) D-dimer concentrations in healthy dogs and dogs with disseminated intravascular coagulation. *Am J Vet Res* **61**:393–398.

CASE 61

1 What is the most likely explanation for the haematological and biochemical abnormalities? Describe the pathomechanism.

Besides a moderate lymphopaenia, the results of the haematology are unremarkable. Lymphopaenia in the absence of other abnormalities most likely indicates a stress (endogenous or exogenous glucocorticoids) response. The borderline increase in MCHC is not clinically significant.

There is a severely increased CK enzyme activity resulting from excessive muscle damage after hypoxia and squeezing while the cat was stuck in the window. ALT enzyme activity is mildly to moderately increased. Muscle damage is the most likely reason for elevated ALT, although hepatocellular damage may contribute.

There is a moderate azotaemia consistent with a reduced GFR because of pre-renal, renal or post-renal causes. A pre-renal cause may be possible because of the hypoxia and/or dehydration. Renal disease may contribute as the accident may have resulted in direct kidney damage.

The slight hyperglycaemia most likely is due to a stress response. Theoretically, diabetes mellitus cannot be excluded, but the history makes this less likely.

Diagnosis: severe muscle damage with azotaemia.

2 What further analyses would you recommend?

Urinalysis to help differentiate pre-renal from renal causes for the azotaemia and evaluate renal function, and repeated glucose measurements and possibly a fructosamine assay to exclude diabetes mellitus.

3 What isoenzymes of creatine kinase (CK) can occur?

CK is necessary for ATP formation, as it transfers the phosphate group from creatine phosphate to adenosine diphosphate. Four isoenzymes have been reported:

- CK-1/CK-BB → located in the brain.
- CK-2/CK-MB → located in cardiac and skeletal muscle.
- CK-3/CK-MM → same location as CK-2.
- CK-Mt → located in the mitochrondria of many tissues.

FURTHER READING

Kaneko JJ, Harvey JW, Bruss ML (2008) *Clinical Biochemistry of Domestic Animals*, 6th edn. Elsevier, London.

Stockham SL, Scott MA (2008) *Fundamentals of Veterinary Clinical Pathology*, 2nd edn. Blackwell Publishing, Oxford.

CASE 62

1 What are the boat-shaped to ovoid structures?

The structures are a rare modification of calcium carbonates; other modifications described include dumbbell-shaped crystals.

2 What is the origin of the spherical structure?

The radially striped spherule is a more common modification of calcium carbonates.

3 What happens when diluted (5–10%) acetic acid is added to the sediment?

Calcium carbonates can only persist in alkaline urine (pH >8.0); they dissolve when diluted acetic acid is added. This can easily be done by adding vinegar to the edge of the cover slip on a urine sediment preparation. The formation of gas bubbles (CO_2) is noted, which only happens when carbonates are present.

4 What is the clinical importance of these structures?

Finding calcium carbonates in horse urine is not of clinical importance; they often form after voiding of the urine.

CASE 63

1 Describe and interpret the present laboratory abnormalities.

There is a mild anaemia based on the decreased number of erythrocytes, decreased haemoglobin concentration and decreased haematocrit. The presence/absence of a regenerative response cannot be judged in equines, as this species does not release polychromatophils from the bone marrow. Mild neutrophilia is accompanied by mild lymphopaenia. The most likely cause is stress response.

Clinical signs point either towards PPID (equine Cushing's disease) or EMS. Clinically, differentiation of both diseases is difficult as clinical signs may be similar (see Table).

COMPARATIVE FEATURES OF PPID AND EMS

Features	PPID	EMS	Miscellaneous Notes/Comments
Age	Usually >15 years (7–>20 years)	>6 years (6–>20 year)	
Cresty neck	Mild	Moderate to severe	
Predisposed to laminitis or laminitis present	Yes	Yes	
Hirsutism/long hair coat	Yes	No	Hirsuitism virtually pathognomonic for PPID
Obesity	No	Moderate/severe	
Abnormal fat deposits (multiple sites)	Yes	Yes	
PU/PD	Yes	No	PU/PD may be difficult to document because of differences in environment, humidity and management, particularly in horses living at pasture. It is more commonly detected in stabled horses because of the wet stall and observed volume of water intake and/or urination
Routine laboratory findings	Common abnormal laboratory findings include mild anaemia, absolute or relative neutrophilia and absolute or relative lymphopaenia (thought to occur in approximately 33% of cases). Mild to moderate hyperglycaemia is seen in 25–75% of cases. Elevated liver enzymes, hypercholesterolaemia and hypertriglyceridaemia also may be seen	Variable. Commonly have increased triglycerides. Glucose concentration usually within reference interval, but some will have increased levels	If hyperglycaemia is detected, it raises concern about the progression of chronic insulin resistance into pancreatic exhaustion and type 2 diabetes mellitus. Type 2 diabetes mellitus is rare in the horse, but occurs occasionally and can be confirmed by detecting glucosuria

The dexamethasone suppression test fails to show suppression after dexamethasone administration. The test is therefore highly suggestive of PPID. False-positive tests may occur in late summer/autumn because of hormonal alterations associated with decreasing day length. The recommended testing time is between mid-November and late June. A negative test result between July and mid-November will help rule out PPID. False positives occur in ~40% of cases when the test is performed in the autumn.

False-negative results may be common in early cases of the disease. In one study, only 56 of 95 (59%) horses with clinical signs consistent with PPID tested positive. Presumably, the majority of the remaining 61% were false-negative test results, because clinical signs are highly predictive of the disease.

2 What laboratory tests may be helpful for further testing?

A TRH stimulation test or an endogeneous ACTH assay may give further information for diagnosing PPID. The TRH stimulation test shows up to a 20% rise in cortisol concentration 15 minutes post TRH stimulation in healthy animals. Cortisol usually returns to baseline at 60 minutes. A 30% or greater increase in cortisol concentration at 15 minutes, often persisting at 60 minutes after administration of TRH, supports a diagnosis of PPID. False-positive tests may occur. In one study, up to 55% (6 of 11) healthy horses tested between mid-July and mid-November had a ~30% increase in serum cortisol, falsely identifying them as having PPID.

Elevated endogenous ACTH levels are considered diagnostic for PPID. Pain or stress may affect ACTH concentrations.

3 Why is time of year an important consideration?

The time of year is important because of seasonal variation in endogenous ACTH assays. TRH stimulation tests and dexamethasone suppression tests should be performed on horses and ponies between mid-July and mid-November in the Northern hemisphere. A negative endogenous ACTH assay (<30 μU/ml or <200 pmol/l) between July and October rules out PPID. A negative dexamethasone suppression test between mid-July and mid-November will help rule out PPID. The use of seasonally adjusted reference intervals may be of benefit in preventing false-positive results from mid-July to mid-November.

4 Why is insulin assay an important part of the work up of this case?

Many horses (25–75%) with PPID will also have insulin resistance, and these horses are more likely to founder. Therefore, measurement of fasting insulin is recommended in horses suspected of PPID for its prognostic rather than diagnostic value.

Alpha-2 agonists such as xylazine or detomidine may falsely increase insulin. Therefore, blood samples should be collected before administering any sedation that may be needed for farriery work or other diagnostic procedures.

CASE 64

1 Are the changes in haematocrit between (1) day 1 and day 3, (2) day 1 and day 7, and (3) day 3 and day 7 likely to represent a significant change based on what we know about biological variation and critical difference (reference change value [RCV]) in the dog?

(1) The change in haematocrit between day 1 and day 3 is a difference of 0.05 l/l or 0.05/0.25 × 100 = 20%. From studies of biological variation in the dog (see Appendix 2, p. 264), we know that intra-individual CV_I = 6.4%. The formula for critical difference or RCV is:

$$RCV = 1.96 \times \sqrt{2 \times \left(CV_I^2 + CV_A^2\right)}$$

CV_I = intra-individual CV; CV_A = analytical CV.

If the CV_A is 1.1%, the RCV would be 18%; if the CV_A is 3%, the RCV would be 19.49%; and if the CV_A is 5%, the RCV would be 22.51%. For these combinations of CV_A and a haematocrit of 0.25 l/l, a significant change in haematocrit is shown in the Table below:

Haematocrit (l/l) that must be attained to represent a significant change from 0.25 when considering CV_I = 6.4% and variable CV_A of 1.1%, 3% and 5%:

	CV_A		
	1.1%	3%	5%
Haematocrit representing significant difference from 0.25 l/l based on intra-individual biological variation (%)	0.295 (18%)	0.299 (19.49%)	0.316 (22.51%)

So, the change from 0.25 to 0.30 l/l is just large enough to be considered a significant change in haematocrit between day 1 and day 3 given a CV_A of 1.1% and 3%, but not at a CV_A of 5%.

(2) Based on the Table above, the change from day 1 to day 7 (0.341 − 0.250 = 0.091 l/l or 0.09/0.250 × 100 = 36.4%) qualifies as a significant change whether the CV_A is 1.1%, 3.0% or 5.0%.

(3) The change from 0.30 l/l (day 3) to 0.341 l/l (day 7) is a change of 0.041 l/l or 0.041/0.30 × 100 = 13.6%. This does

not represent a significant change in haematocrit for any method with a CV_A of 1.1% or greater since it is less than the RCV of 18%.

While the trend in haematocrit is encouraging between days 1 and 3 and days 3 and 7, the degree of change may be significant if the CV_A is <3% but, because of intra-individual biological variation, if the CV_A is 5% or greater, the change in haematocrit is not considered to be of statistical significance. If the CV_A is 5%, then only when the difference between day 1 and day 7 is considered can it be said that the change exceeds that which could be expected based on biological variation within the individual and is likely to represent an evidence-based improvement in the haematocrit. The amount of change in haematocrit needed to provide evidence for a critical difference based on the RCV will vary depending on the CV_A of the instrument/method being used, as illustrated in the Table above. (See Appendix 2, p. 264, for additional information regarding biological variation for various analytes that have been studied in the dog.)

FURTHER READING
Fraser CG (2001) *Biological Variation: From Principles to Practice.* AACC Press, Washington DC.
Walton RM (2012) Subject-based reference values: biological variation, individuality, and reference change values. *J Vet Clin Pathol* 41:175–181.

CASE 65

1 What does the biochemistry profile indicate?
The results of the biochemistry profile indicate the presence of slight hypoalbuminaemia, slight hyperbilirubinaemia, slight hypocholesterolaemia, moderate to marked increases in serum activity of liver enzymes and slight prolongation of plasma coagulation times, along with an increase in the basal concentration of bile acids. These abnormalities support the presence of an hepatic insufficiency. Furthermore, the slight hyperglobulinaemia suggests the presence of a chronic inflammatory process and a neoplasm cannot be ruled out.

2 Why is assessment of coagulation status important in animals with liver disease?
Assessment of the coagulation status is important because the liver is responsible for the synthesis of the majority of coagulation factors. Hepatocytes are also responsible for the clearance and elimination of activated coagulation factors and fibrin degradation products. Haemostatic disorders are therefore a complication of hepatic disease and can lead to clinical signs of bleeding and complicate invasive diagnostic procedures such as fine needle aspiration, biopsy or exploratory laparotomy.

3 On abdominal ultrasound, a large cystic mass was detected in the cranial abdomen, which could originate from the liver. What parasitic disease has to be considered?
Echinococcosis must be considered in the differential diagnoses. Fine needle aspiration of the mass with subsequent cytological evaluation performed after plasma transfusion revealed the presence of parasitic scolices. Care must be taken to avoid human exposure, as there is a zoonotic risk and regulatory authorities must be informed.

FURTHER READING
Chiodini P, Moody A, Manser D (2003) *Atlas of Medical Helminthology and Protozoology*, 4th edn. Churchill Livingstone, Edinburgh.
Ettinger S, Feldman E (2000) *Textbook of Veterinary Internal Medicine*, 6th edn. Elsevier Saunders, St. Louis.

CASE 66

1 What is your assessment of these results?
There is marked pancytopaenia. The anaemia appears to be non-responding, which may be due to acute development and/or decreased marrow production. The possibility of decreased marrow production of all cell types is considered likely since all are markedly decreased. The type of bleeding observed (epistaxis, skin oozing) is consistent with the thrombocytopaenia, although coagulation factor deficiencies cannot be ruled out without further testing for PT and aPTT.

2 What are your differential diagnoses?
These findings support the presence of severe marrow disease with decreased production of all cell types. The bleeding may be contributing to the anaemia, but the amount and type of bleeding is considered unlikely to result in the acute development of the severe anaemia.

Differential diagnoses include severe bone marrow suppression associated with toxin exposure (unknown type), idiopathic bone marrow failure or 'bleeding calf syndrome', also known as bovine neonatal pancytopaenia.

FOLLOW UP
This calf died and postmortem examination showed bleeding into the intestines. There was multifocal haemorrhage in a variety of tissues. The bone marrow showed severe depletion of all cell lineages (marked bone marrow aplasia) and depletion of lymphoid tissue. This is consistent with bovine neonatal pancytopaenia. This poorly understood syndrome occurs sporadically in calves <1 month old. It has been hypothesised to occur in association with vaccination with the Pregsure BVD vaccine, but an aetiology has not been definitively established.

FURTHER READING

Pardon B, Steukers L, Dierick J *et al.* (2010) Haemorrhagic diathesis in neonatal calves: an emerging syndrome in Europe. *Transb Emerg Dis* **57**:135–146.

CASE 67

1 Identify and list the abnormalities, and explain their associations.

Slight normocytic-normochromic, currently non-regenerative anaemia. Slight neutrophilia and monocytosis may in part be stress related, but toxic changes were noted in the neutrophils and this could therefore reflect inflammation/infection.

Marked hyperglycaemia and glucosuria, if persistent and accompanied by clinical signs, are consistent with diabetes mellitus. Slight hyponatraemia and marked hypochloraemia are probably secondary to osmotic diuresis associated with the severe hyperglycaemia. Hyponatraemia may also in part be directly due to the severe hyperglycaemia, which results in osmotic movement of water out of cells into plasma. On average every 5.55 mmol/l (100 mg/dl) increment in serum glucose above the normal range decreases the plasma sodium concentration by 1.1 mmol/l (1.6 mEq/l).

Marked hyperphosphataemia is probably secondary to the moderate to marked azotaemia. Lactic acidosis may also cause hyperphosphataemia. Lactic acidosis is possible in non-ketotic diabetics and may occur because of overproduction as a result of tissue hypoxia (anaerobic glycolysis), deficient removal (hepatic failure), or both, with circulatory collapse. Lactic acid was not measured in this patient. Sample haemolysis or delayed removal of serum or plasma from erythrocytes can also contribute falsely to hyperphosphataemia.

Marked azotaemia is probably consistent with renal disease, but the USG should be interpreted with caution in diabetic patients as osmotic/solute diuresis may contribute to impairment of the kidney's concentration ability, leading to an inappropriate USG. Azotaemia and pancreatitis probably have a compounding effect on each other in this case.

Marked hepatic cholestasis, cellular injury and necrosis may be primary or secondary. There is also evidence of hepatic dysfunction indicated by the increased bile acids. Slight bilirubinuria may be observed in healthy male dogs but in this patient may be due to the hepatopathy. There are slight non-specific muscle changes.

Hypercholesterolaemia may be multifactoral in origin, including its association with diabetes mellitus, acute pancreatitis, cholestasis and decreased lipolysis.

This patient's calculated osmolality is 386 mOsm/kg, exceeding the threshold definition of 350 mOsm/kg. (See calculation in discussion below.)

2 Provide a conclusion for the findings described in question 1 and classify the type of diabetes mellitus.

The severe hyperglycaemia of this degree in a dehydrated patient in the absence of ketosis is consistent with diabetic hyperosmolar non-ketotic syndrome (DHNS). There is concurrent evidence of severe multiple organ involvement including severe cholangiohepatopathy, pancreatitis and probable nephropathy.

3 What is the significance of the occasional hyaline cast?

Up to 2 hyaline casts/lpf (×100) may occur in healthy dogs due to secretion of Tamm–Horsfall mucoproteins by the epithelial cells of the loops of Henle, distal tubules and collecting ducts as well as the normal sloughing of tubular epithelial cells.

4 This is an emergency situation, which should be communicated with the clinician. What is the most important information regarding the treatment of this condition that you need to convey to the clinician?

Fluid therapy is of paramount importance and insulin should not be given in the initial 4–6 hours. This is because insulin would cause a rapid decrease in blood glucose concentration and an increase in extracellular fluid osmolality, changes that promote cerebral oedema in a patient who may already be cerebrally compromised due to severe cellular dehydration.

Despite the severe hyperosmolality, isotonic (0.9%) saline is the initial fluid of choice because it will correct the hydration status and improve blood flow to tissues, thus improving GFR, promoting glucosuria and decreasing blood glucose concentration. The aim is to slowly reduce the extracellular fluid osmolality and minimise brain oedema.

Insulin therapy should only be initiated once dehydration has been corrected, blood pressure has stabilised and there is an improvement in urine production, level of hyperglycaemia and electrolyte abnormalities.

DISCUSSION

DHNS is characterised by severe hyperglycaemia (glucose >33.31 mmol/l [>600 mg/dl]), hyperosmolality (>350 mOsm/kg) and dehydration in the absence of significant ketosis. DHNS is an infrequent complication of diabetes mellitus in the dog and cat. Osmolality can be measured with an osmometer or calculated. When BUN or glucose is increased the formula to use is:

$$\text{mOsm/kg} = 2[Na^+ + K^+(\text{mEq/l})] + [\text{glucose (mg/dl)}/18] + [\text{BUN (mg/dl)}/2.8]$$

All values in SI units must be converted to conventional units before placing them in the formula.

The degree of hyperglycaemia of DHNS tends to be greater than that associated with diabetic ketoacidosis (DKA):

- Glucose in DHNS = 33.06–88.82 mmol/l (600–1600 mg/dl);
- Glucose in DKA = 16.65–44.41 mmol/l (300–800 mg/dl).

Significant ketosis is absent in this syndrome because a small amount of insulin is still produced by the pancreas and that inhibits lipolysis. The limited free fatty acid precursors from the periphery thus restrict the rate at which ketone bodies are formed in the liver. Hepatic resistance to glucagon may also play a role.

FURTHER READING

DiBartola SP (2000) Disorders of sodium and water. In: *Fluid Therapy in Small Animal Practice*, 2nd edn. (ed. SP DiBartola) WB Saunders, Philadelphia, p. 83.

Duncan JR, Prasse KW, Mahaffey EA (1994) Proteins, lipids, and carbohydrates. In: *Veterinary Laboratory Medicine: Clinical Pathology*, 3rd edn. Iowa State Press, Ames.

Feldman EC, Nelson RW (2003) In: *Canine and Feline Endocrinology and Reproduction*, 3rd edn. Saunders, Philadelphia, pp. 613–614.

Stockham SL, Scott MA (2008) *Fundamentals of Veterinary Clinical Pathology*, 2nd edn. Blackwell Publishing, Oxford.

CASE 68

1 Describe the laboratory abnormalities present. Discuss a possible diagnosis and differential diagnoses.

There is a slight mature neutrophilia and a moderate lymphopaenia. Most likely causes are inflammation or glucocorticoid effect. Physiological fight-or-flight reaction may also contribute to the neutrophilia.

Erythrocytes are slightly microcytic (decreased MCV). Possible causes for microcytic RBCs include iron deficiency (mostly in the face of intestinal haemorrhage) or liver insufficiency. These differentials are not supported by the history, physical examination and biochemistry findings. Therefore, biological (physiological) variation may be considered. When in doubt, liver function tests may be performed.

There is a marked azotaemia consistent with a decreased GFR, possibly due to pre-renal, renal or post-renal causes. Marked hyperphosphataemia most likely results from decreased urinary phosphorus excretion as the GFR is decreased. As the cat clinically shows dysuria and stranguria as well as bladder stones, leakage from urine

into the tissues may also be considered. Other potential causes, although less likely, include increased phosphorus absorption from the intestine or hyperthyroidism. However, this cat is quite young and does not show clinical signs consistent with hyperthyroidism.

There is a severe hyperkalaemia present. The most likely cause is decreased renal excretion due to decreased GFR and, potentially, to urinary tract obstruction. Leakage of urine into the abdominal cavity may further exacerbate the condition. In general, tissue necrosis and muscle damage may also lead to hyperkalaemia, but not in this case. There is slight hypernatraemia and slight hyperchloraemia in the face of a normal hydration status (haematocrit and albumin levels are well within their reference intervals). These electrolytes most likely have been lost from the alimentary tract with vomiting. As the cat shows severe dysuria, uroperitoneum may be another differential. As the urine is poor in sodium and chloride, these electrolytes may equilibrate with plasma in the uroperitoneum, thus potentially causing hyponatraemia and hypochloraemia. Moderate hypocalcaemia may result from complex formation with phosphorus, as hyperphosphataemia is present. Renal damage may further impair tubular calcium resorption. Marked hyperglycaemia is present, which may be due to stress-induced hyperglycaemia or diabetes mellitus (DM). As the cat is in pain, stress-induced hyperglycaemia is likely. Nevertheless, DM has to be excluded via follow-up examinations and fructosamine assay. Mild hypocholesterolaemia may result from fasting.

There is a slightly to moderately decreased USG consistent with decreased renal urine concentration ability. The urine is alkaline, which may result from delayed sample analysis, urease-producing bacteria, tubular acidosis or increased pH associated with respiratory alkalosis. The urine test strip is highly positive for erythrocytes and protein. Positivity for erythrocytes may originate from erythrocytes, haemoglobin or myoglobin in the urine. Urine sediment examination should be performed to confirm the presence of erythrocytes. Haemoglobinuria is unlikely, as the plasma is not haemolytic; however, artificial damage to erythrocytes in the urine may have led to leakage of haemoglobin. Myoglobinuria is unlikely in light of the patient's history. Proteinuria may result from pre-renal, renal or post-renal causes. Because of the bladder stones and possible haematuria, a post-renal cause is likely. Nevertheless, renal proteinuria cannot be fully excluded as the patient shows azotaemia in association with decreased renal concentration ability. There is a mild glucosuria. As the cat is markedly hyperglycaemic, the renal tubular transport maximum may have been exceeded, leading to glucosuria. Slight ketonuria may support the suspicion of DM with concurrent ketoacidosis. However, a highly pigmented urine (due to erythrocytes) may lead to a false-positive reaction due to non-specific discolouration.

Diagnoses: renal damage because of post-renal disease (bladder stones) and hyperglycaemia, most likely stress-induced, although DM cannot be fully excluded.

2 What further analyses would you recommend?

Urine sediment examination to evaluate the presence of erythrocytes and leucocytes; microbiological examination of the urine to rule out concurrent urinary tract infection (quantitative urine culture on a cystocentesis or catheterised urine specimen preferred); repeated glucose measurements and fructosamine assay to exclude DM.

FURTHER READING

Kaneko JJ, Harvey JW, Bruss ML (2008) *Clinical Biochemistry of Domestic Animals*, 6th edn. Elsevier, London.

Stockham SL, Scott MA (2008) *Fundamentals of Veterinary Clinical Pathology*, 2nd edn. Blackwell Publishing, Oxford.

CASE 69

1 What is your assessment of the arterial pH?

The arterial pH is increased, therefore this is an alkalaemia.

2 What is your assessment of the likely underlying aetiology for this arterial pH?

The $PaCO_2$ is decreased and no increase in HCO_3^- is present, so this is a respiratory alkalosis.

3 Is there appropriate compensation for this condition, and does it suggest an acute or chronic condition?

If this is an acute respiratory alkalosis, it is expected that a 10 mmHg decrease in $PaCO_2$ would cause a decrease of 2.5 mmol/l HCO_3^-. If this is a chronic respiratory alkalosis, it is expected that a 10 mmHg decrease in $PaCO_2$ would cause a decrease of 5.5 mmol/l HCO_3^-.

In this case, there is a 20 mmHg decrease in $PaCO_2$ from the middle of the reference interval for $PaCO_2$. This would be expected to result in a 5 mmol/l decrease in HCO_3^- in an acute condition and an 11 mmol/l decrease in HCO_3^- in a chronic condition. Based on this data, there is a 4 mmol/l decrease in HCO_3^- from the middle of the reference interval for HCO_3^-. This fits with an acute respiratory alkalosis.

4 What might be the underlying causes for this condition?

Respiratory alkalosis develops when a primary respiratory problem results in too much CO_2 being blown off. Normally, alveolar CO_2 concentration is around 40 mmHg and is in equilibrium with pulmonary capillary blood CO_2, giving arterial blood a normal CO_2 concentration

of about 40 mmHg. If alveolar CO_2 concentration decreases, blood CO_2 concentration decreases, producing respiratory alkalosis. Except in artificial situations, such as gas anaesthesia, decreased alveolar CO_2 concentration is always due to increased ventilation (hyperventilation). Hyperventilation and the resulting respiratory alkalosis can be caused by intrathoracic or extrathoracic problems.

Intrathoracic respiratory alkaloses are caused by increased ventilation in response to hypoxaemia resulting from decreased pulmonary perfusion or impaired oxygen diffusion (ventilation/perfusion imbalance or mismatch) and can be further investigated by evaluation of the thoracic cavity (e.g. auscultation, radiographs).

Extrathoracic respiratory alkaloses are caused by increased ventilation either in response to tissue hypoxia resulting from conditions such as anaemia or in response to CNS stimulation unrelated to hypoxaemia (e.g. fear, pain, head trauma). Extrathoracic respiratory alkaloses generally are further investigated by evaluation of the patient's CNS, emotional state and/or haemoglobin concentration or haematocrit.

Intrathoracic respiratory alkaloses can be differentiated from extrathoracic respiratory alkaloses by evaluation of arterial blood oxygen concentration. Intrathoracic respiratory alkaloses result from a decrease in blood oxygen concentration and, therefore, are always associated with low PaO_2, whereas, extrathoracic respiratory alkaloses are associated with normal or increased PaO_2. Anaemia, which can cause extrathoracic respiratory alkalosis, causes normal to increased PaO_2 rather than decreased PaO_2 because PaO_2 is measured in the plasma and thus represents only the PaO_2 of the plasma, not the actual blood oxygen content.

Therefore, this dog has an extrathoracic respiratory alkalosis. This dog should be evaluated to determine if this might be a neurological condition, if pain or fear is present or if there is anaemia, which may drive increased respiration, and therefore blowing off of CO_2.

FURTHER READING

Dibartola SP (2012) *Fluid, Electrolyte and Acid-Base Disorders in Small Animal Practice*, 4th edn. Elsevier Saunders, St. Louis.

CASE 70

1 Describe how leucocytes are differentiated by the ADVIA® Haematology System and where various cell types can be seen on physiological scattergrams.

The ADVIA® peroxidase cytogram depicts nucleated cells differentiated by size of the cells (y-axis) and intensity of stained intracellular peroxidase granules (x-axis). After lysis of RBCs, the remaining cells are stained with 4-chloro-1-naphthol which, together with hydrogen peroxide, results in a dark precipitate. Light absorbance of stained peroxidase is finally performed by the ADVIA® and the cells differentiated via cluster analysis:

- Neutrophils (pink) contain the highest amount of peroxidase and are of medium size. They are therefore located on the higher right side of the peroxidase cytogram.
- Canine eosinophils (but not feline ones) also contain peroxidase granules and are located in the cluster below the neutrophils (yellow).
- Monocytes are of similar size to neutrophils but their intracellular peroxidase concentration is lower. Cells are therefore located in the cluster to the left of the neutrophils (green).
- Lymphocytes do not contain, peroxidase and are small. They are depicted in blue and located in the lower left area of the scattergram.
- In the higher left corner, large unstained cells (LUCs) are depicted (light blue). These cells may include medium-sized to large lymphocytes/lymphoblasts or activated macrophages.
- Debris is indicated by a black colour and is located below the lymphocytes.
- The basophil cytogram depicts leucocytes differentiated after lysis of RBCs and platelets, as well as after stripping of the cytoplasm of leucocytes in a chemical reaction. The y-axis shows the cell size, while the x-axis displays nuclear configuration (e.g. mononuclear cells [lymphocytes and monocytes, in blue] versus polymorphnuclear cells [neutrophils and eosinophils, in pink]). Basophils and lysis-resistant cells are located in the upper cluster (orange).

2 What abnormalities are visible in this ADVIA® cytogram, and what is the most likely diagnosis based on the haematological results?

In the peroxidase cytogram a large cell cluster is visible expanding from the lymphocytes (blue) into the area of the LUCs (light blue). A few cells of this cluster are in the monocyte scatter; however, as they are part of the large cell cluster originating from the lymphocytes, it is unlikely that these are real monocytes. Based on the ADVIA® cytogram, acute lymphoblastic leukaemia or lymphoma stage 5 are highly likely.

Further results of the haematology show a normocytic-normochromic, non-regenerative slight anaemia. In this situation, anaemia of chronic disease or bone marrow infiltration with lymphoblasts is possible. Marked thrombocytopaenia is present. Platelet clumping should be ruled out by examination of the blood smear. However, platelet clumping resulting in such a marked thrombocytopaenia is rare in dogs and real thrombocytopaenia should

be considered. The most likely cause is decreased production of platelets in the bone marrow. Increased platelet destruction due to primary or secondary immune-mediated mechanisms or increased consumption of platelets, such as with DIC, is a further differential.

Bone marrow evaluation and evaluation of peripheral lymphatic organs are warranted to distinguish leukaemia from lymphoma. However, frequently discrimination of these diseases is not possible at this stage.

3 How do you interpret the basophilia reported by the ADVIA® Haematology System?

As lymphoblasts are as lysis resistant as basophils, lymphoblasts will also extend in the basophil cluster in the basophilic channel of the ADVIA®. Cells therefore are misdiagnosed. Such highly abnormal results produced by the haematology analyser have to be verified by evaluation of the blood smear.

FURTHER READING

Stockham SL, Scott MA (2008) *Fundamentals of Veterinary Clinical Pathology*, 2nd edn. Blackwell Publishing, Oxford.

Weiss DJ, Wardrop KJ (2010) (eds) *Schalm's Veterinary Hematology*, 6th edn. Blackwell Publishing, Ames.

CASE 71

1 Describe the cells on the blood smear and give a morphological diagnosis as well as possible differentials.

On an eosinophilic background, several medium-sized to large round cells are visible in addition to several erythrocytes. The 'round cells' display moderate amounts of basophilic cytoplasm and occasionally contain a few indistinct azurophilic small granules and a perinuclear halo. These cells are mononuclear with a round to oval or indented nucleus with a rough chromatin pattern. Nucleoli are only indistinct. The larger cells display moderate variation in the shape of the nuclei. The smaller cells look similar to granular lymphocytes. The morphology of the larger round cells may comprise lymphoblasts suggestive of lymphoma stage V or acute lymphoblastic leukaemia, with the perinuclear halo pointing to B cells and plasma cells, but the azurophilic granules suggest large granular lymphocytes. Additional differentials for 'round cells' include precursors of other haematopoietic lineages, histiocytes or mast cells.

2 What immunocytochemical markers would you apply to help identify more specifically the cells visible on the blood smear?

The immunocytochemical markers in the Table below may be applied to help identify the 'round cells' visible on the blood smear from this dog.

Marker	Interpretation of Cells Positive for the Marker
CD34	Immature cells
CD21, CD79a	B lymphocytes
CD3, CD4, CD8	T lymphocytes
Ig kappa/lambda chain	Plasma cells
CD117	Mast cells
CD18, CD45	Leucocytes
CD41, CD61	Megakaryocytes
CD11c, CD11d	Histiocytes, lymphatic tissue

FOLLOW UP

Cells stained positive for CD3 and CD4 and negative for CD79a. This finding is consistent with T-cell neoplasia. The dog developed non-regenerative anaemia and the thrombocytopaenia and neutropaenia worsened. Bone marrow examination revealed severe infiltration of lymphatic blasts with replacement of haematopoietic precursors. Acute lymphoblastic leukaemia of T cell origin was diagnosed.

FURTHER READING

Raskin RE, Meyer D (2010) *Canine and Feline Cytology*, 2nd edn. Saunders Elsevier, St.Louis.

Stockham SL, Scott MA (2008) *Fundamentals of Veterinary Clinical Pathology*, 2nd edn. Blackwell Publishing, Oxford.

CASE 72

1 What do you need to do in order to investigate a possible underlying cause for the increased number of high calcium results?

The first place to look is at the results of your quality control evaluation and recent external quality assessment performance. You should be looking for any out-of-control results, abnormal external quality assessment performance or other abnormalities that may indicate a system problem that could result in the observed increase in abnormal results.

2 A review of recent quality control shows that the level 1 control ('normal') is within normal limits. The level 2 control ('abnormal' high) shows a shift in the data with the last four results exceeding +1 SD above the mean. What might this mean?

The shift in the results for the 'abnormal' control material suggests that there may be a systematic error that is affecting the high results. This may be related to deterioration in the lamp (light source) for the analyser. The lamp should be checked first.

3 If you consistently have a high percentage of increased calcium results and the clinical conditions diagnosed do not correspond to conditions where high calcium is expected, **no abnormal control material performance is identified and external quality assessment performance is acceptable, what else should you consider?**

If a high percentage of increased calcium results is consistently obtained but other findings do not suggest underlying disease that may result in this alteration and quality control and external quality assessment performance are acceptable, it may be that the reference interval is not appropriate for the population seen in your practice. Inquiry as to the number and type of reference individuals and the pre-analytical standardisation of conditions and statistical methods used to establish the reference intervals should be conducted. Reference interval transference validation may be needed to determine if the reference interval is suitable for use in your practice. This involves testing a minimum of 20 healthy individuals in order to determine if the reference interval is likely to be applicable to the population of animals in your practice (see Further reading).

FURTHER READING

Friedrichs KR, Harr KE, Freeman KP *et al.* (2012) ASVCP reference interval guidelines: determination of *de novo* reference intervals in veterinary species and other related topics. *J Vet Clin Pathol* **41**:441–453.

Westgard JO (2002) *Basic QC Practices: Training in Statistical Quality Control for Healthcare Laboratories*, 2nd edn. Westgard QC, Madison.

CASE 73

1 Which proteins do the most rapid tests detect?

The majority of the ELISA in-house tests detect p24, the major capsid protein of the retrovirus, or the protein p15.

2 How would you interpret the positive ELISA result?

The prevalence of FIV in cats in central Europe is low, making a true positive result test less likely. However, this cat is a male stray, prone to cat fights and bites, increasing the risk of FIV infection. Therefore, the cat may be part of a high-risk population and the result may be truly positive.

As no test has a sensitivity and specificity of 100%, false-positive results have to be expected. Therefore, in a low prevalence population, every positive ELISA result has to be verified by a reference method, at best a Western blot.

3 What other tests for FIV do you know? Describe their advantages and disadvantages, if any.

- Virus isolation. This is considered the gold standard in FIV diagnostics. However, it is laborious, time consuming and expensive, making it less applicable for routine examinations.

- PCR. The sensitivity and specificity of PCR assays range from around 40% to 100%. Possible reasons for this variation may lay in the assay itself. Most PCR assays detect clade A, the dominant subtype of FIV in the UK and also present in the USA. However, other FIV clades exist and are not detected by PCR.
- Western blot. This technique is currently used to distinguish false- and true-positive ELISA results and is frequently available in reference laboratories.
- ELISA. Several ELISA tests exist, also available as bedside tests. All but one cannot reliably differentiate between a natural infection and patients vaccinated against FIV. However, the test differentiating between these circumstances is not widely available.

FOLLOW UP

Western blot analysis was performed and turned out positive in this cat.

FURTHER READING

Hosie MJ, Addie D, Belák S *et al.* (2009) Feline immunodeficiency. ADCD guidelines on prevention and management. *J Feline Med Surg* **11**:575–584.

Levy JK, Crawford PC, Kusuhara H *et al.* (2008) Differentiation of feline immunodeficiency virus vaccination, infection, or vaccination and infection in cats. *J Vet Intern Med* **22**:330–334.

CASE 74

1 Describe and interpret the laboratory abnormalities.

There is a moderate azotaemia, which generally indicates decreased glomerular perfusion rates due to pre-renal, renal or post-renal disease. Given the history, this is strongly suggestive of AKI due to lily intoxication. Other differentials include grape/raisin, EG or NSAID toxicity.

The exact mechanism of toxicity associated with lilies (e.g. Easter lily [*Lilium langiflorum*]) is not known. Pre-renal azotaemia seems unlikely as albumin and sodium are within normal limits. Post-renal disease can also be excluded, as no signs of inflammation are present in the urine sediment.

Moderate hyperglycaemia is present, which is most likely a stress response. A differential diagnosis would be diabetes mellitus. Repeated analysis after recovery from the AKI may be of benefit. A slight increase in CK indicates muscle damage.

Urinalysis reveals decreased renal concentration ability (isosthenuria) consistent with AKI. Glucosuria and proteinuria are present. In the case of lily intoxication, both abnormalities point towards tubular deficits. Since hyperglycaemia is present, glucosuria may be present if the renal tubular transport maximum for glucose is exceeded.

In cats, the transport maximum is approximately 16 mmol/l, which is not reached in this case. Therefore, a renal tubular defect/deficiency in absorption of glucose is supported. Proteinuria may also be associated with a pre-renal abnormality (muscle disease leading to myoglobinuria, haemolysis leading to haemoglobinuria, neoplasia leading to paraproteinuria). Myoglobinuria may be expected as increased CK enzyme activity indicates muscle damage. However, myoglobinuria leads to red discolouration of the urine, which is not present in this case. Post-renal disease (e.g. inflammation) as a cause for proteinuria can be excluded as further results of urinalysis are unremarkable.

2 What kind of clinical signs might you expect from lily toxicity in this cat?

Clinical signs associated with lily toxicity in the cat develop within 2 hours after lily ingestion and include vomiting, depression and PU/PD. Renal failure typically develops over the next few days.

3 What histological findings might be present if this cat dies from lily toxicity?

Expected histological findings include necrosis of the proximal convoluted tubules of the kidney and degeneration of pancreatic acinar cells

4 What is the treatment and prognosis for lily toxicity?

Early treatment with diuresis over 48 or more hours is the recommended treatment. Oliguria or anuria are poor prognostic indicators. If there is minimal or no elevation in creatinine with diuresis at 24–48 hours post exposure, the prognosis is usually good.

FURTHER READING

Fitzgerald KT (2010) Lily toxicity in the cat. *Top Compan Anim Med* **25**:213–217.

CASE 75

1 How would you describe this anaemia, and what are possible causes?

There is evidence of a moderate anaemia with no evidence of regeneration, considering the normal MCV and only slightly decreased MCHC (normocytic-normochromic to slightly hypochromic RBCs) and the absence of polychromatophils on blood film examination. Considering the concurrent thrombocytopaenia and neutropaenia, there is evidence of pancytopaenia, which is the reduction in the number of two or more cell populations. The main differential diagnosis for pancytopaenia is a primary bone marrow dysfunction (primary or metastatic neoplasia,

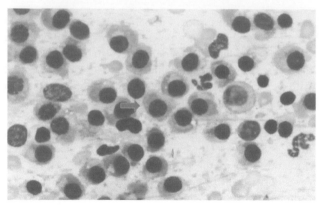

FIG. 75.1 Bone marrow aspirate, mature plasma cells (orange arrow). Modified Wright–Giemsa, ×50 (oil).

aplastic anaemia, myelofibrosis). Bone marrow cytology and core biopsy are recommended in order to investigate this (**Fig. 75.1**).

2 How would you explain the presence of rouleaux?

Rouleaux are aggregates of erythrocytes resembling a pile of coins. Their formation involves interactions between erythrocyte membranes and other plasma molecules (albumin, globulins). Therefore, increased rouleaux formation frequently occurs if there is hyperglobulinaemia or hyperfibrinogenaemia.

3 How would you explain the high serum protein? What test would you suggest to investigate this?

There is a marked hyperglobulinaemia, which may be due to increased production secondary to chronic inflammation (*Ehrlichia* spp. or *Leishmania* spp. or other infections). The antigenic stimulation caused by the infectious agent causes an increased release of cytokines (IL-6) and a consequent increased production of globulin by the hepatocytes and immunoglobulin by B-cell lymphocytes.

B-cell neoplasia (multiple myeloma, extramedullary plasmacytoma, B-cell lymphoma, B-cell leukaemia) may also cause gammopathy. Neoplastic cells produce high quantities of immunoglobulin. These proteins are electrophoretically, structurally and antigenically homogeneous because they are produced by a single clone of neoplastic cells. Serum protein electrophoresis (SPE) may be helpful because in this case it results in a monoclonal gammopathy. Hyperproteinaemia caused by infectious agents commonly results in a polyclonal gammopathy, although ehrlichiosis and leishmaniasis may also cause a monoclonal gammopathy. Low albumin may reflect a negative acute-phase protein response, caused by a decreased production by hepatocytes during acute inflammation. Mild to moderate hypoalbuminaemia

may also be caused by a negative feedback mechanism involving an oncotic pressure receptor on hepatocytes (downregulation of albumin synthesis).

4 How would you explain the proteinuria?

The presence of high amounts of protein in the urine likely reflects significant protein loss, although a urinary protein:creatinine ratio is recommended to confirm this. Renal protein loss is commonly caused by glomerular damage, which may occur with myeloma, ehrlichiosis and leishmaniasis or other infections resulting in antigen–antibody complex formation.

Analysis of urine for Bence-Jones proteins may be useful if there is suspicion of a lymphoproliferative disease. These are light chains of immunoglobulin produced by lymphocytes and plasma cells and are frequently observed in association with B-lymphocyte or plasma cell neoplasia.

5 What are the differential diagnoses for this case? What test would you suggest to confirm your diagnosis?

The main differentials in this case are B-cell neoplasia or an infectious disease (ehrlichiosis or leishmaniasis). Radiographs revealed the presence of multiple areas of osteolysis in the spinal column, suggesting a multiple myeloma, likely to be the cause of the clinical signs (lameness and back pain). Bone marrow cytology and histology were performed and showed high numbers of mature plasma cells with only a few erythroid and myeloid precursors left, confirming the suspicion of multiple myeloma. SPE was also performed and showed the presence of a monoclonal gammopathy.

FURTHER READING

Stockham SL, Scott MA (2008) *Fundamentals of Veterinary Clinical Pathology*, 2nd edn. Blackwell Publishing, Oxford, pp. 379–385 and 460–462.

CASE 76

1 What test would be suitable for diagnosis of equine pregnancy approximately 60 days post breeding?

Pregnant mare serum gonadotropin (PMSG) is most suitable for diagnosis of pregnancy approximately 60 days post breeding. PMSG is produced by the endometrial cups and is detected between 40 and 120 days of pregnancy.

2 What is a pitfall of this test?

A pitfall of PMSG is that it may be positive (false positive for pregnancy) if the foal is lost between the time that the endometrial cups develop and the time that they regress.

3 What other laboratory test can be used for equine pregnancy during late gestation (>100 days)?
Another laboratory test for equine pregnancy that is useful at >100 days of pregnancy is oestrone sulphate. If the foal dies during late gestation, this hormone decreases rapidly. Therefore, oestrone sulphate can be used for pregnancy diagnosis and for determination of a live foal in a mare with known pregnancy between 100 days of pregnancy and foaling.

CASE 77

1 What crystal is shown in Fig. 77.1?
The crystal is a sulpha crystal, resembling sheaves of needles with eccentric binding. The referring veterinarian confirmed that the dog was treated with sulphamethoxazole/trimethoprim, which was one of the antibiotics recommended after the microbial sensitivity test.

2 What test can be performed to verify the nature of these crystals?
The presence of sulpha drugs in urine can be confirmed by a lignin test. Several drops of urine and several drops of hydrochloric acid are added to a piece of lignin-containing paper (cheap newspaper). A positive reaction is indicated by an orange–yellow staining (**Fig. 77.2**). This test is fairly specific and based on the reaction of arylamide groups in sulfa drugs with cellulose.

3 Do they have any clinical significance?
The clinical significance is controversial. One opinion is that sulpha crystals form in the bladder, not the renal tubules, and this suggests there is no reason to stop the therapy. However, there is evidence from a recent study that even the latest generation of sulpha drugs may cause renal damage, so discontinuance of the sulpha drug should be considered, particularly if impaired renal function is identified.

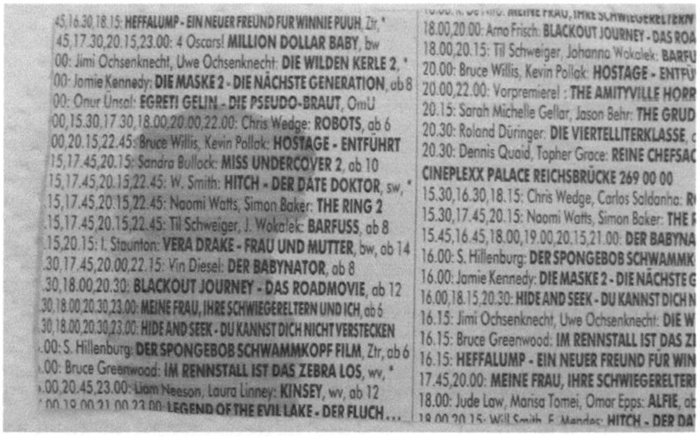

FIG. 77.2 Positive (left) and negative (right) lignin test. (Courtesy Dr Judith Leidinger)

FURTHER READING
Osborne CA, Stevens JB (1999) *Urinalysis: A Clinical Guide to Compassionate Patient Care.* Bayer Corporation, Shawnee Mission.
Väth T (2005) *Die cerebrale Toxoplasmose bei AIDS: Untersuchungen zur Pharmakokinetik von Sulfadiazin unter Urinalkalisierung. (Cerebral toxoplasmosis in AIDS: studies of the pharmocokinetics of sulfadiacine influenced by the alkalisation of urine).* PhD Thesis, Würzburg.

CASE 78

1 Describe and discuss the significant haematological and biochemistry findings as well as the urinalysis.
Haematology is unremarkable apart from a significantly decreased MCV. The decreased MCV is further supported by the microscopic evaluation of the blood smear revealing microcytic-normochromic erythrocytes. Decreased MCV/microcytic erythrocytes may be due to iron deficiency because of chronic gastrointestinal haemorrhage or severe infestation with ectoparasites (fleas, ticks), or liver failure. The latter is more likely given the absence of anaemia and the history. Moreover, in iron deficiency erythrocytes tend to be microcytic-hypochromic rather than microcytic-normochromic and hypochromasia will occur prior to development of microcytosis. Microcytosis of erythrocytes in liver failure is not due to a decreased total body iron. It is considered to be caused by a functional iron deficiency due to defective hepatic protein synthesis resulting in an impaired iron transport.

The biochemical profile shows a mild to moderate decrease in urea concentration suggestive of decreased protein uptake due to vomiting/anorexia or decreased albumin synthesis due to liver failure. Given the presence of microcytic-normochromic erythrocytes and the history, the latter is the most likely cause, although vomiting may contribute. Hypocholesterolaemia gives further support of liver failure ressulting in decreased production. A slight increase in ALT activity is indicative of hepatocellular damage.

The slight increase in ALP activity is most likely due to an increase of the bone isoenzyme in a young growing animal (Maine Coon cats may grow until the age of 4 years).

There is a mild hypernatraemia and hyperchloraemia, which is suggestive of hypertonic dehydration due to pure water loss or loss of a hypotonic fluid via the gastrointestinal tract or the kidneys. A slightly increased calcium concentration is also commonly seen in young growing cats.

2 What further tests are required given the history and the haematological/biochemistry abnormalities?
The overall picture is suggestive of severe liver failure, so that an assessment of liver function is indicated.

Liver function tests include measurement of a basal bile acid test or basal ammonia concentration. An ammonia tolerance test should be performed if basal values are normal. According to the literature, in dogs normal basal bile acids do not rule out liver failure and gallbladder contraction has to be stimulated either with food or intramuscular administration of 0.3 μg/kg of a synthetic cholecystokinin analogue (e.g. ceruletide [Takus®]). Cats, however, demonstrated no significant changes of serum bile acid concentrations after stimulation with the same dosage of ceruletide, so that measurement of basal bile acid concentration is sufficient.

In a cat of this age, congenital diseases such as portosystemic shunt and arterioportal fistulae can be suspected. The latter, however, is extremely rare in cats. Acquired extrahepatic shunts are less likely but may occur in young animals in conditions that are characterised by high portal pressure (i.e. severe chronic hepatitis, liver cirrhosis). Portosystemic shunts can be detected via (spleno-) portography and ultrasound. The diagnostic use of sonography, however, is highly dependent on the experience of the operator. Prior to portography, a coagulation profile should be performed, as the majority of coagulation factors are synthesised in the liver.

In a cat with non-specific clinical signs such as underdevelopment, intermittent gastrointestinal signs and ataxia, feline leukaemia virus infection (FeLV) and feline infectious peritonitis (FIP) should be ruled out.

FOLLOW UP
Liver function tests

Analyte (units)	Result	Reference Interval
Basal serum bile acids (μmol/l)	**16**	<15
Fasted ammonia (μmol/l)	**122**	<59

Basal serum bile acid concentrations are slightly increased and the fasted ammonia concentration is moderately increased, which is diagnostic of liver insufficiency.

FeLV antigen testing and FIP antibody titre are both negative.

Coagulation profile

Analyte (units)	Result	Reference Interval
PT (seconds)	9.7	7–10 (<15)
aPTT (seconds)	**26.4**	9.5–10.5
Fibrinogen (g/l)	**1.2**	2–4

There is a prolongation of aPTT compatible with disorders of the intrinsic or common coagulation pathway. In this case, impaired synthesis of coagulation factors due to severe liver insufficiency is most likely.

Splenoportography
Splenoportography revealed a portophrenico shunt.

Diagnosis
Severe liver failure due to a portophrenico shunt.

OTHER COMMENTS
In contrast to dogs, in which portosystemic shunts are generally associated with decreased urea plasma concentrations, cats are often presented with a slight azotaemia.

Compared with basal ammonia plasma concentrations, basal bile acids were only slightly increased in this cat. However, studies in dogs have demonstrated that measurement of ammonia is more sensitive and specific for diagnosis of portosystemic shunting. In this patient, diagnosis of liver failure was based on moderately increased plasma fasted ammonia concentration. An ammonia tolerance test would not have provided any further information and is contraindicated owing to the risk of causing a hepato-encephalic syndrome. Ammonia is not stable in plasma as it evaporates rapidly. Thus, measurement has to be performed directly after sampling. For this reason, point-of-care tests have been developed and evaluated for use in veterinary medicine.

Copper-coloured irises are often associated with the presence of portosystemic shunts in cats.

FURTHER READING
Bauer NB, Schneider MA, Neiger R *et al.* (2006) Liver disease in dogs with tracheal collapse. *J Vet Intern Med* **20**:845–849.

Bridger N, Glanemann B, Neiger R (2008) Comparison of postprandial and ceruletide seum bile acid stimulation in dogs. *J Vet Intern Med* **22**:873–878.

Gerritzen-Bruning MJ, van den Ingh TS, Rothuizen J (2006) Diagnostic value of fasting plasma ammonia and bile acid concentrations in the identification of portosystemic shunting in dogs. *J Vet Intern Med* **20**:13–19.

Jacob I (2000) *Der Ceruletid-Test zur Diagnostik von Lebererkrankungen im Blutserum von Katzen (Diagnostic use of the ceruletide stimulation test for diagnosis of liver diseases in the blood serum of cats).* PhD Thesis, University of Giessen.

Rufer M, Grunbaum EG (1997) Bile acid stimulation test with ceruletide. *Tierarztl Prax* **25**:80–84.

CASE 79

1 Describe and discuss the haematological abnormalities.
There is a moderate leucocytosis based on a moderate neutrophilia with left shift and moderate signs of toxicity. Mild monocytosis is present. Given the history of a chronically infected wound, these changes are consistent

with chronic active inflammation, most likely due to the infected wound on the leg. Band neutrophils indicate that the need for neutrophils in the periphery exceeds the bone marrow storage pool capacity for neutrophils.

2 What aetiologies do you suspect for the development of toxic neutrophils?

Toxic neutrophils develop during accelerated myelopoiesis and therefore are consistent with a maturation disorder. They have nothing to do with some kind of intoxication, but it is known that inflammatory mediators such as cytokines lead to their development. Furthermore, various infectious diseases are accompanied by toxic neutrophils, most likely due to products from infectious agents.

3 What signs of toxicity can be seen in neutrophils, and what do they indicate?

Toxic signs have to be differentiated based on features of the cell, nucleus and cytoplasm. A macrocytic cell, a swollen and/or hypolobulated nucleus as well as a nucleus with less condensed chromatin may be observed.

The colour of the cytoplasm may change and appear more basophilic as a result of an increased staining of RNA. A foamy or vacuolated cytoplasm may occur if cytoplasmic granules burst. Döhle bodies are frequently visible as a sign for toxic neutrophils. They occur if the proteins producing rough endoplasmatic reticulum aggregates are stained. Note that Döhle bodies in small numbers are physiological in cats. Large Döhle bodies should not be confused with morulae from *Anaplasma* spp., distemper inclusions in dogs or inclusions present in patients with Chediak–Higashi syndrome. Finally, toxic granulation may be visible as a sign of severely toxic neutrophils. Small magenta granules are visible in the cytoplasm. These granules are consistent with primary granules. As the granule membrane becomes permeable, acidic stains can diffuse in and stain the granules. Although rarely observed in dogs and cats, similar granules may be found in some Birman cats or in patients with some lysosomal storage diseases. These have to be kept in mind as differentials.

FURTHER READING

Stockham SL, Scott MA (2008) *Fundamentals of Veterinary Clinical Pathology*, 2nd edn. Blackwell Publishing, Oxford.

Weiss DJ, Wardrop KJ (2010) (eds) *Schalm's Veterinary Hematology*, 6th edn. Blackwell Publishing, Ames.

CASE 80

1 What is your assessment of these laboratory findings?

There is slight neutrophilia that is likely due to the presence of inflammation. The slight increases in MCV and MCH

are unlikely to be of significance in the absence of other erythroid abnormalities.

There is a moderate increase in total protein with a borderline decrease in albumin and a moderate increase in globulins, resulting in a decreased A:G ratio. The increase in globulins may be due to inflammation and/or increased gamma globulins associated with immune stimulation or lymphoid neoplasia. The albumin may be decreased as a negative acute-phase reactant protein, but the possibility of decreased hepatic production or increased loss (gastrointestinal or renal) cannot be ruled out entirely. The results of the SPE (see below) are likely to help define these components and may help determine an underlying cause.

The marked increases in ALP and GGT, with slight increase in GLDH, AST and LDH, all suggest hepatobiliary disease. The absence of an increase in total bilirubin suggests cholestasis is unlikely and that this is a chronic condition. The slight decrease in urea in conjunction with these findings suggests decreased hepatic production. The increased bile acids supports the presence of hepatic dysfunction and increases the probability that the alterations in total protein, albumin and globulins are due to the presence of ongoing hepatic disease. This may result in the reported ataxia and apparent blindness, due to hepatic encephalopathy.

The slight increase in CK may be due to muscle catabolism associated with weight loss and the reported thin body condition. The increase in LDH may also be contributed to by elevation in the muscle enzyme component. The decrease in phosphorus suggests decreased intestinal absorption, which may be associated with decreased intake.

The SPE shows slight increases in all globulin fractions except for alpha-1 globulins. The increases in alpha-2 and beta globulins most likely reflect inflammation and the increase in gamma globulins reflects immune stimulation associated with decreased clearance of metabolites, bacterial endotoxins or other metabolic by-products by the liver.

2 What is the significance of the increased prominence of the 'shoulder' on the albumin peak and of the decreased definition between the beta-2 and gamma globulins apparent in the electrophoretic densitometry tracing?

The presence of increased prominence of the albumin 'shoulder' supports the presence of inflammation. In North America it is more common to include this 'shoulder' within the alpha-1 globulin fraction, while in Europe it is more commonly left within the albumin fraction when demarcating the various fractions. The decreased definition between the beta-2 and gamma globulin fractions is known as beta-gamma bridging. It is classically associated with hepatic disease, but may also occur with inflammatory or infectious disease or with neoplasia. These findings are consistent with the hepatobiliary disease noted above. In the study by Keav and Doxey (1981/82), the positive predictive value of beta-gamma bridging for hepatic disease was 32% (95% confidence interval = 15–53.5%).

3 What are likely differential diagnoses, and what further tests may be indicated?

The disproportionate increases in ALP and GGT compared with other hepatic enzymes suggests that biliary involvement is more prominent than hepatocellular damage. This is a common finding with ragwort toxicity, but may occur with other chronic hepatobiliary conditions, such as biliary lithiasis or liver damage with biliary proliferation (reactive or neoplastic). The increase in bile acids to >50 µmol/l is a poor prognostic indicator if due to ragwort toxicity. Hepatic biopsy may be useful in demonstrating megaloblastic hepatopathy typical of ragwort toxicity or may help determine if other conditions are present. Hepatic aspirates may be useful for demonstration of megaloblastic features associated with ragwort toxicity, but may not be sensitive in the detection of other inflammatory conditions or for assessment of hepatic architecture.

REFERENCE AND FURTHER READING

Camus MS, Krimer PM, Leroy BE *et al.* (2010) Evaluation of positive predictive value of serum poretin electrophresis beta-gamma bridging for hepatic disease in three species. *Vet Pathol* 47:1064–1070.

Keay G, Doxey DL (1981/1982) Species characteristics of serum proteins demonstrated after agarose gel electrophoresis. *Vet Res Commun* 5:263–270.

CASE 81

1 What is the most likely explanation for the hyperchloraemia? Describe the mechanism for this finding.

Chloride is measured via potentiometry and an ion-sensitive electrode. This dog is being treated with potassium bromide. As bromide is another hyalide with a negative charge, it is also detected by the chloride assay and thereby interferes with the result. This leads to a false hyperchloraemia.

Other differentials that should be considered are:

- Decreased chloride excretion can be excluded as no physical or laboratory renal abnormalities are detected, which makes this possibility highly unlikely. In addition, the degree of hyperchloraemia is not

plausible as electrolyte concentrations are maintained in a narrow range by the body. However, urinary fractional excretion of chloride may be assessed to definitively rule out this possibility.
- NaCl infusion had not been reported by the owners. In the face of normal renal function no hyperchloraemia should develop after such an infusion, especially if hypernatraemia is missing.
- Phenobarbitone could be considered as another interferent. However, as such an interference has not been reported for the chloride assay, this can also be excluded.

2 What is the most likely explanation for the increased ALP and ALT enzyme activities?

Phenobarbitone leads to toxic damage of hepatocytes and therefore to leakage of cytoplasmic ALT into the serum. ALP is altered because phenobarbitone induces increased production of this enzyme. Because of this, previous hypoxic damage is unlikely as a cause, but is a possibility.

CASE 82

1 What is your assessment of these findings?

The slightly high haematocrit with increased plasma protein by refractometry and increased albumin are consistent with dehydration. Dehydration is also the most likely cause for the increase in urea and creatinine, with high normal phosphorus, although renal or post-renal contributions cannot be ruled out completely. Globulins are increased because the plasma protein measured by refractometry is increased, and serum albumin is only slightly increased.

Correlation with clinical assessment of hydration status and USG should be considered to determine if renal compromise may be present. The clinical signs are highly suggestive of traumatic reticuloperitonitis and when plasma protein is >100 g/l, it is highly likely that this condition is present. In cows with suspected traumatic reticuloperitonitis, approximately 80% with total plasma protein >100 g/l were confirmed with this condition.

The slight alterations in MCV and MCH are likely due to the fact that these are calculated values and are unlikely to be of significance owing to their mild nature and absence of anaemia.

The leucocytosis with neutrophilia, left shift and lymphopacnia is supportive of acute inflammation, as is the moderate increase in fibrinogen and the fibrinogen:plasma protein ratio of >10%.

The low sodium and chloride may be contributed to by partial anorexia (decreased intake), as well as sequestration of HCl in the rumen associated with ruminal stasis or vagal indigestion. These findings, with increased TCO_2, are suggestive of metabolic alkalosis, and an arterial blood gas analysis should be considered to confirm whether this is present. The low potassium may be due to decreased intake, but may also occur with a shift of potassium ions into the intracellular compartment in exchange for hydrogen ions when alkalosis is present. The shift of potassium ions is usually minor with alkalosis, so decreased intake due to anorexia is suspected. The sodium, chloride and potassium may be lower than indicated because of the concurrent dehydration.

The slight decrease in anion gap is likely due to decreased negative charges associated with hyperglobulinaemia.

The slight increase in CK may be due to muscle damage or catabolism and is relatively mild. The slight increase in ALP without an increase in GGT may be due to hepatobiliary insult and/or decreased hepatic blood flow associated with partial anorexia, but there are no other laboratory results supporting hepatocellular insult. The possibility of intestinal or bone components contributing cannot be ruled out.

The elevated abdominal fluid total protein is supportive of protein exudation and the cloudy character supports increased cells and/or protein within the abdominal fluid. Collecting from the ruminal–reticular recess increases the probability of obtaining a representative sample, since acute reticuloperitonitis may be localised to this area.

2 What is the most likely clinical diagnosis/differential diagnosis?

The most likely diagnosis is acute traumatic reticuloperitonitis. Differential diagnoses include a perforating abomasal ulcer and ketosis. Total plasma protein tends to be less elevated (<100 g/l) in cows with a perforating abomasal ulcer and not elevated in cows with ketosis.

Acute reticuloperitonitis is more likely than chronic reticuloperitonitis due to the presence of fever and elevated HR, which often return to within normal limits with chronicity. The left shift also provides further support for an acute inflammatory condition. Diffuse peritonitis is less likely since it is often a fulminating condition with progression to prostration and recumbency and death within a few days.

FOLLOW UP

A 'pole test' (putting pressure on the cranial abdomen with a pole beneath the cow) elicited a positive pain response, providing further support for traumatic reticuloperitonitis. Confinement, depositing a magnet into the reticulum and antibiotic treatment resulted in resolution of clinical signs.

FURTHER READING

Dubensky RA, White ME (1983) The sensitivity, specificity and predictive value of total plasma protein in the diagnosis of traumatic reticuloperitonitis. *Can J Comp Med* **47**:241–244.

Orpin P (2008) Clinical management of traumatic reticuloperitonitis in cattle. *In Practice* **30**:544–551.

Ward JL, Ducharme NG (1994) Traumatic reticuloperitonitis in dairy cows. *J Amer Vet Med Assoc* **204**:874–877.

CASE 83

1 List the main target autoantigens on the erythrocyte surface.

Target autoantigens on the erythrocyte surface include: band 3, anion exchange molecule; spectrin, part of the cytoskeleton; and glycophorins.

2 Which type of hypersensitivity is responsible for development of immune-mediated haemolytic anaemia? Describe the pathogenesis.

Immune-mediated haemolytic anaemia (IMHA) develops as primary (idiopathic) or secondary disease. Autoreactive antibodies or antibodies directed against drugs or microbes adhere to the erythrocyte surface and initiate a type II hypersensitivity reaction. The antibodies mostly involved are IgM or IgG. They initiate the classical complement pathway, resulting in formation of the membrane attack complex, which creates a pore in the erythrocyte membrane. Through this pore the erythrocyte is osmotically destroyed, resulting in intravascular haemolysis. If the immune complexes or complement components bind to the Fc-receptor on phagocytes (e.g. in the spleen), damage or destruction of erythrocytes takes place. Damage of the erythrocyte membrane or just puncture of the membrane results in a shape change from biconcave to round (spherical) and therefore spherocytes develop. The cell may also directly be engulfed (erythrophagocytosis), which results in extravascular haemolysis.

3 What diseases may lead to secondary IMHA?

Diseases leading to secondary IMHA include: neoplasia (e.g. lymphoma, myeloproliferative disease, various types of sarcoma); infectious disease (especially babesiosis, ehrlichiosis, anaplasmosis, leishmaniasis, rickettsiosis); and drugs (e.g. sulphonamides, possibly cephalosporins and carprofen).

FURTHER READING

McGavin MD, Zachary JF (2006) *Pathologic Basis of Veterinary Disease*, 4th edn. Mosby Elsevier, Philadelphia.

Weiss DJ, Wardrop KJ (2010) *Schalm's Veterinary Hematology*, 6th edn. Blackwell Publishing, Ames.

CASE 84

1 Discuss the laboratory findings and their physiological significance.

The haematological findings are moderate neutrophilia with a left shift and monocytosis. These findings support an acute inflammatory condition with possible necrosis.

The combination of high ALP, GGT and GLDH confirm cholestasis and hepatocellular damage. The increased bile acids indicate impaired hepatic function and are expected with the increase in total bilirubin and the clinically visible icterus. The predominance of unconjugated bilirubin is expected in this mare and does not suggest acute haemolysis, as it might in dogs or cats. An increase in total bilirubin of up to three times the upper limit of the reference interval may occur with partial or complete anorexia and is thought to be contributed to by poor hepatic blood flow associated with anorexia. In this case, the 4–5 times elevation compared with the upper reference limit of total bilirubin supports a cholestatic component.

2 What are your differential diagnoses based on these findings?

The primary consideration in this case is cholangiohepatitis. This is not a common diagnosis in the horse, but may be associated with cholelithiasis. This condition also may result in colic, as described in the history. Ascending infection from the intestine is a possibility, as is chronic and active hepatitis/cholangiohepatitis. Ragwort toxicity rarely causes the marked jaundice and haematological features seen in this case, so is considered unlikely.

3 What tests should be carried out next in this mare?

Evaluation of platelets and whole blood clotting time or aPTT and PT is recommended prior to obtaining a liver biopsy.

CASE 85

1 Have a look at the blood smear. What are the inclusions in the neutrophils?

The inclusions in the neutrophils of this dog are consistent with morulae. Morulae present in canine neutrophils include *Anaplasma phagocytophila* and *Ehrlichia ewingii*. The latter organism, however, is generally seen in the southern and mideastern United States, whereas *Anaplasma phagocytophila* is endemic in Germany. Morulae of *Ehrlichia canis* are similar, but present in monocytes.

2 Describe and discuss further abnormalities present on the smears.

There is a severe thrombocytopaenia. Platelets are mainly giant (of the same size as erythrocytes; **Fig. 85.2**, upper right), which is considered a sign of regeneration. In the current case, thrombocytopaenia is most likely due to immune-mediated destruction of platelets and/or megakaryocytes induced by *Anaplasma phagocytophila* infection. However, examination of a bone marrow aspirate is indicated if thrombocytopaenia fails to respond to treatment.

The neutrophils are toxic and display a foamy, basophilic cytoplasm. They tend to be giant (>14 µm, which approximates to more than twice the diameter of a canine erythrocyte). Toxic changes in neutrophils result from developmental abnormalities in early neutrophil precursors due to a particularly intense inflammatory process. Giant neutrophils suggest myelodysplasia, which in this case is most likely due to inflammation.

3 Describe and discuss the haemogram.

There is slight leucopaenia based on a moderate lymphopaenia suggestive of stress/corticosteroid effect. Neutrophils and bands are within the reference interval; however, in a febrile patient the absence of neutrophilia is considered an inadequate response. This inadequate response may be due to an acute demand in the periphery exceeding the storage pool and regeneration capacity of the bone marrow. Moreover, *Anaplasma/Ehrlichia* organisms are known to induce an immune-mediated destruction of bone marrow precursors, which may result in bone marrow hypoplasia in chronically infected animals.

There is a severe thrombocytopaenia, which is also most likely caused by immune-mediated destruction of megakaryocytic precursors and/or platelets due to anaplasmosis.

4 Discuss the pattern of dysproteinaemia.

A mild hyperproteinaemia characterised by a mild hypoalbuminaemia and hyperglobulinaemia is present. In this patient, hyperglobulinaemia is most likely due to a subacute to chronic systemic inflammation and immunological stimulation. Whereas inflammation is generally associated with a polyclonal gammopathy, neoplasia (multiple myeloma, B-cell lymphoma) induces a monoclonal or, rarely, a biclonal gammopathy. However, it should be considered that ehrlichiosis/anaplasmosis may also cause an oligoclonal gammopathy in rare cases.

Electrophoresis should be considered to further characterise the pattern of protein response in the current patient.

In this patient, hypoalbuminaemia is most likely due to decreased hepatic production induced by an inflammatory process, as albumin is a negative acute-phase protein.

5 What recommendations do you have regarding treatment and prophylaxis?

The drug of choice for treatment of anaplasmosis and all forms of ehrlichiosis is doxycycline (10 mg/kg body weight PO q24h for at least 28 days). There should be dramatic clinical improvement within 24–48 hours following initiation of treatment in dogs with acute-phase or mild chronic-phase disease. As previous infection does not confer lifelong immunity, tick control is the main prevention of canine ehrlichiosis/anaplasmosis.

FURTHER READING

Neer TM, Breitschwerdt EB, Greene RT et al. (2002) Consensus statement on ehrlichial disease of small animals from the infectious disease study group of the ACVIM. American College of Veterinary Internal Medicine. J Vet Intern Med 16:309–315.

Silaghi C, Gilles J, Hohle M et al. (2008) Anaplasma phagocytophilum infection in Ixodes ricinus, Bavaria, Germany. Emerg Infect Dis 14:972–974.

CASE 86

1 Describe and discuss the significant laboratory abnormalities, and indicate the most likely diagnosis.

The erythrocytes are slightly microcytic and borderline hypochromic. Differential diagnoses for microcytosis include iron deficiency (mostly in association with hypochromasia) and liver insufficiency.

The slightly decreased urea concentration associated with moderately increased pre-prandial bile acids, slight hypocholesterolaemia and borderline hypoalbuminaemia are indicative of impaired liver function. The history, age of the patient and degree of elevation in the pre-prandial bile acids are most suggestive of a portosystemic shunt. However, the absence of an increase in the post-prandial bile acids is not typical of this diagnosis. Possible reasons for this absence in the face of impaired liver function are contraction of the gallbladder prior to the test, not ingesting the entire test meal (did not stimulate gallbladder contraction), delayed gastric emptying, delayed intestinal transit time or delayed intestinal absorption. The bile acid stimulation test should be repeated.

One differential for decreased urea concentration in a young dog may be urea cycle enzyme deficiencies, but this condition is very rare. Hypoalbuminaemia may also occur because of decreased dietary protein intake, decreased intestinal absorption of protein or increased loss via the intestines, kidneys or skin. As no diarrhoea has been reported, no proteinuria is detected and no skin burns are present, these differentials can be excluded. Differential diagnoses for hypocholesterolaemia are few apart from impaired hepatic function. Protein-losing enteropathy associated with lymphangiectasia could lead to hypocholesterolaemia due to loss of lipids by damaged enterocytes. Furthermore, dogs with hypoadrenocorticism are described as showing

decreased cholesterol concentrations, but the underlying pathophysiology is not established.

ALT enzyme activity is slightly increased, pointing to hepatocellular damage. As functional hepatic mass is diminished in patients with liver insufficiency, the number of hepatocytes is often just too low to lead to a prominent increase in ALT. Therefore, in end-stage liver disease, the liver enzyme concentrations may not be diagnostically useful. A decreased urea concentration subsequently leads to decreased renal medullary concentration ability and decreased USG. Polyuria and polydipsia are frequently noted clinically in these patients. Moderate hyperphosphataemia, mild hypercalcaemia and a moderate increase in ALP enzyme activity (bone ALP isoenzyme) are physiological in a growing young dog and exemplify ongoing growth with increased bone turnover.

2 What further tests would you recommend, and why?

Further recommended tests include:

- Ultrasonographic evaluation, by an experienced ultrasonographer, of the portal vessels to definitively confirm the diagnosis of portosystemic shunt.
- Basal ammonium concentration to further confirm the diagnosis may be considered.

FURTHER READING

Adam FH, German AJ, McConnell JF et al. (2012) Clinical and clinicopathologic abnormalities in young dogs with acquired and congenital portosystemic shunts: 93 cases (2003–2008). J Am Vet Med Assoc 241:760–65.

Ruland K, Fischer A, Hartmann K (2010) Sensitivity and specificity of fasting ammonia and serum bile acids in the diagnosis of portosystemic shunts in dogs and cats. J Vet Clin Pathol 39:57–64.

CASE 87

1 Identify and list the abnormalities and explain their associations.

Slight macrocytic-hypochromic anaemia with marked regeneration. The degree of regeneration is excessive for this slight anaemia.

Hyperkalaemia might be an artefact with release of K^+ from platelets or increased due to the very high number of reticulocytes. Immature reticulocytes have a higher K^+ concentration compared with mature erythrocytes because they still have the Na^+/K^+ pump in the cell membrane. Hyperkalaemia can occur with severe muscle damage, but the current CK increase is slight and non-specific. (**Note:** Phosphofructokinase (PFK)-deficient

Whippets have marked clinical signs of exertional myopathy similar to those seen in PFK-deficient humans. In contrast, PFK-deficient English Springer and Cocker Spaniels have relatively mild muscle signs.) The mild non-specific increased CK could be an artefact if the sample is haemolysed.

Increased NT-proBNP if accompanied by clinical signs is consistent with congestive cardiac disease.

The increased urine protein:creatinine ratio is consistent with proteinuria, which, if pre-renal causes can be ruled out, may be due to tubular or glomerular pathology. Slight bilirubinuria may be found in healthy male dogs.

2 Is the automated low MCHC reported by the analyser genuine or not? Provide an explanation for your answer.

This could be genuine or an artefact. If genuine, polychromatophils are larger than mature erythrocytes and do not contain their complete haemoglobin complement. Marked polychromasia may have a concomitant increased MCV and decreased MCHC. If the automated MCHC is accurate, then hypochromasia has been missed on blood film evaluation.

If an artefact, RBCs swell in transit (samples posted to a laboratory), which may produce an erroneously increased MCV, which in turn leads to an erroneous calculated MCHC (see equations below). This concurs with the absence of hypochromasia observed on blood film.

$$MCV = \frac{Hct(\%) \times 10}{RBC} \qquad HCT = \frac{MCV \times RBC}{1,000}$$

$$MCHC = \frac{Hgb \times 1,000}{MCV \times RBC}$$

3 Two further samples over the following 3 months revealed similar findings. (1) Is the degree of regeneration appropriate for the degree of anaemia? (2) Is the number of nucleated RBCs appropriate for the degree of reticulocytosis?

(1) Unlikely. The degree of regeneration is far greater than that expected with this mild anaemia. (2) Yes. There are very high numbers of nucleated erythrocytes but they are proportional in number to the extremely high number of reticulocytes.

4 Why is immune-mediated haemolytic anaemia (IMHA) not a consideration with this set of laboratory results?

The combination of no spherocytosis, no agglutination and a negative Coombs test indicates that IMHA is unlikely.

5 Lead is within reference interval, but which part of the haematological report may have prompted the veterinarian to request analysis of lead?

Presence of nucleated RBCs.

6 What is the most likely diagnosis with the excessive degree of erythrocyte regeneration, the mild degree of anaemia and evidence of clinical disease, particularly after exercise, along with this patient's breed?

PFK deficiency.

7 What tests would be helpful in confirming a diagnosis?

Absence of increased erythrocyte osmotic fragility (increased with IMHA); negative Coombs test; increased alkaline fragility; low 2,3-diphosphoglycerate concentration (rule out pyruvate kinase deficiency); measure PFK enzyme activity in dogs >3 months of age. Definitive test: DNA test (PCR) can distinguish between normal, carrier and affected dogs; requires a cheek brush or EDTA sample sent by regular post; can be used at any patient age.

FURTHER READING

Gerber K, Harvey JW, D'Agorne S *et al.* (2009) Hemolysis, myopathy, and cardiac disease associated with hereditary phosphofructokinase deficiency in two Whippets. *J Vet Clin Pathol* **38**:46–51.

Giger U, Harvey JW (1987) Hemolysis caused by phospho-fructokinase-deficient English Springer spaniels: seven cases (1983–87). *J Am Vet Med Assoc* **191**:453–459.

CASE 88

1 How would you interpret this anaemia?

There is evidence of a severe anaemia, which is non-regenerative considering the absence of polychromatophils on the blood film and the low reticulocyte count. The concurrent neutropaenia and thrombocytopaenia are indicative of pancytopaenia, which is a reduction of two or more cell lines. This is likely to be due to bone marrow dysfunction.

2 What further tests would you suggest? What is your diagnosis?

FeLV and FIV testing is recommended because myeloproliferative and lymphoproliferative diseases are frequently associated with retroviral infections in cats. A SNAP test has been performed and the cat is FeLV positive.

Because of the pancytopaenia, a bone marrow aspirate was performed (**Fig. 88.1**). There is evidence

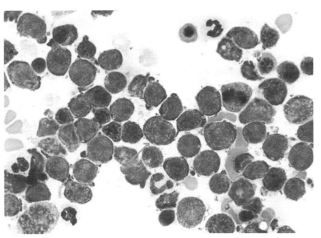

FIG. 88.1 Bone marrow aspirate. Note the monomorphic population of blastic cells (orange arrow). Wright–Giemsa, ×50 (oil).

of a monomorphic population of blasts, which have completely effaced the bone marrow parenchyma with only occasional erythroid and myeloid precursors left. This has caused insufficient production of erythroid and myeloid cells and caused the pancytopaenia.

The morphological features are suggestive of a lymphoid cell population, although immunophenotyping is necessary in order to characterise the lesion. Immunocytochemistry was performed. Cells reacted positively for CD79, which is a cluster of differentiation molecules expressed by B-lymphoid cells. The cytological features and the immunocytochemistry results are suggestive of a B-ALL (acute lymphoid leukaemia). Unfortunately, CD34, which is a marker of early haematopoietic cells, has not been validated in the cat and the acute origin of the leukaemia cannot be confirmed.

The presence of neoplastic cells in the bone marrow is indicative of leukaemia, although considering the absence of these cells in the peripheral blood, the term aleukaemic leukaemia can also be used. This condition is uncommon but has been described in dogs and cats.

FURTHER READING

Weiss DJ, Wardrop KJ (2011) *Schalm's Veterinary Hematology*, 6th edn. Wiley-Blackwell, Ames.

CASE 89

1 What is your assessment of the arterial pH?
The pH is increased, therefore this is an alkalaemia.

2 What is your assessment of the likely underlying aetiology for this arterial pH?
The HCO_3^- is increased, so the alkalaemia is due to a metabolic alkalosis.

3 Is there appropriate compensation for this condition, and what does it suggest?
Metabolic alkalosis gives a variable response and no reliable formula is available to calculate an appropriate response. However, an increase in $PaCO_2$ is expected and it is not increased in this case. Therefore, a mixed acid–base disorder with a metabolic alkalosis (bicarbonate increased) and a respiratory alkalosis ($PaCO_2$ decreased over what is expected) is considered likely.

4 What might be the underlying causes for this condition?
Metabolic alkaloses can be subclassified as chloride responsive or chloride resistant by evaluating urine chloride concentration. Chloride-responsive metabolic alkaloses result from excess chloride loss in gastric fluid (likely present here as the dog is vomiting), sweat or saliva (in the horse) and results in an extremely low urine chloride concentration (<10 mEq/l). Chloride-resistant metabolic alkaloses result from excess plasma concentrations of aldosterone or aldosterone agonists, which cause excess renal chloride excretion and a high urine chloride concentration (>20 mEq/l). Treatment of chloride-responsive metabolic alkalosis is aimed at finding the source of the chloride loss and providing an adequate source of chloride, whereas treatment of chloride-resistant metabolic alkalosis is aimed at finding the source of excess aldosterone or the aldosterone agonist.

Paradoxical aciduria may develop with chloride-responsive metabolic alkalosis. Often, when paradoxical aciduria develops the potassium deficiency must be corrected for complete correction of the acid–base imbalance.

Because the PaO_2 is slightly increased (not decreased), an extrathoracic problem resulting in the respiratory alkalosis component is an underlying cause. Extrathoracic respiratory alkaloses occur as a result of hyperventilation caused by CNS lesions, emotional stress or decreased oxygen carrying capacity of the blood and are associated with normal or slightly increased arterial blood oxygen concentrations. It is easy to understand how hyperventilation resulting in decreased arterial blood CO_2 concentration and normal or increased arterial blood oxygen concentration can result from CNS and emotional conditions. In this patient, the painful lesion in the abdomen led to stress and hyperventilation.

However, the development of decreased arterial blood CO_2 concentration with normal or increased arterial blood oxygen concentration caused by decreased blood oxygen carrying capacity may, at first, be confusing. In blood, most oxygen is carried bound to haemoglobin. Oxygen bound to haemoglobin is in equilibrium with oxygen in plasma and provides a reservoir of oxygen. As oxygen diffuses from plasma into tissues, plasma oxygen is replenished from the oxygen reservoir provided by haemoglobin-bound oxygen. Decreased haemoglobin concentration (classic anaemia) or decreased haemoglobin oxygen carrying capacity (cyanide toxicity, nitrate toxicity, carbon monoxide toxicity) decreases the haemoglobin-bound oxygen reservoir. As a result, plasma and functional haemoglobin are normally saturated, or slightly supersaturated, with oxygen when the blood leaves the lungs. However, plasma and haemoglobin are quickly depleted of oxygen (PaO_2 decreases) after blood enters the tissues. Whether or not anaemia or decreased haemoglobin oxygen carrying capacity is present in this patient must be elucidated by evaluation of a blood smear and exclusion of, for example, Heinz bodies by new methylene blue staining.

The final diagnosis was a mixed acid–base disorder with metabolic alkalosis due to loss of Cl^- and H^+ via gastric fluids and respiratory alkalosis owing to a painful abdomen and subsequent hyperventilation.

FOLLOW UP
A severely painful cranial abdomen associated with vomiting is highly suggestive of acute pancreatitis, which could be verified by a markedly increased cPLI concentration and supported by ultrasound examination. Biochemistry showed hypertriglyceridaemia, which in this breed is suggestive of familial hypertriglyceridaemia of Miniature Schnauzers. However, whether the increased triglyceride concentration was the cause or a consequence of the pancreatitis could not be determined. Haematology revealed mild to moderate non-regenerative anaemia contributing to the combination of a decreased arterial blood CO_2 concentration with normal/increased arterial blood oxygen concentration.

FURTHER READING
Dibartola SP (2012) *Fluid, Electrolyte and Acid-Base Disorders in Small Animal Practice*, 4th edn. Elsevier Saunders, St. Louis.

CASE 90

1 Discuss the laboratory findings and their significance.
The marked increase in GGT confirms cholestasis, but there is little hepatocellular damage (mild GLDH). The GGT is disproportionately high compared with ALP, suggesting the hepatic problem may be at a relatively early stage or might be due to ragwort ingestion (bile duct duplication resulting in the disproportionately increased GGT compared with ALP).

Bile acids are at the top of the reference interval, suggesting little or no impairment of hepatic function; continued monitoring is required to determine if these

may continue to rise. The albumin is at the bottom of the reference interval, which may be insignificant but could indicate that it is falling and hepatic function may soon be compromised. Continued monitoring is required to determine if there is a continued decline in albumin. If a continued decline in albumin is observed, this is an indicator of a poor prognosis.

The PT (extrinsic pathway) is markedly increased, which likely explains the haematoma. PT is relatively prolonged compared with aPTT; this may be due to higher sensitivity of PT and short half-life of factor VII compared with other factors. The platelets are not low enough to have contributed to the formation of the haematoma and haematomas are not typical of primary haemostatic problems; the slightly low value may be an artefact (collection into glass container, time before sample analysis, presence of platelet clumping) or may be due to slightly increased consumption by the haematoma. Haematoma formation is more characteristic of abnormalities of secondary haemostasis (factor deficiencies) rather than primary haemostasis (platelet deficiency or dysfunction or vascular wall abnormalities).

2 What are your differential diagnoses?
Overall, the results might suggest early ragwort poisoning (GGT is very sensitive to this), although it was unusual that the PT was so impaired when other indicators of liver functions were not.

FOLLOW UP
A recent massive access to ragwort was subsequently confirmed by the owner. After removal from the pasture, GGT was used to monitor progress. This gradually returned to normal and no further bleeding was observed.

CASE 91

1 What is the likely defect?
With a prolonged PT and a normal aPTT it could be very early warfarin poisoning, but the TEG analysis rules this out, since it would be severely affected. The most likely diagnosis is factor VII deficiency. This was confirmed on a factor VII clotting activity (FVII:C) assay, which showed the dog had less than 2% factor VII activity.

2 What is the usual clinical severity of the defect in Beagles?
Canine factor VII deficiency is best characterised in Beagles. Factor VII-deficient Beagles rarely experience bleeding, even after surgery or trauma. In contrast, factor VII-deficient Malamutes typically experience more severe signs including haematomas and prolonged post-traumatic bleeding. Clinical severity may also vary in individuals within a single breed.

3 What advice would you give the owner regarding breeding?

Factor VII deficiency is a recessive trait. A missense mutation in exon 5 of the factor VII gene was first identified in Beagles and has subsequently been found in Alaskan Klee Kais and Deerhounds. Heterozygous carriers have FVII:C values that are intermediate between affected and wild-type dogs, but there is an overlap between homozygotes and heterozygotes. FVII:Ag analysis is more precise than FVII:C analysis for detecting carriers, but direct detection with DNA analyses is preferable. This dog has very low FVII:C values and it is therefore very likely that it is a homozygote and therefore will pass the trait on to all its offspring and so should not be used for breeding.

FURTHER READING

Brooks MB (2010) Hereditary coagulopathies. In: *Schalm's Veterinary Hematology*, 6th edn. (eds DJ Weiss, KJ Wardrop) Blackwell Publishing, Ames, pp. 661–667.

Callan MB, Aljamali MN, Margaritis P *et al.* (2006) A novel missense mutation responsible for factor VII deficiency in research Beagle colonies. *J Thromb Haemostasis* **4**:2616–2222.

Knudsen T, Kjelgaard-Hansen M, Tranholm M *et al.* (2011) Canine-specific ELISA for coagulation factor VII. *Vet J* **190**:352–358.

Lubas G, Caldin M, Wiinberg B *et al.* (2010) Laboratory testing of coagulation disorders. In: *Schalm's Veterinary Hematology*, 6th edn. (eds DJ Weiss, KJ Wardrop) Blackwell Publishing, Ames, pp. 1082–1100.

CASE 92

1 What is the most likely diagnosis?

This dog presented with a marked hypovolaemic crisis. The lack of a stress leucogram with a mild lymphocytosis suggests a lack of cortisol production. The biochemistry profile indicates the presence of marked azotaemia. The presence of moderate hyponatraemia and marked hyperkalaemia, along with a reduced Na:K ratio (16), mild hyperchloraemia and marked metabolic acidosis, indicates aldosterone deficiency. Considering the presence of hypovolaemia, pre-renal causes of azotaemia seem likely in this case. Therefore, the most likely diagnosis is acute primary hypoadrenocorticism, a condition rarely described in cats.

2 What are the differential diagnoses for marked hyperkalaemia?

Other possible causes for marked hyperkalaemia include AKI, urinary tract obstruction, severe gastrointestinal diseases, hepatic failure, severe metabolic or respiratory acidosis with subsequent shift of K^+ from the intracellular to the extracellular pool, massive cellular injury with subsequent release of intracellular potassium in blood, chylous effusions and iatrogenic or severe leucocytosis/thrombocytosis.

3 Why does metabolic acidosis develop in the condition diagonised in this cat?

Metabolic acidosis is a common finding in hypoadrenocorticism. This is principally related to the aldosterone deficiency impairing renal tubular secretion of H^+. A decreased GFR can also contribute to metabolic acidosis.

FURTHER READING

Ettinger S, Feldman E (2000) *Textbook of Veterinary Internal Medicine*, 6th edn. Elsevier Saunders, St. Louis.

Ilkiw JE, Rose RJ, Martin IC (1991) A comparison of simultaneously collected arterial, mixed venous and cephalic venous blood samples in the assessment of blood gas and acid-base status in the dog. *J Vet Intern Med* **5**:294–298.

Stockham SL, Scott MA (2008) *Fundamentals of Veterinary Clinical Pathology*, 2nd edn. Blackwell Publishing, Oxford.

CASE 93

1 What is the nature of the crystals shown above?

The morphology of the crystals, particularly the protrusions seen on the spherulith in the centre ('thorn apple' forms), and the yellow–brownish colour provide strong evidence for ammonium urate (syn.: ammonium biurate).

2 What other crystals show a similar morphology?

Xanthine crystals. They look similar and cannot be distinguished from ammonium urate by microscopy.

3 What do they indicate?

Ammonium urates are associated with hepatic insufficiency, especially congenital portosystemic shunts. However, ammonium urate crystals are common in Dalmatians and English Bulldogs without liver insufficiency. Since Miniature Schnauzers have not been identified as a breed in which ammonium urate crystals are normally expected, investigation for hepatopathy is indicated.

Note: For interpretation of the + proteinuria detected by dipstick and by the sulphasalicylic acid test, the USG of 1.048 must be taken into consideration. A urinary protein:creatinine ratio from several urine samples could be used to quantify the extent of the proteinuria.

FURTHER READING

Osborne CA, Stevens JB (1999) *Urinalysis: A Clinical Guide to Compassionate Patient Care.* Bayer Corporation, Shawnee Mission.

CASE 94

1 Describe the abnormalities detected.
Based on the decreased RBC count, haemoglobin concentration and haematocrit, there is a moderate normocytic-normochromic anaemia. As the reticulocyte count is not increased, the anaemia is non-regenerative.

2 List possible causes for the finding and briefly describe the pathological mechanisms.
There are several different causes for a non-regenerative anaemia:

- Acute (less than 3–4 days) blood loss or haemolysis. After the acute onset of blood loss/disease, the bone marrow needs time to react to the diminished erythrocyte number. Therefore, in a time frame of 3–4 days, no increased reticulocyte count is expected. During this time, no exact statement can be given concerning the nature of the anaemia (regenerative versus non-regenerative).
- Bone marrow disease (decreased production). Precursors of erythropoiesis may be damaged or replaced in the bone marrow, leading to hypoplastic/aplastic erythropoiesis. Causes that should be considered include bone marrow necrosis or fibrosis and (metastatic) neoplasia in the bone marrow.
- Infectious disease. Ehrlichiosis in dogs or feline leukaemia virus (FeLV) infection in cats. FeLV subtype C binds to its receptor (which is also a haeme exporter) on the colony-forming unit for erythrocytes. As cytotoxic haeme can no longer be exported out of the cell, the cell is destroyed and erythropoiesis is inefficient/ineffective in maintaining the erythron.
- Drugs. Several drugs may cause aplastic anaemia or generalised bone marrow hypoplasia. Special attention should be taken in the administration of trimethoprim/sulphadiazine, phenylbutazone (dogs, possibly horse), albendazol (dogs, cats), griseofulvin (cats) or chemotherapy. In dogs, endogenous or exogenous oestrogen intoxication may also lead to erythroid hypoplasia/aplasia.
- Anaemia of chronic disease. Several different mechanisms, mostly including an iron distribution disorder (e.g. due to the acute-phase protein hepcidin, which leads to iron retention in macrophages), ineffective erythropoiesis and shortened erythrocyte survival time.

FOLLOW UP
Biochemistry was performed and revealed markedly increased liver enzymes as well as impaired hepatic function. Ultrasonography of the liver showed a likely tumour, probably causing anaemia of chronic disease.

CASE 95

1 Discuss the laboratory findings and their significance.
The erythrocyte parameters are indicative of haemoconcentration. The neutropaenia is due to margination of neutrophils in the capillary (especially pulmonary) beds (endotoxin and TNF effect). The increased PT and low platelets suggest consumption due to a hypercoagulable state such as DIC.

The serum proteins and urea are also suggestive of haemoconcentration, but as the disease progresses the proteins are likely to fall due to extravascular leakage (the limb oedema) and protein-losing enteropathy. The hyperglycaemia is consistent with increased gluconeogenesis, which is a TNF-mediated effect.

Triglycerides are in the range expected for inappetence rather than the hyperlipaemia syndrome, although developing hyperlipaemia cannot be discounted (less likely in a horse as opposed to a pony) as endotoxin inhibits lipoprotein lipase activity (clears VLDL from circulation).

The electrolyte changes suggest enteric loss. Although an acid–base balance was not assessed, acidosis is likely to occur in this case due to the degree of bicarbonate loss. Decreased GFR will decrease the kidneys' ability to compensate by increasing urinary H^+ excretion. Hypoxaemia and a resulting increase in peripheral anaerobic metabolism also result in increased lactate production, exacerbating acidosis.

2 What is your interpretation and any recommendations?
The history, clinical signs and clinicopathological findings all indicate endotoxaemia due to acute colitis.

Evaluation of FDPs should be considered if further confirmation of DIC is desired. Blood gas analysis will likely confirm the presence of acidosis and an increased anion gap is expected because of increased levels of lactate/lactic acid associated with shock and poor tissue perfusion.

CASE 96

1 Interpret any abnormal laboratory results and discuss any pathophysiological mechanisms that could be causing changes in the laboratory values.
Slight non-regenerative anaemia, usually associated with chronic/inflammatory disease. The leucogram suggests stress. Acanthocytes and cell fragments can be seen in cats associated with a microangiopathy, lipid abnormalities or hepatic lipidosis.

Cats can have up to 5% Heinz bodies normally. When these are mildly increased, this can be associated with chronic metabolic conditions such as diabetes mellitus, lymphoma, hyperthyroidism and chronic renal or hepatic/pancreatic disease. These animals are usually not anaemic or they exhibit very slight anaemia. Higher levels of Heinz bodies in cats shorten the life span of red cells, which may result in anaemia. They are associated with exogenous oxidants such as dietary onions, garlic, propylene glycol (found in some commercial cat food), zinc, naphthalene (moth repellent) and following acetaminophen administration.

Glucose is low and can be associated with inappetence.

Increase in urea (with normal creatinine) is most likely pre-renal and can be seen with heart disease, gastrointestinal tract haemorrhage, other catabolic conditions such as hyperthyroidism (this cat may be a little young to see hyperthyroidism at this stage), anorexia, infection and pyrexia. Steroids and catabolic drugs (tetracycline) may also cause mild increases in urea.

This combination of hyperbilirubinaemia and increased ALT/AST and ALP activities with a 'normal' GGT is characteristic of hepatic lipidosis in cats.

The hepatocellular injury evidenced by the ALT/AST increase and the cholestasis indicated by ALP leads to decreased bilirubin clearance, resulting in hyperbilirubinaemia with resultant hyperbilirubinuria. This degree of increase in ALP activity is uncommon in cats other than in association with lipidosis. Lipidosis can occur as a result of substantial fat mobilisation from adipocytes secondary to anorexia over several days or of acute diabetes (the latter is not evident in this case).

If the GGT was also increased, other causes of cholangiohepatitis should be considered. These include bacterial or cellular infiltrates (e.g. plasmacytic/lymphocytic infiltrates), hepatic lymphoma or other neoplasia, extrahepatic biliary obstruction (bacterial, extrahepatic space-occupying lesion, choleliths), idiopathic cirrhosis or amyloidosis.

Marked hypokalaemia and hypophosphataemia at low levels may be associated with erythrocyte haemolysis (hypophosphataemia), hypokalaemic myopathy, enteric atony and vomiting, ventroflexion of the head or neck, and neurobehavioural changes that can mimic hepatic encephalopathy.

Slight increases in creatinine kinase are not an uncommon finding and can be seen with a struggling animal, difficult bleed, prior injections, etc and are generally not considered to be clinically significant.

A single lowered USG is not necessarily significant (especially in a well-hydrated animal), but the recommendations are to repeat this to see if it is reproducible. Lowered USG can also be associated with urinary tract infection despite a lack of active sediment. The 1+ proteinuria is likely due to the pH/blood. Lipiduria is a common finding in hepatic lipidosis.

In summary, the changes in biochemistry are characteristic of hepatic lipidosis. Hepatic lipidosis in cats is a common disease syndrome in North America and other countries in the northern hemisphere. It can be fatal if not treated rapidly. Overweight cats are at increased risk.

2 What further tests, laboratory or otherwise, are indicated in this case?

Confirmation of hepatic lipidosis can be made by means of liver ultrasound and fine needle aspiration (FNA) of the liver. A full coagulation screen is recommended prior to liver biopsy or FNA. Bile acids will not add anything to the clinical information at this stage as there is cholestasis, and this in itself will increase the bile acids.

FURTHER READING

Center SA (2005) Feline hepatic lipidosis. *Vet Clin North Am Small Anim Pract* **35**:225–269.

CASE 97

1 Discuss the laboratory findings and their significance.

The history is suspicious for HAC, although clearly not specific. GGT and GLDH are moderately increased, suggesting a degree of cholestasis and hepatocellular damage, although the bile acids are just within the normal range so there is no severe impairment of hepatic function. However, these kind of results for liver parameters are very common in apparently normal older horses and, on their own, should be interpreted with caution.

There is no evidence for impaired renal function. There is a moderate, mature neutrophilia, also consistent with HAC. There is significant hyperglycaemia, which is high enough to exceed the renal threshold and cause osmotic diuresis. Hyperglycaemia (secondary diabetes mellitus) is common in late-stage hyperadrenocorticalism and may be accompanied by glycosuria. Primary diabetes mellitus and hyperglycaemia associated with hepatic failure are rare in horses.

The urinary cortisol:creatinine ratio can be a useful screening test, although it is better used to eliminate the diagnosis (normal result) than to confirm it. However, the overnight dexamethasone suppression test is confirmatory. This test was previously considered to be the 'gold standard' test for HAC in the horse, although other tests (endogenous ACTH, insulin assay, TRH stimulation test, combined dexamethasone suppression/TRH stimulation) may also be used.

The ACTH assay is currently considered to be the standard for the diagnosis of HAC.

2 What is your interpretation, and what is the underlying cause for this condition?
It is consistent with equine HAC. This is most likely due to hyperplasia or adenoma of the pituitary gland resulting in PPID.

CASE 98

1 This haematology case is referred to you for review because your technician says that the Rule of 3 has been violated. What is the Rule of 3?
The Rule of 3 for veterinary haematology refers to the following:

$$\text{haemoglobin (g/l)} \times 0.003 = \text{haematocrit (l/l)} \pm 0.03$$

$$\text{Or haemoglobin (g/dl)} \times 3 = \text{haematocrit (\%)} \pm 3.$$

Haemoglobin is usually an accurate reflection of the oxygen carrying function of the blood. It is measured directly. Usually, the relationship between haemoglobin and haematocrit is maintained according to the above formula. For example:

If the haemoglobin is 86 g/l, then the haematocrit
$= 86 \times 0.003 = 0.258 \pm 0.03 = 0.228 - 0.288 \text{ l/l}.$

Or, if haemoglobin is 8.6 g/dl, then the haematocrit
$= 8.6 \times 3 = 25.8 \pm 3 = 22.8 - 28.8\%.$

If the haematocrit reported by automated analysis falls outside this interval, this represents a haemoglobin–haematocrit mismatch or violation of the Rule of 3. In this cat, the haemoglobin is 54 g/l, so the haematocrit = 54 × 0.003 = 0.162 l/l. As the given haematocrit is markedly higher than the haematocrit given by the Rule of 3, the rule has been violated.

2 What should be done if the Rule of 3 is violated?
If the Rule of 3 is violated (i.e. a haemoglobin–haematocrit mismatch is present):

● Look at the plasma to see if haemolysis is present. If so, this can result in a higher haemoglobin reading compared with the haematocrit because of *in-vivo* or *in-vitro* destruction of erythrocytes. If haemolysis is observed, determine if it is likely to be *in vivo* (true intravascular haemolysis) or *in vitro* (artefactual due to unbalanced centrifugation, excessively hot or cold temperatures, concurrent lipaemia or other factors) in origin. With haemolysis,

the MCHC is also often increased: MCHC (g/l) = haemoglobin (g/l)/haematocrit (l/l).
● Perform a spun PCV (microhaematocrit) to more accurately determine the haematocrit.

FOLLOW UP
Close observation of the patient's samples revealed haemolysis as the cause for the haemoglobin–haematocrit mismatch. A repeat sample was drawn, which did not show these alterations.

CASE 99

1 Describe and discuss the significant haematological findings based on the results provided and present in the blood smear.
There is a markedly regenerative, severe, macrocytic-hypochromic anaemia that likely accounts for the lethargy and reluctance to get up. Causes for regenerative anaemia include haemolytic anaemia (e.g. immune-mediated disorders, infectious disease, oxidative damage to erythrocytes, intravascular coagulation) or blood loss anaemia. Numerous poikilocytic erythrocytes, a marked anisocytosis, few to moderate polychromatic RBCs, moderate spherocytes and one nucleated RBC are shown on the smear. Spherocytes support an immune-mediated basis for the anaemia.

The anaemia is associated with a marked thrombocytopaenia. As no platelet clumps are reported, true thrombocytopaenia is likely. Possible causes include decreased platelet production in the bone marrow, shortened platelet survival due either to accelerated platelet destruction or platelet consumption or to infectious diseases (e.g. anaplasmosis, babesiosis, ehrlichiosis).

Moderate leucocytosis based on a moderate neutrophilia with regenerative left shift and moderate monocytosis is present. This pattern points to an active inflammatory disease (e.g. infection, inflammation, IMHA, necrosis).

2 What further tests would you recommend, and why?
To definitively diagnose the cause of the present finding and to gain insights into the cause of the immune-mediated disease, several further diagnostic tests should be performed:

● Blood smear evaluation to rule in/out immune-mediated disease. Erythrocytes have already been examined and spherocytes have been detected. Special attention should be made to the possible presence of erythrocyte agglutination or signs of oxidative damage of erythrocytes (e.g. eccentrocytes). New methylene blue staining may be necessary to evaluate

Heinz bodies, which are also a sign of oxidative damage. Platelets and leucocytes should also be evaluated. The size of the platelets may be important, as large platelets are a sign of platelet regeneration. Neutrophils may show signs of toxicity, which would point to an infectious disease. Finally, special attention should be taken in the search for infectious agents (e.g. *Babesia* spp., *Anaplasma* spp. or *Ehrlichia* spp. [minimum 15 minutes search]).

- Test for autoagglutination and/or a Coombs test to support immune-mediated disease. If autoagglutination is detected, a Coombs test is unnecessary. A negative Coombs test does not rule out the possibility of immune-mediated disease, but a positive test provides support for it.
- Tests for infectious agents: *Anaplasma*, *Ehrlichia* and *Babesia* PCR/antibodies.
- Others:
  ❏ Based on the haematological findings, immune-mediated destruction of erythrocytes is likely. IMHA should be further evaluated with the analyses recommended above. IMHA is often associated with marked leucocytosis with left shift. The left shift does, therefore, not necessarily point to inflammatory disease. However, as immune-mediated destruction of RBCs may also occur secondarily (e.g. due to neoplasia), the patient should be screened for further diseases via radiological and/or ultrasonographic examinations.
  ❏ Patients with IMHA are prone to thromboemboli or DIC. Thrombocytopaenia may be either a sign of an immune-mediated destruction of platelets in conjunction with immune-mediated erythrocyte destruction (Evans' syndrome) or a sign of coagulopathy with increased platelet consumption. Therefore, PTT and PT, as well as D-dimers, should be evaluated. If available, thrombelastography would give detailed information about the coagulation status of the patient.

CASE 100

1 Describe and discuss the significant biochemistry findings as well as the results of the urinalysis and measurement of the PTH serum concentration.

The most significant findings are a marked hypocalcaemia and a moderate hyperphosphataemia. In the absence of azotaemia, the combination of hypocalcaemia and hyperphosphataemia is strongly supportive of hypoparathyroidism, as PTH promotes absorption of calcium from the intestine, calcium resorption from the bone and phosphaturia. Hyperphosphataemia further enhances hypocalcaemia by inhibition of renal formation

of 1,25-dyhydroxycholecalciferol (calcitriol), which results in a decreased resorption of calcium from the intestine and absorption from the bone.

EG intoxication may also cause hypocalcaemia due to chelation and calcium deposition in the soft tissues. However, hypocalcaemia tends to develop later when hyperphosphataemia is severe. Moreover, EG intoxication causes a marked increase in osmolal gap (i.e. the difference between calculated and measured osmolality). A rough calculation of osmolality is made by the equation:

$$\text{Calculated osmolality} = 2 \times Na^+ = 2 \times 148 \text{ mmol/l}$$
$$= 296 \text{ mmol/l}$$

Thus, the osmolal gap = measured osmolality – calculated osmolality = 306 mmol/l – 296 mmol/l = 10 mmol/l (reference interval, near 0).

EG intoxication would be expected to cause a severe increase (>40–50 mmol/l).

Common causes for hypocalcaemia are laboratory errors such as mixing of the sample with air resulting in decreased ionised calcium concentrations or contamination of the specimen with EDTA because EDTA chelates calcium.

A slight hypomagnesaemia is also present. Hypomagnesaemia may be associated with hypoparathyroidism, which is the most likely diagnosis in this dog given the calcium/phosphate abnormalities. Increased diuresis results in hypomagnesaemia and is also possible in this dog as there is a decreased USG.

There is a slight increase in liver enzyme activities indicative of hepatocellular damage. The >2-fold increase in pancreas enzyme activities is suggestive of pancreatitis at the time of sample taking. Pancreatitis may also result in a hypocalcaemia and hypomagnesaemia; however, this would not explain the hyperphosphataemia. A borderline hyperalbuminaemia suggests slight dehydration.

The USG of 1.023 is considered to be too low in a slightly dehydrated patient. Decreased USG is indicative of impaired renal function. In this context it should be considered that there is evidence of inflammation of the urogenital tract (pyuria, microhaematuria, bacteruria, proteinuria). Bacterial toxins may interfere with the action of arginine vasopressin (AVP) at the V_2 receptor of the renal collecting tubule, resulting in reduced concentration of the urine. Thus, urine culture testing and antibiotic treatment should be performed.

The serum PTH concentration was 25 pg/ml (reference interval, 8–45 pg/ml). For interpretation it has to be taken into account that increased PTH concentrations would be expected in the face of a severe hypocalcaemia. Thus, plasma levels within the reference range are considered to be decreased in relation to the actual demand.

2 What diagnosis can be made based on the clinical and laboratory findings, and what is the prognosis?

The findings are consistent with relative primary hypoparathyroidism. The prognosis is excellent with proper treatment and management. Treatment is performed with dihydrotachysterol, a synthetic vitamin D analogue. Correct management of the patient requires close monitoring of calcium plasma concentrations every 1–3 months once the dog is stabilised.

Relative hypoparathyroidism is diagnosed if the PTH concentration is inappropriately low but remains within the reference interval. Absolute hypoparathyroidism is present if PTH concentrations below the reference interval are detected simultaneously with hypocalcaemia.

In people, hypomagnesaemia was reported to cause functional hypoparathyroidism; however, its significance is not known in dogs. In this dog, magnesium is slightly decreased. Slight hypomagnesaemia stimulates PTH secretion; however, a severe depletion results in a decreased PTH secretion, increases end-organ resistance to PTH and impairs calcitriol synthesis.

FURTHER READING

DiBartola SP (2005) *Fluid, Electrolyte and Acid-base Disorders in Small Animal Practice*, 3rd edn. WB Saunders, Philadelphia.

Feldman EC, Nelson RW (2004) Hypocalcemia and primary hypothyroidism. In: *Canine and Feline Endocrinology and Reproduction*, 3rd edn. Saunders, St. Louis, pp. 716–741.

Ralston S, Boyle IT, Cowan RA *et al.* (1983) PTH and vitamin D responses during treatment of hypomagnesaemic hypoparathyroidism. *Acta Endocrinol.(Copenh)* **103:**535–538.

CASE 101

1 Compare and contrast AKI and chronic renal failure in the horse with regard to common clinical presentation, common clinicopathological findings and prognostic indicators. (See Table below.)

Condition	Common Clinical Presentation	Categorisation of Mechanisms	Common Clinicopathological Findings	Prognostic Indicators
Acute kidney injury (AKI)	Usually referred for some other primary problem such as enterocolitis, colic, sepsis or rhabdomyolysis. Renal disease detected with laboratory work up for these conditions. May be oliguric, anuric or polyuric	Pre-renal: due to renal hypoperfusion. Renal: tubular necrosis, toxic insult, infectious, pigmentary nephroses (haemoglobin or myoglobin), vascular/ thromboembolic. Post-renal: obstructive urolithiasis or urinary bladder rupture with uroperitoneum	Increased urea, creatinine and phosphorus. Decreased USG (prior to fluid therapy), usually isosthenuric or <1.020. Increased renal fractional excretion of electrolytes. Hypocalcaemia. Hyponatraemia, hypochloraemia, particularly with polyuria; variable K+: oliguric or anuric, more likely hyperkalaemic; polyuric and anorexic, more likely hypokalaemic or normokalaemic	Response to therapy with resolution of laboratory abnormalities and clinical improvement
Chronic renal failure	Poor performance, dull hair coat may be early indicators. With progression, chronic weight loss, lethargy, anorexia, ± polydipsia/ polyuria, ± ventral oedema. GI/oral ulceration, soft faeces, increased dental tartar, uraemic (fishy) odour may develop late in course of disease with increasing azotaemia	Developmental or congenital disease: agenesis, hypoplasia or dysplasia; polycystic kidney disease: glomerular and/or tubular abnormalities. Glomerulonephropathy: immune-mediated, ischaemic, toxic, infectious, post infectious. Tubular and/or interstitial nephropathy: ischaemic, toxic, infectious, post infectious, pigmentary nephrosis, obstructive urolithiasis, idiopathic. Neoplastic (rare, usually unilateral). End-stage renal disease: usually not possible to determine initiating cause	Anaemia (usually mild and non-responding). Increased creatinine and urea. Decreased USG (prior to fluid therapy), usually isosthenuric or <1.020. Increased renal fractional excretion of electrolytes. Hypoalbuminaemia (<25 g/l). Hyponatraemia, hypochloraemia, hyperkalaemia, hypercalcaemia, hypophosphataemia. Increased urine protein:creatinine ratio (>3)	Good initial response to treatment and ability to maintain body weight or reverse weight loss usually good prognostic indicators. More favourable if initial creatinine <440 μmol/l at initial presentation. Often can be managed successfully for months to years. Guarded prognosis if creatinine >440 μmol/l but <880 umol/l at initial presentation. Indicative of significant decline in renal function. Variable outcomes. Poor prognosis if creatinine >880 μmol/l at initial presentation; generally do not survive for more than a few weeks

According to this classification, the veterinarian was correct and the horse most likely has chronic renal failure.

2 What is the underlying mechanism for development of hypercalcaemia in chronic renal disease in the horse?

Unlike dogs, horses do not develop renal secondary hyperparathyroidism with chronic renal failure. Horses absorb large amounts of dietary calcium in the intestinal tract and eliminate the excess as calcium carbonate (and to a lesser extent as calcium oxalate) urinary crystals. In horses with chronic renal failure, urinary calcium excretion is reduced and the magnitude of hypercalcaemia varies with the amount of calcium in the diet. Changing from a high calcium diet (such as alfalfa hay) to a lower calcium diet (pasture or grass hay) can help return serum calcium concentration to within the reference interval.

FURTHER READING

Geor RJ (2007) Acute renal failure in horses. *Vet Clin North Am Equine Pract* **23**:577–591.

Schott HC (2007) Chronic renal failure in horses. *Vet Clin North Am Equine Pract* **23**:593–612.

CASE 102

1 What is your analysis of these results?

The slight increase in RBC count, haemoglobin and haematocrit are consistent with dehydration and/or splenic contraction with excitement. Dehydration is considered likely based on the history of poor appetite and dysphagia, although nothing is noted in the history regarding water consumption. If dehydration is present, the total protein and albumin may be elevated, but rehydration is unlikely to drop these below reference interval.

The slight increase in CK without an increase in AST suggests acute muscle damage. With the history of colic this is likely due to rolling or recumbency.

The increase in total bilirubin is likely to be due to anorexia associated with poor appetite and dysphagia. Total bilirubin may increase up to 3 times the upper limit of the reference interval because of anorexia alone. The possibility of hepatic disease or post-hepatic disease appears unlikely owing to the absence of other abnormalities pointing to the liver. The slight increase in ALP may be due to continued bone growth in this relatively young horse or to intestinal disease associated with colic, weight loss and dysphagia.

The increase in urea may be pre-renal (dehydration), renal and/or post-renal in origin. The history of urinary tenesmus with increased urea suggests that post-renal origin should be a primary consideration. The absence of a concurrent increase in creatinine may reflect the extremely thin body condition with loss of muscle mass.

The low chloride is suggestive of sequestration of chloride because of poor stomach emptying associated with the dysphagia and colic.

2 What is your primary diagnosis?

Given the combination of severe weight loss, dysphagia, colic and urinary tenesmus, chronic grass sickness (also known as equine dysautonomia) is the primary consideration. Chronic grass sickness is a disease primarily of young horses (most aged 3–5 years) at grass and most presentations are in the spring. There is high mortality (approx 90%). This condition has been reported in multiple countries within northern Europe and in South America. There may be difficulty swallowing, colic, reflux of stomach contents, excessive salivation, muscle tremors and patchy sweating. Horses with less severe forms of the condition may suffer severe weight loss, dry mucous membranes and difficulty in swallowing. There is an increased prevalence of *Clostridium* spp. in the gastrointestinal tract of horses with this condition, but it is not certain whether this is a cause or a result of the disease. The condition arises because of paralysis of the autonomic nervous system of the gastrointestinal tract.

FURTHER READING

Mars J, Milne EM, John HA (2001) Liver and biliary system pathology in equine dysautonomia (grass sickness). *J Vet Med Series A* **48**:243–255.

Milne EM (1996) Clinical diagnosis and management of acute and sub-acute grass sickness; *Equine Vet Educ* **8**:71–73.

CASE 103

1 Why do these results rule out rodenticide toxicity?

The absence of prolongation in PT rules out rodenticide toxicity. Factor VII has the shortest half-life, approximately 6 hours, and as a result the extrinsic pathway (measured by PT) will be the first to show prolonged clotting time. Since the PT is not prolonged, rodenticide (anticoagulant) toxicity is ruled out.

The half-life of the other necessary factors are factor II = 41 hours, factor IX = 13.9 hours and factor X = 16.5 hours. As the toxicity progresses, the extrinsic, intrinsic and common pathways become affected and the partial thromboplastin time (aPTT) becomes prolonged as well. Because the circulating vitamin K-independent factors are not affected, there is a time lag of anywhere from 12 hours up to 7 days between exposure to the toxin and development of bleeding, which may be internal or external, including bleeding into joints, thoracic and abdominal cavities, the urinary system and/or the gastrointestinal tract.

2 What are your differential diagnoses, and why?
Differential diagnoses include:

- Haemophilia. Very rare in the cat and unlikely in a cat of this age without previous clinical signs related to bleeding.
- Factor XII (Hageman factor) deficiency. This condition does not result in clinical signs of bleeding, but may result in prolongation of aPTT. It is thought to be an inherited incompletely dominant trait.

FOLLOW UP
Factor analysis confirmed the presence of factor XII deficiency.

FURTHER READING
Green RA, White F (1977) Feline factor XII (Hageman) deficiency. *Am J Vet Res* **38**:893–895.

CASE 104

1 Describe and discuss the significant haematological and biochemistry findings, as well as the results of the fluid analysis.
Haematology is unremarkable apart from a slight lymphopaenia and monocytosis. With neutrophils being at the upper limit of the reference range, this pattern suggests corticosteroid effect (stress).

Biochemistry shows a slight hypernatraemia and hyperchloraemia, which are indicative of hypertonic dehydration, most likely due to pure water loss or loss of hypotonic fluid. There is a borderline increase in urea concentration. In the face of normal creatinine concentration, this finding is suggestive of gastrointestinal haemorrhage or pre-renal azotaemia due to dehydration.

A slight hyperproteinaemia is present and characterised by a slight hyperglobulinaemia. In a cat of this age, chronic inflammation is the most likely aetiology. Neoplasia (multiple myeloma, B-cell lymphoma) may result in hyperglobulinaemia, but this is less likely in a kitten than inflammation. Albumin plasma concentration is within the reference interval; however, given the evidence of dehydration in this patient it might be even lower. Albumin is a negative acute-phase protein and its hepatic production is downregulated in inflammatory processes. The albumin:globulin ratio is very low in this cat (0.45;

reference limit >0.8), further supporting a diagnosis of chronic inflammation.

A moderate increase in liver enzyme activities is indicative of hepatocellular damage. As GLDH is located within the mitochondria of hepatocytes, this enzyme leakage is indicative of hepatic necrosis. The SG and protein concentration of the thoracic effusion are compatible with an exudate or modified transudate. The nucleated cell count is low, resulting in final classification as a modified transudate. Non-degenerate neutrophils in low numbers suggest the absence of bacterial leucotoxin and therefore a sterile fluid.

2 What diagnosis can be made based on the clinical and laboratory findings, and what is the prognosis?
The overall picture is consistent with feline infectious peritonitis (FIP). The diagnosis was supported by a coronavirus RT-PCR from effusion fluid. Other features supportive of FIP are the lymphopaenia and decreased A:G ratio (<0.8). Protein electrophoresis was not done in this cat, but would be expected to demonstrate a polyclonal gammopathy in both the serum and the abdominal fluid.

The prognosis is poor as no successful treatment exists. Treatment has been proposed with recombinant feline interferon and prednisolone; however, this therapy scheme has proven to be ineffective in a controlled clinical study.

FOLLOW UP
Treatment was performed with drainage of the thoracic effusion, recombinant interferon omega and prednisolone, as reported previously. After 3 months, the cat developed signs of a non-effusive ('dry') form of FIP and was euthanised due to the poor prognosis. Diagnosis of FIP was confirmed by histopathological examination. Typical granulomas were present in all organs.

FURTHER READING
Ishida T, Shibanai A, Tanaka S *et al.* (2004) Use of recombinant feline interferon and glucocorticoid in the treatment of feline infectious peritonitis. *J Feline Med Surg* **6**:107–109.

Ritz S, Egberink H, Hartmann K (2007) Effect of feline interferon-omega on the survival time and quality of life of cats with feline infectious peritonitis. *J Vet Intern Med* **21**:1193–1197.

CASE 105

1 What is your analysis of these results?
The marked increases in muscle enzymes (CK and AST) support the presence of muscle damage. The absence of anaemia suggests that the red–brown discolouration

of the urine is more likely due to myoglobinuria than haemoglobinuria. Evaluation of the serum or plasma for discolouration suggestive of haemolysis is recommended. If the serum or plasma does not have red discolouration, this supports the presence of myoglobinuria. Electrophoresis of the urine may be considered to confirm myoglobinuria.

The slight increase in GLDH suggests slight hepatocellular insult. The moderate hyperglycaemia suggests severe stress and/or altered metabolism. Evaluation for possible lipaemia is recommended to determine if hyperlipidaemia may be present. The slight hypocalcaemia may be due to nutritional imbalance, decreased intestinal absorption or calcium binding by other toxins or plants or dystrophic mineralisation.

2 What are your differential diagnoses?

A variety of differential diagnoses, including bacterial toxins, plant intoxication, mycotoxins, rhabdomyolysis, ionophore (monensin) toxicity, nutritional (vitamin E/ selenium) myopathy or the acute form of grass sickness (dysautonomia), should be considered. However, given the history of involvement of multiple animals with acute death, the absence of exercise and high muscle enzymes with hypocalcaemia, hyperglycaemia and myoglobinuria are highly suggestive of atypical myopathy.

The condition of atypical myopathy is a frequently fatal sporadic myopathy of unknown origin in grazing horses. It may occur simultaneously with grass sickness. It appears to be triggered by climatic conditions, with cold and stormy weather. It has a rapid onset and typically involves multiple horses, although with varying morbidity and mortality. There is usually recumbency, stiffness or weakness and myoglobinuria.

CASE 106

1 What is your assessment of the arterial pH?

The arterial pH is decreased, therefore this is an acidaemia.

2 What is your assessment of the likely underlying aetiology for this arterial pH?

The HCO_3^- is decreased, so this is a metabolic acidosis.

3 Is there appropriate compensation for this condition, and what does it suggest?

Appropriate compensation for metabolic acidosis is predicted by the formula:

$$PaCO_2 = 1.54 (HCO_3^-) + 8.4 \pm 1.1$$
$$PaCO_2 = 1.54 (10) + 8.4 \pm 1.1$$
$$= 15.4 + 8.4 \pm 1.1 = 23.8 \pm 1.1 = 22.7 \text{ to } 24.9$$

The $PaCO_2$ is not decreased and is not in the range of 22.7 to 24.9, as would be expected if appropriate compensation is present. This supports the presence of a mixed acid–base disorder – a combined metabolic acidosis and respiratory alkalosis.

4 What might be the underlying causes in this patient?

Because of the increased anion gap, a titrational acidosis with loss of bicarbonate or introduction of an exogenous acid is suspected. The respiratory alkalosis component is likely due to an intrathoracic condition because of the low PaO_2. Therefore, we are looking for multiple problems in this patient that would result in loss of bicarbonate or a poisoning/ toxicity with concurrent ventilation/perfusion mismatch.

The respiratory alkalosis with low PaO_2 is consistent with intrathoracic origin. There are two general situations that result in development of intrathoracic respiratory alkaloses: (1) impaired diffusion of oxygen and CO_2 and (2) impaired pulmonary perfusion.

Equilibration of oxygen and CO_2 is impeded by conditions that alter the thickness or quality of the alveolar/ capillary barrier (e.g. pulmonary oedema, pneumonia). Unless very severe, impairment of oxygen and CO_2 diffusion results in CO_2 equilibrating between alveoli and blood while oxygen does not. As a result, oxygen concentration of arterial blood decreases, stimulating oxygen-sensitive chemoreceptors, which increase respiratory rate and depth. The increased rate and depth of respiration increases alveolar ventilation, decreasing alveolar CO_2 concentration. Increased alveolar ventilation does not significantly increase alveolar oxygen concentration because normal alveolar oxygen concentration is very close to that of ambient air. As alveolar CO_2 concentration decreases and equilibration of blood and alveolar CO_2 concentration continues, $PaCO_2$ decreases and respiratory alkalosis develops.

Also, when perfusion of the lungs is impaired, intrathoracic respiratory alkalosis develops unless perfusion is severely impaired, in which case respiratory acidosis develops. Decreased pulmonary perfusion results in decreased contact between pulmonary blood and the capillary/alveolar barrier and, hence, decreased CO_2 and oxygen equilibration. As a result, CO_2 (because of its more rapid equilibration) completely equilibrates but oxygen does not fully equilibrate, causing decreased PaO_2 and, subsequently, respiratory alkalosis, as described above for impeded oxygen and CO_2 perfusion.

FOLLOW UP

Thoracic and abdominal radiographs revealed severe pleural effusion as well as a broken pelvis, most likely resulting from the trauma of the car accident. Clinical chemistry revealed marked azotaemia, which may be accounting for the metabolic acidosis in this case. Unfortunately, the dog died before further examination could be carried out.

FURTHER READING

Dibartola SP (2012) *Fluid, Electrolyte and Acid-Base Disorders in Small Animal Practice*, 4th edn. Elsevier Saunders, St. Louis.

CASE 107

1 Describe and discuss the significant laboratory abnormalities, and discuss possible diagnoses.

The most striking finding is the moderate to marked hyperglycaemia, which is consistent with diabetes mellitus (DM). A differential diagnosis is stress hyperglycaemia, which, however, is not as common in dogs and does not result in such a high magnitude. Moderate glucosuria is consistent with hyperglycaemia. The concurrent ketonuria and acidaemia are consistent with DM and ketoacidosis. Moderate hyponatraemia is due to increased renal sodium excretion in conjunction with ketonuria (excretion of cations is increased because of the presence of non-absorbable anions in the tubular lumen). Shifting of water from intracellular fluid to extracellular fluid owing to hyperglycaemia leading to a dilutional hyponatraemia should also be considered. Slight hypokalaemia is most likely caused by increased renal potassium excretion due to ketonuria (same mechanism as sodium). Increased loss due to vomiting and decreased intake due to anorexia are also possible. Slight hypercholesterolaemia is described in patients with DM. Other causes could be cholestasis, but with normal ALP levels this is less likely. ALT and GLDH are mildly increased and indicate hepatocellular injury with leakage of cytosolic and mitochondrial enzymes out of the cells.

Blood gas analysis reveals a severe metabolic acidosis with respiratory compensation.

2 How is the anion gap (AG) calculated, and how do you interpret the AG in this case? What differential diagnoses do you have for the increased AG detected in this dog?

The body is always eager to maintain electroneutrality in the body fluids. Therefore, anions and cations are present in equilibrium. Diagnostically, several anions (most importantly Cl^- and HCO_3^-) and cations (most importantly Na^+ and K^+) can be routinely detected. There are several anions and cations that are not routinely checked. Therefore, a theoretical AG is present. The AG is calculated as follows:

$$AG = (Na^+ + K^+) - (Cl^- + HCO_3^-)$$

The AG in this patient is:

$$(Na^+ + K^+) - (Cl^- + HCO_3^-) = (139 + 3.1) - (106 + 9)$$
$$= 142.1 - 115 = 27.1$$

In health the AG ranges from 12–24 mmol/l in dogs. Calculation of the AG is useful to detect unmeasured anions leading to metabolic acidosis. An increased AG may be observed due to unmeasured lactate in the face of massive rhabdomyolysis, phosphate in renal insufficiency or ketone bodies in ketoacidosis. The latter is the cause for the increased AG in this patient. Foreign substances may also lead to an increased AG, such as EG intoxication, whereby glycolate and oxalate are formed by the liver and bicarbonate is consumed, leading to metabolic acidosis with increased AG. Intoxication with methanol, paraldehyde, methaldehyde or high dosages of penicillin are further examples of causes for increased AG acidosis.

CASE 108

1 Describe the laboratory abnormalities present as well as the bases for these. What clinical signs do you expect in association with this history?

Often, vomiting is the first clinical sign with xylitol toxicity. Moderate hypoglycaemia is present, which may lead to lethargy and weakness between 30 and 60 minutes following ingestion, although development of hypogly-caemia may be delayed up to 12 hours in some cases. Hypoglycaemia is due to rapid absorption of xylitol in dogs, with marked insulin release and subsequent hypogly-caemia. Rarely, some cases may present early with hypo-glycaemia, followed by hyperglycaemia. This is thought to be due to a Samogyi-overswing reaction that occurs with insulin overdoses. There may be subsequent diarrhoea, collapse and seizures associated with the hypoglycaemia.

There is a slight hypokalaemia (insulin-mediated shift of K^+ with glucose into the cell) and hyperphosphataemia (insulin increases cellular permeability to phosphate).

The increase in ALT indicates hepatocellular damage. If acute liver failure develops, this usually is within 12–24 hours of xylitol ingestion, but sometimes extending up to 72 hours following ingestion. Some dogs may not show hypoglycaemia prior to development of liver failure. The mechanism for development of liver failure is poorly understood, but has been hypothesised to be due to xylitol or its metabolites resulting in decreased ATP within the liver or production of reactive oxygen compounds that may cause cellular damage.

Dogs typically develop lethargy and vomiting, as well as petechiation or ecchymoses and gastrointestinal haemorrhage in association with a marked increase in ALT, a slight to moderate increase in total bilirubin, a slight increase in ALP and moderate hypoglycaemia (due to hepatic failure rather than xylitol effect) and slight to moderate hyperphosphataemia. Hyperphosphataemia appears to be a poor prognostic indicator.

Further laboratory abnormalities exemplifying coagulopathies are moderate to marked thrombocytopaenia and markedly prolonged PT and aPTT.

2 Would you expect this amount of ingestion to be toxic?

It is estimated that one or two pieces of gum could cause hypoglycaemia in a 10 kg (20 lb) dog. For granulated (baking) xylitol, one cup weighs about 190 grams. Dogs ingesting >0.1 g/kg of xylitol should be considered at risk for hypoglycaemia. At doses exceeding 0.5 g/kg there is risk of liver failure. It is possible that this dog has ingested a toxic dose of xylitol, so veterinary attention is needed.

CASE 109

1 What is your assessment of the fluid protein electrophoresis results?

There is a high concentration of total protein in the effusion, a large proportion of which is due to gamma globulin. There is a narrow band in the beta-2 region of the trace consistent with a 'point of insertion' artefact.

2 What is the most likely clinical diagnosis?

The most likely clinical diagnosis is feline infectious peritonitis (FIP). When gamma globulins are >32% of the total globulins and the total protein is >75 g/l, there is a high probability of FIP. Albumin <40% of total globulins and A:G ratio <0.81 also support FIP but have lower positive predictive values.

Other findings supportive of FIP include a polyclonal gammopathy in serum and lymphopaenia. A definitive antemortem diagnosis, however, requires biopsy of affected tissues ± immunostaining for feline coronavirus. Other possible causes of a pleural effusion should be ruled out.

FOLLOW UP

In this case, feline coronavirus RNA was identified in the pleural fluid, supportive of FIP.

FURTHER READING

Shelley SM, Scarlett-Kranz J, Blue JT (1988) Protein electrophoresis as a diagnostic test for feline infectious peritonitis. *J Am Anim Hosp Assoc* **24**:495–500.

CASE 110

1 What is your interpretation of these test results?

These test results are consistent with the presence of an ovarian remnant. The hCG has stimulated ovarian activity and ovulation, resulting in increased progesterone levels associated with the presence of a corpus luteum.

2 How does the hCG protocol and testing differ in the dog and the cat?

hCG protocols for ovarian remnant testing in the dog and cat are given below. Oestradiol is the hormone assayed in the dog, while progesterone is assayed in the cat.

Dog	Interpretation Guidelines
Testing should be done when clinical signs of oestrus are present.	
Take basal sample.	Basal oestradiol <10.0 pmol/l
Inject 200–500 IU hCG IV.	
Take second sample at 90–120 minutes following hCG administration.	Oestradiol >10.0 pmol/l suggestive of an ovarian remnant

Cat	Interpretation Guidelines
Testing should be done 1–3 days after onset of oestrus behaviour.	
Take basal sample.	Basal progesterone <3.0 nmol/l
Inject 500 IU hCG IM.	
Take second sample at 7 days following hCG administration.	Progesterone >5.0 nmol/l suggestive of an ovarian remnant (is often >15.0 nmol/l)

Note: Serum gel tubes should not be used because of possible interference/adsorption of hormones. Use plain red top tube for blood collections and promptly spin down and separate serum following clotting.

3 What result would you expect in this cat if you performed vaginal cytology?

Vaginal cytology showing progressive keratinisation of the squamous epithelium in dogs or cats exhibiting clinical signs of oestrus is consistent with oestrogen effect and provides strong support for the presence of ovarian activity if access to exogenous hormones has been ruled out.

FURTHER READING

Wallace MS (1991) The ovarian remnant syndrome in the bitch and the queen. *Vet Clin North Am Small Anim Pract* **2**:501–507.

CASE 111

1 What is the most likely explanation for the microcytic RBCs (decreased MCV)?

The MCV describes the size of the erythrocytes. The decreased MCV indicates that microcytic (too small) erythrocytes are present. Microcytic RBCs most commonly occur in patients with liver insufficiency (e.g. patients with portosystemic shunt) or in the face of iron deficiency. Microcytosis due to iron deficiency often has concurrent hypochromasia (decreased MCHC) and most commonly results from intestinal bleeding.

In this case, the cat shows slightly microcytic RBCs and slight to moderate thrombocytopaenia. As the MCV describes the mean cellular volume, the majority of RBCs already have to be microcytic for the MCV to be decreased. Therefore, small changes in the MCV may be important. Hepatic failure is unlikely in this patient, as no abnormalities in the biochemistry profile have been detected. In addition, the history and physical examination did not reveal melaena and hypochromasia is absent.

To find the reason for the microcytosis, it is necessary to look at the methodology of the haematology analyser, the impedance method (**Fig. 111.1**).

In an isotonic bath, blood cells pass through a small aperture from the anode side towards the cathode side, thereby displacing electrons. The electrons normally maintain a current through the aperture. If a blood cell displaces an electron, the current is interrupted, which creates a detectable voltage peak.

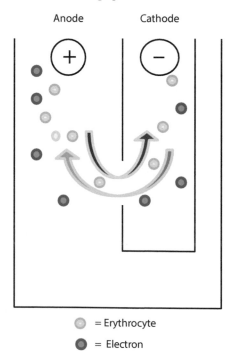

FIG. 111.1 Principle of impedance measurement.

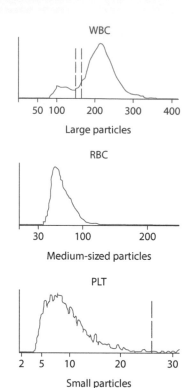

FIG. 111.2 Histogram of WBCs, RBCs and platelets in a cat.

An unremarkable graph displayed by an impedance analyser is shown (**Fig. 111.2**). The analyser differentiates the cells based on their size. WBCs, RBCs and platelets are displayed in separate graphs divided according to their size.

If microcytic RBCs are present, the shape of the RBC curve is no longer more or less bell-shaped but displays a dislocation to the left, where smaller particles are detected. Platelets are normally very small and displayed in the graph on the far right side. Especially in cats, platelets often tend to clump. Platelet clumps are larger in size than single platelets. As they do not have the right size to be recognised as platelets by the analyser, a false thrombocytopaenia results. Furthermore, platelet clumps may have the size of microcytic RBCs or even leucocytes and are therefore misclassified in this example as small RBCs by the analyser. This results in a falsely low MCV, as the analyser has detected microcytic 'erythrocytes' (which are really platelet clumps).

2 What further diagnostics can you perform to detect the cause of the microcytic RBCs?

In every case of thrombocytopaenia, the sample should be checked for the presence of platelet clumps. While some analysers are able to report clumps, the majority do not. Therefore, it is of central importance to evaluate a blood smear and search for platelet clumps. It is important to look for platelet clumps, which might indicate that the platelet

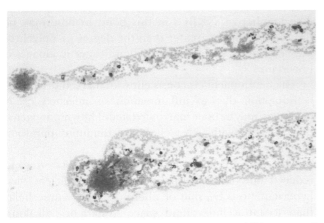

FIG. 111.3 Blood smear, feathered edge. In addition to small erythrocytes and moderate numbers of different leucocytes, several large platelet aggregates are visible. May–Grünwald–Giemsa, ×10.

count is artefactually decreased. Most often these are located in the feathered edge (**Fig. 111.3**) but they may also be present throughout the smear. If platelet clumps are seen, usually this is an indication that there are 'adequate' platelets. This means that platelet numbers may be within or slightly below the reference interval, but a marked decrease in platelet count that may result in spontaneous haemorrhage (usually $<20 \times 10^9$/l) is unlikely. The number of platelets can be estimated from the following:

Average number of platelets per hpf (×100 [oil]) × 20 = estimated number of platelets.

Or, if the average number of platelets per hpf (×100 [oil]) = >20, increased number; if 10–20, within expected limits; if 5–10, slightly decreased; if 2–5, moderately decreased; if <2, marked decrease.

In addition to searching for platelet clumps, the size of the RBCs should be evaluated and the pathologist should look for microcytosis.

FURTHER READING

Stockham SL, Scott MA (2008) *Fundamentals of Veterinary Clinical Pathology*, 2nd edn. Blackwell Publishing, Oxford.

CASE 112

1 How would you classify this anaemia? Give a possible explanation for this classification.

The decrease in RBC count, haemoglobin and haematocrit are indicative of a moderate anaemia. MCV and MCHC are within normal limits and there is no evidence of polychromasia. This is consistent with a normocytic-normochromic anaemia, which is commonly observed in pre-regenerative conditions (acute blood loss)

or in truly non-regenerative anaemia (bone marrow dysfunction, anaemia of chronic disease). Considering the history (no evidence of blood loss) and the results of the haematology (no evidence of pancytopaenia), an anaemia of chronic disease is the most likely differential. However, repeating the FBC in 3–4 days to assess the regeneration is recommended because reticulocytes are expected in peripheral blood about 3–4 days after erythropoetin stimulates marrow.

Anaemia of chronic disease is frequently observed in domestic mammals and is secondary to any chronic disorder with an inflammatory component. The main causes of this condition are:

- Shortened survival of RBCs.
- Impaired iron mobilisation or utilisation because of an increase in iron storage due to alteration of ferritin production and alterations in transferrin receptors. Moreover, there is internalisation of the protein ferroportin by cytokines with a consequent inability of macrophages to export iron.
- Impaired production of erythrocytes, which become refractory to increased erythropoietin because of the effects of inflammatory cytokines on precursors.

2 Give a possible explanation for the lymphocytosis.

There is a mild lymphocytosis and the lymphoid cells do not display any features of atypia. This may be a physiological lymphocytosis due to the shifting of lymphocytes from the marginated lymphocytes pool to the circulating pool or, more likely, may be due to chronic inflammation in response to chronic antigenic or cytokine stimulation.

3 Give a possible explanation for the thrombocytopaenia.

Thrombocytopaenia and macrothrombocytosis are frequently observed in this breed. It is an inherited platelet disorder, which is commonly not associated with any clinical bleeding problem. Platelet concentrations $<250 \times 10^9$/l may be observed in healthy CKCSs and be clinically not significant.

4 What is the microorganism in the BAL?

Pneumocystis carinii, an extracellular opportunistic pathogen, now classified as a fungus. It has been reported in humans, particularly associated with acquired immunodeficiency virus infection. It has also been reported in dogs, particularly in Miniature Dachshunds and CKCSs, as a cause of pulmonary infections. Several lightly basophilic cysts that contain up to eight intracystic basophilic bodies are shown in the cytology images. BAL cytology also showed a concurrent mixed inflammation.

5 What further investigations would you recommend?

Several studies show that there is a defect in immunity in CKCSs that underlies the susceptibility of these dogs to pneumocystosis. For this reason, measurement of immunoglobulins is recommended. A low IgG combined with a high IgM is a frequent finding in dogs with *Pneumocystis* infection. This is likely due to a selective defect in IgG production and to the inability of antigen-activated B lymphocytes to switch immunoglobulin class to IgG production.

IgM and IgG were measured on serum:

Analyte (units)	Result	Reference Interval
IgG (g/l)	**0.72**	10–20
IgM (g/l)	**2.3**	1–2

6 What is your overall interpretation?

There is evidence of bronchopneumonia caused by *Pneumocystis carinii* with a concurrent anaemia of chronic disease and lymphocytosis likely secondary to chronic inflammation. There is an underlying immunodeficiency disease with decreased production of IgG.

FURTHER READING

Stockham SL, Scott MA (2008) *Fundamentals of Veterinary Clinical Pathology*, 2nd edn. Blackwell Publishing, Oxford.

Watson PJ, Wotton P, Eastwood J *et al.* (2006) Immunoglobulin deficiency in Cavalier King Charles Spaniels with *Pneumocystis* pneumonia, *J Vet Intern Med* **20**:523–527.

CASE 113

1 Describe the abnormalities observed in these photomicrographs of the blood film.

The marked reduction in erythrocyte density is consistent with severe anaemia. Anisocytosis 3+, including macrocytes and rare microcytes. An abnormal erythrocyte morphology, including dacrocytes (tear drop-shaped cells), spindle-shaped erythrocytes and uneven distribution of haemoglobin in the RBCs, is observed. Numerous metarubricytes are seen. These changes can be seen with iron deficiency as well as with other causes of anaemia. Rare dyserythropoiesis is suggested by the nuclear/cytoplasmic asynchrony (i.e. large nuclei present in a fully haemoglobinised erythrocyte).

2 List the abnormalities detected in the laboratory profile and their potential associations.

There is a severe normocytic-normochromic regenerative anaemia. May be due to blood loss or haemolysis.

The number of NRBCs at this point in time may be disproportionately greater than the degree of polychromasia for other species, but the significance in alpacas is uncertain.

The neutropaenia is consistent with marked peripheral consumption due to inflammation or infection or, if persistent, may be bone marrow related. The lymphopaenia is consistent with stress/steroids. Immunosuppression cannot be ruled out.

The marked hypophosphataemia may be due to reduced intestinal absorption (phosphate-deficient diet, hypovitaminosis D), shift of phosphate from extracellular fluid to intracellular fluid space (respiratory alkalosis) or defective mobilisation of phosphate from bone (postparturient paresis [cattle], eclampsia [bitches] or renal disease [horses]).

The slight hypomagnesaemia may be due to hypoproteinaemia, inadequate intestinal absorption (including prolonged anorexia or poor feed intake, grass tetany in cattle) or excessive urinary loss. The slight hepatocellular necrosis is probably secondary. There is a slight non-specific hyperbilirubinaemia. The marginal hypoalbuminaemia may be due to an acute-phase response (inflammation), protein-losing condition, acute blood loss or a hepatopathy. Note that the combination of anaemia and hypoproteinaemia in camelids is less likely to be due to haemorrhage than in other species because both anaemia and hypoproteinaemia are common non-specific findings in most sick camelids.

Iron is increased but the farmer had already supplemented iron.

3 List differentials for regenerative anaemia in an alpaca.

The differentials for regenerative anaemia in alpacas are: chronic blood loss (e.g. parasitism); immune-mediated haemolytic anaemia; haemoparasite (*Candidatus Mycoplasma haemolamae*); haemolysis secondary to hypophosphataemia; bone marrow disorder.

Low plasma copper levels have been associated with anaemia in llamas, where the anaemia resolved with copper supplementation.

4 Explain the pathophysiological mechanism by which hypophosphataemia causes haemolysis.

The pathophysiological mechanism by which hypophosphataemia causes haemolysis is by impairment of the erythrocyte glycolytic pathway by depletion of ATP (phosphorus is needed to produce ATP in RBCs). Without energy from ATP the erythrocyte is unable to maintain its membrane pumps, shape or integrity. Increased fragility leads to erythrocyte haemolysis.

5 What other laboratory test would you like to perform to determine a potential cause of hypophosphataemia in this type of animal in the winter?

The further laboratory test to elucidate this condition would be serum vitamin D. Follow-up results (20.0 nmol/l [reference interval for adult alpaca, 39–437]) confirmed severe hypovitaminosis D.

DISCUSSION

The criteria for defining regenerative and non-regenerative anaemia are not yet clear in camelids. Anisocytosis, polychromasia, reticulocytosis and increased numbers of metarubricytes may all be seen with regenerative anaemia, but they are not consistently present (Tornquist, 2009). Mean reticulocytes for healthy normal alpacas are reported to be 1.4% or range from 12,000–79,000/µl. Up to 2–3 metarubricytes/100 WBCs may be seen in non-anaemic llamas. In an experimental model of regenerative anaemia, metarubricyte numbers were reported as high as 20/100 WBCs. But in another experimental regenerative anaemia study there was no increase in reticulocytes or metarubricytes.

Myelodysplastic syndrome is one of the differentials in this case given the involvement of multiple cell lines. Myelodysplastic syndrome can occur with an altered bone marrow environment. Human studies have identified that vitamin D plays a role in differentiating haematopoietic cells in the bone marrow and the production of cytokines by several cells in the bone marrow including mesenchymal, lymphoid and myeloid lineages. Hypovitaminosis D has been postulated to be the cause of myelodysplastic syndrome in an alpaca reported in the literature in Australia, where this case also originated.

The marked hypophosphataemia in this case is probably due to vitamin D deficiency. Vitamin D is necessary to facilitate intestinal absorption of phosphate and salivary-intestinal phosphorus recycling.

Exposure of the skin to ultraviolet light is necessary to produce vitamin D from cholesterol metabolites. Surplus vitamin D is then stored in the liver and used in the winter when ultraviolet light intensity may decline, particularly at the most distant latitudes in the northern and southern hemispheres. In humans, where populations with different skin types have migrated to different geographic locations, vitamin D deficiency is becoming an even greater problem. Iron deficiency can further exacerbate the problem because this can impair iron absorption of fat, vitamin A and vitamin D.

Hypophosphataemia is documented to cause haemolytic anaemia in cattle (post-parturient haemoglobinuria), dogs, cats and horses.

REFERENCE AND FURTHER READING

De Luca HF (1998) Vitamin D. In: *The Vitamins: Fundamental Aspects in Nutrition and Health*, 2nd edn. (ed. GF Combs). Academic Press, New York, pp. 155–187.

Judson GL, Feakes A (1999) Vitamin D doses for alpacas (*Lama pacos*). *Aust Vet J* **77:**310–315.

Manolagas SC, Yu XP, Bellido T *et al.* (1994) The role of vitamin D: a pluripotent steroid hormone: structural studies, molecular endocrinology and clinical implications. *Proceedings of the Ninth Workshop on Vitamin D*, Orlando, Florida, pp. 675–689.

Murray SL, Lau KW, Begg A *et al.* (2001) Myelodysplasia, hypophosphataemia, vitamin D and iron deficiency in an alpaca. *Aust Vet J* **29:**328–331.

Smith BB (1996) Hypophosphatemic rickets in south American camelids: interaction of calcium, phosphorus, and vitamin D. *Proceedings Postgraduate Foundation in Veterinary Science*, University of Sydney, **278:**202–217.

Tornquist SJ (2009) Clinical pathology of llamas and alpacas. *Vet Clin North Am Food Animal Pract* **25:**311–322.

Van Saun RJ (2006) Nutritional diseases of South American camelids. *Small Ruminant Res* **61:**153–164.

Van Saun RJ, Smith BB, Waltrous BJ (1996) Evaluation of vitamin D status of llamas and alpacas with hypophosphatemic rickets. *J Am Vet Med Assoc* **209:**1128–1133.

CASE 114

1 What is your assessment of these results?

The initial AST and CK results are consistent with the history of equine rhabdomyolysis syndrome (also known as azoturia). The declining results over the next week are consistent with the half-lives of these enzymes and the response to fluid therapy.

The biochemistry and urine results indicate AKI, with significant loss of tubular reabsorptive function resulting in the production of dilute urine and significant urinary loss of serum sodium and chloride and retention of serum calcium. While no myoglobinuria was noted at this time, it was considered most likely that the AKI occurred secondary to the rhabdomyolysis, with deposition of pigment casts within the renal tubules. The urea and creatinine declined with fluid therapy.

Further testing

Renal ultrasonography identified significant bilateral renomegaly with reduced corticomedullary definition in the right kidney. No evidence of hydronephrosis or urolithiasis was noted. The maximal renal arteriolar velocity was 60 cm/sec in both kidneys with a renal resistive index of 0.5 (60 cm/sec systolic, 30 cm/sec diastolic), indicating normal renal blood flow. No bacteria were isolated from a sterile catheterised urine sample obtained prior to starting antimicrobial therapy.

After 5 days the serum sodium and chloride concentrations had normalised, although the USG remained at 1.008. Further salt supplementation was then given in the feed as the mare had regained a moderate appetite. On day 7, the urea and creatinine concentrations had normalised and the intravenous fluid therapy (IVFT) was gradually reduced and stopped 24 hours later. Unfortunately, after a further 72 hours the mare was mildly dehydrated (PCV = 41%) and the serum creatinine had increased to 229 μmol/l. Furthermore, while the AST was still gradually decreasing, a second peak of CK activity was evident (4,289 U/l). No further abnormalities were detected on urinalysis with the urinary fractional excretion % for Na⁺, Cl⁻ and K⁺ all returning to normal; renal ultrasonography showed improved corticomedullary definition in the right kidney. Because of the increased creatinine concentration, IVFT was reinstated for a further 72 hours at maintenance rate and salt supplementation was withheld. After this second period of IVFT, the creatinine concentration returned to normal limits and was found to have stabilised, with normal values recorded 20 days from presentation.

Histopathological examination of muscle biopsies from the sacrocaudalis dorsalis medialis and the semitendinosus muscles demonstrated mild muscle fibre necrosis, consistent with recurrent exertional rhabdomyolysis. Periodic acid–Schiff staining was normal, with no evidence of polysaccharide storage myopathy.

The mare was discharged 21 days after presentation with strict exercise and dietary control instructions; the majority of the calorific content of the feed to be derived from fats rather than carbohydrate. It was recommended that, after a short reintroduction to light exercise, a serum sample be obtained to re-assess the muscle enzymes and the renal parameters, at which point further advice could be given as to the ongoing management of this case.

2 What is the most likely cause of the continued inappetence and lethargy in this mare?

The cause of the inappetence and lethargy was the development of AKI following an episode of severe exertional rhabdomyolysis.

3 What is the pathophysiological basis for myoglobinuric nephrosis?

The increased concentration of myoglobin in the blood following the rhabdomyolysis is thought to cause an obstructive form of nephropathy where the accumulation of pigment and sloughed tubular cells causes obstruction of the renal tubules, rather than true tubular necrosis. Furthermore, the pigment also has direct vasoconstrictory effects on the renal vasculature, further reducing renal

blood flow. By the time of presentation, because of the extent of the tubular damage, the mare had entered into a polyuric state, producing isosthenuric urine. The use of furosemide was indicated because of its effects at promoting renal clearance of the pigment, and so long as the fluid demands were met with IVFT, this was of no detriment to the mare. Ultimately, after a prolonged period on IVFT, the mare was able to regain sufficient renal function to maintain urea and creatinine within reference intervals. While this represents sufficient renal function, it does not give indications as to any resultant renal damage. Therefore, although the short-term prognosis in this case is favourable, the long-term prognosis will be more guarded, particularly if further episodes of rhabdomyolysis occur.

CASE 115

1 How would you describe the RBC morphology?

Erythrocytes are normocytic-normochromic. Marked spherocytosis is present (this may be difficult to judge in the cat, but the erythrocytes are very round and dense and smaller than the other erythrocytes). There are moderate 'ghost cells' indicative of haemolysis. There are a few Heinz bodies (which may be within normal limits for cats).

2 What is a strong indication for an immune-mediated anaemia in this case?

Erythrocyte phagocytosis by neutrophils.

3 What additional test could be useful?

Coombs test. A positive test provides support for an immune-mediated basis; a negative test does not rule out an immune-mediated anaemia.

CASE 116

1 Describe and discuss the laboratory abnormalities present. What are the bases for the changes that are present? How will the laboratory abnormalities change over the next few days if this is EG toxicity and it is left untreated?

Antifreeze contains EG, which is highly toxic for cats. Increased levels of EG within the blood are therefore expected with peak levels usually reached between 1 and 4 hours post ingestion. There is a moderate hyperglycaemia owing to inhibited glycolysis by EG metabolites. This abnormality occurs early after ingestion and persists if left untreated, as in this case.

Moderate hypocalcaemia is present. The mechanism here is chelation by metabolites of EG. In association with this, calcium oxalate monohydrate crystalluria is often present. Both findings may occur early after ingestion and persist if left untreated.

Moderate hyperphosphataemia is present, indicating that the antifreeze contains phosphate-containing rust inhibitors. In this case, hyperphosphataemia is seen early after ingestion. If the product does not contain the rust inhibitors, hyperphosphataemia may be seen within 24–72 hours following ingestion if the patient is left untreated and progresses to renal failure. Increased urea and creatinine concentrations, indicating decreased GFR and associated with renal failure and decreased elimination of waste products, are also present at this later stage of disease. AKI with oliguria/anuria is then often also accompanied by hyperkalaemia, as potassium excretion is impaired.

2 What findings would you expect in a blood gas analysis over the same time frame?
Decreased pH and decreased bicarbonate will result in metabolic acidosis in the blood gas analysis. Furthermore, an increased anion gap will be present. Both findings occur because of the presence of EG, which is an unmeasured anion/toxin. Multiple metabolites further contribute to the metabolic acidosis. These findings may also develop early after ingestion and persist if left untreated.

Within 1 hour of ingestion an increased serum osmolality and osmol gap can also be encountered.

3 What findings would you expect in an urinalysis over the same time frame?
Isosthenuria (USG = 1.008 – 1.015) or close to it can be expected within 3 hours of ingestion due to the PU/PD induced by EG within the blood. Granular casts originating from acute tubular necrosis are variably present.

As stated above, calcium oxalate monohydrate crystalluria is often present due to chelation of calcium and the effects of EG and its metabolites. Crystals develop within 3 hours (cats) and 5 hours (dogs) of ingestion. Monohydrate crystals are more frequently observed than calcium oxalate dihydrate crystalluria.

4 What is the prognosis for EG toxicity?
The prognosis is usually good with aggressive treatment following early detection (<8 hours post ingestion); if untreated, the prognosis is poor.

FURTHER READING
Stockham SL, Scott MA (2008) *Fundamentals of Veterinary Clinical Pathology*, 2nd edn. Blackwell Publishing, Oxford.

CASE 117

1 What are the crystals in focus in Figs. 117.1 and 117.2?
The focus is on large, colourless, 'battle-axe'-shaped crystals. They are a more rare modification of calcium oxalate monohydrate. Other modifications are boat-shaped, picket-shaped or Maltese cross-shaped crystals.

2 What are the crystals in focus in Fig. 117.3?
The focus is on calcium oxalate dihydrate crystals, which appear as very small to small colourless double pyramids ('envelope shapes').

3 What is clinically the most important cause of the concurrent occurrence of the two crystals?
The mixture of the two types of calcium oxalate crystals together with the clinical signs is highly indicative for EG intoxication. EG is an antifreeze with a sweetish taste. It causes AKI with hypocalcaemia and metabolic acidosis.

FURTHER READING
Ettinger SJ, Feldman EC (2010) *Veterinary Internal Medicine*, 7th edn. Saunders Elsevier, St. Louis.
Osborne CA, Stevens JB (1999) *Urinalysis: A Clinical Guide to Compassionate Patient Care*. Bayer Corporation, Shawnee Mission.

CASE 118

1 Describe the present laboratory abnormalities. What is the most likely diagnosis?
The most striking finding is moderate hypokalaemia. In association with the history, clinical signs and ultrasonography this is most likely due to increased aldosterone concentration and hyperaldosteronism. Normokalaemia may occur earlier in the disease or in cats with less severe hyperaldosteronism.

Mild hypernatraemia is present as water resorption occurs in conjunction with aldosterone-driven sodium resorption. Therefore, sodium may be normal or only mildly increased.

There is a mild azotaemia based on increased urea, creatinine and phosphorus concentration, reflecting pre-renal, renal or post-renal disease. Hypertension is frequently present in cases with hyperaldosteronism. This may lead to concurrent renal damage.

The mildly increased CK enzyme activity most likely reflects hypokalaemic myopathy.

2 What further laboratory findings are expected in this disease? What are their pathophysiological bases?
Further laboratory abnormalities that are expected with feline hyperaldosteronism include: increased urinary fractional excretion of K (aldosterone-driven loss of potassium); increased or high normal plasma/serum aldosterone in conjunction with hypokalaemia, systemic hypertension and an adrenal mass; increased urine aldosterone:creatinine ratio.

Blood gas analysis often shows metabolic alkalosis, which may result from increased hydrogen ion loss in the urine and movement of hydrogen ions from extracellular to intracellular space because of loss of K^+ ions.

3 What other disease(s) or condition(s) is (are) commonly associated with this condition in cats?

Hypertension, which may result in cardiac hypertrophy and renal damage; renal damage, which may result from hypertension; hypokalaemic polymyopathy from hypokalaemia.

FURTHER READING

Shulman RL (2010) Feline primary hyperaldosteronism. *Vet Clin North Am Small Anim* **40**:353–359.

CASE 119

1 Based on this history, how would you differentiate vomiting from regurgitation?

Vomiting: food is digested/partially digested, pH acidic (gastric juices), there is bile present. Regurgitation: food is normally undigested, pH usually alkaline, usually occurs immediately after eating. The history should confirm that the patient is truly vomiting and that the signs described are not associated with gagging, coughing, dysphagia or regurgitation, which may appear to the client as vomiting.

2 Give a list of possible differentials for the dog's chronic vomiting.

Gastrointestinal causes of chronic vomition include: dietary indiscretion (overeating or ingestion of rotten food/toxins); dietary intolerance or allergy/dietary changes; chronic gastritis/enteritis; gastric or duodenal ulcer; inflammatory bowel disease; intussusception; pyloric hypertrophy; gastric or duodenal neoplasia; gastric hypomotility disorder; maldigestion and/or malabsorption; hiatal herniation; gastric outflow obstructions occurring from space-occupying gut lesions (e.g. gastric or duodenal foreign body, mucosal hypertrophy, tumours [neoplasia] or polyps).

Infectious causes: *Helicobacter* spp. are commonly found in the stomachs of healthy dogs and cats and those with clinical signs of vomiting; *Salmonella* spp., *E.coli*, *Campylobacter* spp; viral (parvovirus or distemper); *Physlaloptera*; worms.

Systemic/metabolic diseases that may cause chronic vomiting include: chronic renal disease; hepatic diseases (hepatitis, cholangitis, cholangiohepatitis, hepatic neoplasia); diabetes mellitus (with/without ketoacidosis); hypoadrenocorticism (Addison's disease); acute/chronic pancreatitis or pancreatic neoplasia; megaoesophagus (congenital or acquired), oesophageal foreign body, oesophagitis,

or an oesophageal stricture; gastro-oesophageal intussusception; hypercalcaemia (toxic/humoral hypercalcaemia of malignancy) peritonitis; pyometra; septicaemia; drugs (digoxin, chemotherapy drugs, NSAIDS).

Miscellaneous causes: autonomic or visceral epilepsy arising from the limbic region; motion sickness, inflammation of the labyrinth or lesions of the cerebellum; blood-borne substances stimulating the chemoreceptor trigger zone, including certain drugs (apomorphine or cardiac glycosides), uraemic toxins, bacterial toxins, electrolyte, osmolar and acid–base disorders as well as a number of metabolic abnormalities.

3 Evaluate the laboratory data and give explanations for the abnormalities seen.

FBC parameters are within reference intervals. There is a lowered plasma protein, along with decreased total protein and albumin, which may suggest either decreased protein production from the liver, or a protein-losing nephropathy (PLN: e.g. amyloidosis and glomerulonephritis), or a protein-losing enteropathy (PLE: e.g. worms, bacterial infections [*Campylobacter*, *Salmonella*], protozoa [*Giardia*], inflammatory bowel disease, neoplastic bowel disease). Third-space shifting (into large body compartments such as chest and abdomen or gastrointestinal tract) is another consideration.

The simplest way to differentiate PLE from third spacing or PLN is to do a dipstick examination on the urine looking for proteinuria. The lowered total protein and albumin and negative proteinuria makes PLN less likely, although with the dilute USG (1.010) this cannot be completely ruled out; a urine protein:creatinine ratio may be considered to rule this out.

Slightly increased ALP, bilirubin and ALT can be seen in primary liver disease (cholangiohepatitis) and, possibly, gastrointestinal disease or pancreatitis. Differentials include hepatic neoplasia (especially lymphoma), chronic active hepatitis (Dobermanns), bile duct obstruction (extrahepatic mass, choleliths), amyloidosis and idiopathic hepatic cirrhosis.

Repeating liver parameters in approximately 5–7 days would help assess progress and may influence prognosis. Liver or abdominal ultrasound with aspiration or biopsy of abnormal areas may also be useful. A coagulation screen prior to liver biopsy is strongly recommended.

Bile acids may not add anything to the clinical information at this stage, as there is cholestasis, and this in itself will increase the bile acids. The bilirubinuria reflects the increased serum bilirubin.

A single lowered USG is not necessarily significant (especially in a well hydrated animal), but it is always recommended that this is repeated to see if the lowered USG is persistent. Lowered USG can also be associated with urinary tract infection, despite lack of active sediment, particularly with the few cells seen, as usually with dilute urine there is little sediment activity evident. Lowered USG may also be associated with gut/liver disease.

Overall, the results suggest PLE.

4 Discuss a diagnostic plan.

- Check for faecal occult blood, faecal floatation for parasites, wet preparations, faecal culture/serology/PCR for specific pathogens.
- TLI (fasted sample) to determine if pancreatic insufficiency may be present.
- Radiology – plain and contrast studies.
- Ultrasound.
- Endoscopy.
- Dietary trial: dietary intolerance or hypersensitivity has effects on mucosa, and affects the microbial flora.
- In cases of hypersensitivity, dietary trials for at least 4 weeks should be undertaken with hypoallergenic diets, which contain hydrolysed protein. Commercial diets are available that are less than 10 kd in size – this is below the molecular weight that triggers the immune response (e.g. Hills Z/D or equivalent). If there is no improvement after 4 weeks, then the problem is probably not hypersensitivity, but it may still be a sensitivity or intolerance. In these cases, a dietary trial with restricted-protein diets with increased soluble fibre may help with large intestinal diarrhoea. (e.g. Hills I/D or W/D or equivalent).
- Faecal alpha-1-protease inhibitor (α_1PI) activity is useful to rule in/out PLE; both dogs and cats with gastrointestinal protein loss have increased faecal α_1PI concentrations.

Dogs with gastrointestinal tract signs and slight hypo-proteinaemia (55–59 g/l) should be carefully monitored, and dogs with a total protein of <55 g/l should undergo intestinal biopsy. Biopsy may be contraindicated when there is severe hypoalbuminaemia (<15 g/l), as there is increased risk of biopsy site dehiscence of the intestinal mucosa.

PLE can be associated with a variety of disorders such as idiopathic inflammatory gastroenteropathies:

- Small intestinal bacterial overgrowth, now referred to as antibiotic-responsive diarrhoea.
- Foreign bodies.
- Gastrointestinal neoplasia (lymphoma or other).
- Intussusceptions (chronic lesions are often missed, and this is an important cause of PLE in juvenile animals).
- Infectious enteritis (i.e. viral, bacterial, parasitic and fungal, especially histoplasmosis and pythiosis).

- Intestinal lymphangiectasia. Chronic PLE of the dog characterised by insufficiency and marked dilation of the intestinal lymphatics. Impaired intestinal drainage caused by obstruction to normal lymphatic flow leads to stasis of chyle within dilated lacteals and lymphatics of the bowel wall and mesentery. Overdistended lacteals then release intestinal lymph into the gut lumen by rupture or extravasation, causing loss of plasma proteins, lymphocytes and lipid (chylomicrons).
- Adverse reactions to food.
- Sepsis.
- Hypoadrenocorticism.
- Immune-mediated diseases.

FOLLOW UP

On further work up the dog was found to have an intestinal lymphoma.

FURTHER READING

Elwood C (2003) Investigation and differential diagnosis of vomiting in the dog. *In Practice* **25**:374–386.

Graham KL, Buss MS, Dhein CR *et al.* (1998) Gastroesophageal intussusception in a Labrador retriever. *Can Vet J* **39**:709–711.

von Werthern CJ, Montavon PM, Fluckiger MA (1996) Gastro-oesophageal intussusception in a young German shepherd dog. *J Small Anim Pract* **37**:491–494.

CASE 120

1 Describe the findings visible on the blood smear. What is the most likely diagnosis in this patient?

The blood smear shows moderate anisocytosis (variable size of the erythrocytes) with several macrocytic-normochromic RBCs. Mild to moderate poikilocytosis (abnormal shape of the erythrocytes) based on some acanthocytes (arrows) is present. Furthermore, some Howell–Jolly bodies (small, eccentrically placed blue remnants of erythrocyte nuclei) can be seen. Macrocytic-normochromic erythrocytes in a male stray cat are highly suspicious for feline leukaemia virus (FeLV) infection.

2 State the underlying pathophysiological mechanism for the development of the non-regenerative anaemia.

The exact cause of the macrocytosis is not known, but accelerated erythroid regeneration, myeloproliferative disease or myelodysplasia are current theories. One differential for the normocytic-normochromic anaemia may therefore be FeLV-induced dyserythropoiesis. The only FeLV subtype responsible for abnormal/ineffective erythropoiesis is FeLV-C. The FeLV-C receptor is a haeme transporter, which physiologically exports free haeme out of the cell, as this would be cytotoxic if not included in haemoglobin. Binding of FeLV-C to the haeme transporter on colony-forming units (erythroid precursor cells) in the bone marrow inhibits haeme export. Subsequently, free haeme is trapped in the cell, leading to cellular destruction and loss of differentiation in the subsequent erythroid precursors. The final event may include erythroid aplasia. Less severe forms may include dysplasia of erythroid and myeloid precursors.

Howell–Jolly bodies are nuclear remnants in the RBC cytoplasm. This is mostly associated with dyserythropoiesis or accelerated erythropoiesis. Acanthocytes occur in the face of metabolic disease (renal, hepatic) or due to mechanical destruction of RBCs, such as microangiopathy. A biochemical analysis may be beneficial to gain further insight into the cause of the acanthocytes.

3 What diagnostic test can you perform to confirm the suspicion raised by the finding on the blood smear?

The most rapid and convenient test for evaluation of FeLV infection is an ELISA that detects the nucleocapsid protein p27 in plasma. The sensitivity and specificity of the test varies from 40% to 53% and 100%, respectively. While a positive test will confirm infection, a negative test may be false negative due to absent viraemia. These cases warrant further diagnostics to definitively exclude disease. PCR is generally used and is available in at least two variants: real-time DNA (provirus)-PCR or RNA-PCR. The first can quantify FeLV pro-viral DNA in a highly sensitive and specific way. Using RNA-PCR quantification of free viral particles is also possible.

FURTHER READING

Kaneko JJ, Harvey JW, Bruss ML (2011) *Clinical Biochemistry of Domestic Animals*, 6th edn. Elsevier, London.

Lutz H, Addie D, Belák S *et al.* (2009) Feline leukemia ABCD guidelines on prevention and management. *J Feline Med Surg* **11**:565–574.

Stockham SL, Scott MA (2008) *Fundamentals of Veterinary Clinical Pathology*, 2nd edn. Blackwell Publishing, Oxford.

Sykes JE (2010) Immunodeficiencies caused by infectious diseases. *Vet Clin North Am Small Anim Pract* **40**:409–423.

Thrall MA, Baker DC, Lassen ED (2004) *Veterinary Hematology and Clinical Chemistry*. Lippincott Williams & Wilkens, Baltimore.

Weiss DJ, Wardrop KJ (2010) *Schalm's Veterinary Hematology*, 6th edn. Blackwell Publishing, Ames.

CASE 121

1 What is your assessment of these findings?

The findings are consistent with marked hypomagnesaemia with moderate hypocalcaemia, moderate hyperkalaemia and borderline hyponatraemia.

2 What is the most likely clinical diagnosis?

The most likely clinical diagnosis is hypomagnesaemic tetany.

3 What are the physiological bases for these findings?

Hypomagnesaemic tetany in lactating cows is a complex disorder that occurs when cows graze lush green pasture with magnesium concentrations <0.2%, calcium concentration <0.3%, sodium concentration <0.15% and potassium concentration >3.0% on a dry matter basis. This occurs most frequently when pastures have been fertilised using potassium and nitrogen and when soils are naturally high in potassium and low in sodium. It may be exacerbated by previous feeding of hay or silage with a low magnesium content and minimal or no concentrates.

CSF Mg^{2+} concentrations are maintained relatively constant despite wide variations in serum or plasma magnesium concentrations. Hypomagnesaemia of <0.5 mmol/l may result in a decrease in the concentration of magnesium in the CSF to below 0.5 mmol/l and lead to hyperexcitability, muscle spasms, convulsions and death.

Magnesium is primarily absorbed from the rumen. Increased K^+ concentrations in the reticulorumen may result in decreased Mg^{2+} absorption. Intraruminal K^+ concentrations increase if herbage with high K^+ and low Na^+ concentrations are fed when cattle are deficient in sodium and the diet is changed from hay or silage or dry feed to lush pastures. High intraluminal ammonium ion concentration may also reduce Mg^{2+} absorption independent of that of K^+. High intraluminal ammonium ion concentrations occur following ingestion of herbage with high nitrogen and low soluble carbohydrate concentrations.

Many cows do not develop hypomagnesaemic tetany until blood calcium levels fall below 2.0 mmol/l. Other factors that may contribute include lack of shelter or husbandry that may result in reduced food intake in high-risk cows.

CASE 122

1 What is your analysis of these findings?

The slight increase in MCHC may be due to inaccuracies in haemoglobin or haematocrit determinations. (**Note:** MCHC = haemoglobin/haematocrit and/or slight haemolysis resulting in a lower than expected haematocrit compared with the haemoglobin.) It is unlikely to be of clinical significance, since the other measurands of the erythron are within expected limits.

The borderline leucocytosis is also unlikely to be of clinical significance, since the concentrations of the leucocytes in the differential are still within expected limits, but the possibility of developing or resolving inflammation cannot be ruled out.

Platelet clumping affects the platelet count, which should be considered as a minimal concentration. Platelet estimation on the blood film examination appears adequate.

The marked hyperproteinaemia and hyperglobulin-aemia may reflect inflammation, immune stimulation and/or neoplasia. The serum protein electrophoresis pattern is suggestive of acute and delayed (chronic) inflammation. Mildly decreased albumin represents a negative acute-phase response and, together with the marked increase in alpha-2 fraction, is often associated with acute inflammation. Marked increase in beta globulins also indicates an inflammatory response. The marked polyclonal gammopathy suggests chronic antigenic stimulation. In cats this is often associated with feline infectious peritonitis, feline immunodeficiency virus, inflammatory hepatopathy and enteropathies, parasitic infection or chronic infection. The possibility of an underlying neoplasia is not ruled out, although a monoclonal gammopathy that would provide the strongest support for B-cell-derived neoplasia is not seen.

The moderate increase in ALT and bilirubin supports the presence of hepatic insult. The increased bilirubin is most likely of hepatic or post-hepatic origin since no haemolytic disorder resulting in anaemia is identified. In this context, the marked increase in bile acids may reflect the cholestasis (downregulation/decrease of bile acids transport proteins on the canalicular membrane) and may not provide a reliable indication of the liver function.

The marked increase in CK supports muscle damage or catabolism.

The slight increase in amylase may be due to pancreatitis (although no increase in lipase is present), intestinal disease and/or decreased GFR (although no increase in urea or creatinine supporting decreased GFR is detected).

The high Na:K ratio with low normal K suggests there may be impending total body depletion of K^+ due to decreased intake (inappetence reported) and/or increased loss (not investigated above).

2 What additional testing might be of benefit in this case?
- Ultrasound evaluation of the liver and kidneys (evaluation of architectural features, possible focal abnormalities, portosystemic shunt, or other abnormalities).
- Aspirates of any abnormal areas detected on ultrasound evaluation.
- If renal enlargement is confirmed by additional imaging, aspiration of the kidney (investigate possible inflammation or neoplasia).

- Urinalysis (investigation of renal abnormalities, USG and possible PU/PD).
- Feline pancreatic lipase (investigation of possible pancreatitis).

CASE 123

1 How do you interpret the laboratory findings?
There is a mild normocytic-normochromic anaemia. The absence of significant anisocytosis based on normocytic-normochromic erythrocytes suggests a non-regenerative anaemia. Possible causes include acute blood loss anaemia (less than 3–4 days ago) or reduced or inefficient erythropoiesis. As no blood loss has been reported, this differential is unlikely. Reduced erythropoiesis takes place in the face of decreased erythropoietin concentration or bone marrow disorders. Ineffective erythropoiesis, in contrast, may occur in the face of destruction of erythroid precursors in the bone marrow or defective erythrocytes. Ineffective erythropoiesis may occur due to missing nutrients (e.g. iron, copper) or folate or cobalamin deficiencies. As cobalamin concentration is markedly decreased in this dog and required for DNA synthesis, this is the most likely reason for the anaemia. In addition, inherited cobalamin malabsorption due to a deficiency in the cobalamin/intrinsic factor complex receptor is reported in Giant Schnauzers.

Hereditary cobalamin deficiencies have been reported in Beagles, Border Collies and Shar Peis and in familial cobalamin malabsorption in Giant Schnauzers. Decreased cobalamin concentrations may also be seen with exocrine pancreatic insufficiency, intestinal bacterial overgrowth or ileal disease.

2 Describe the process from cobalamin ingestion to cobalamin absorption.
Cobalamin is a water-soluble vitamin and originally involves a group of substances with a porphyrin-like corrin ring that are bound to cobalt. What is normally referred to as 'cobalamin' is actually the substance 'cyanocobalamin'. Cobalamin is ingested with the food and thus enters the acidic environment of the stomach. There it binds to the R protein, also known as cobalophilin or haptocorrin. As this complex enters the small intestine, it also enters an alkaline environment. This increase in pH leads to a separation of the complex. Intrinsic factor, which then rapidly binds to free cobalamin, is secreted from pancreatic cells and in dogs also from gastric cells. In the face of exocrine pancreatic insufficiency, intrinsic factor is not adequately synthesised, leading to decreased cobalamin concentrations in serum. Intestinal bacteria may further consume cobalamin. This explains diminished cobalamin

levels in patients with small intestinal bacterial overgrowth. The cobalamin–intrinsic factor complex finally binds to its receptors (cubulin) in the ileum. A wide variety of ileal diseases (e.g. inflammation, villous atrophy or resection) therefore also lead to cobalamin deficiency in the body. Binding to the cubulin (the intestinal cobalamin receptor) leads to entrance of cobalamin into enterocytes and the portal blood, where cobalamin binds to its transport protein transcobalamin 2. Cobalamin is thus transported throughout the body. The basis for cobalamin deficiency in Border Collies has been shown to be due to cubulin deficiency.

3 How do cobalamin and folate interact?

Cobalamin acts as an important cofactor for methionine synthase, an enzyme that converts N^5-methyltetrahydrofolate to tetrahydrofolate. The latter is necessary for DNA synthesis. After uptake of dietary folate in the brush border of the small intestine, folate is converted to N^5-methyltetrahydrofolate in the blood. Commonly, N^5-methyltetrahydrofolate is abbreviated to folate in daily use.

Editors' note: There are commercially available genetic tests for hereditary cobalamin deficiencies for several breeds. Use of these tests may be of benefit in determining carriers and affected individuals and in making decisions regarding informed breeding of these individuals.

FURTHER READING

Fyfe, JC, Jezyk, PF, Giger, U *et al.* (1989) Inherited selective malabsorption of vitamin B12 in giant schnauzers. *J Am Anim Hosp Assoc* **25**:533–539.

Owczarek-Lipska M, Jagannathan V, Drögemüller C *et al.* (2013) A frameshift mutation in the cubilin gene (*CUBN*) in Border Collies with Imerslund–Gräsbeck syndrome (selective cobalamin malabsorption). *PLoS ONE* **8**:e61144. doi:10.1371/journal.pone.0061144.

Stockham SL, Scott MA (2008) *Fundamentals of Veterinary Clinical Pathology*, 2nd edn. Blackwell Publishing, Oxford.

CASE 124

1 How would you explain the initial high calcium?

There is a moderate increase in total calcium, confirmed by the concurrent increase in ionised calcium (the fraction of calcium that is not protein bound). Increases in ionised calcium may be due to: increased mobilisation from bone or absorption in intestine (primary hyperparathyroidism); increased vitamin D activity (hypervitaminosis D); decreased urinary excretion of calcium (renal failure); or idiopathic conditions (in the cat).

2 What additional test would you do?

PTH measurement may be helpful in order to identify primary hyperparathyroidism. This condition is frequently caused by a neoplastic condition of the parathyroid glands (commonly adenoma, rarely carcinoma), which induces an increase in PTH secretion. Increase in PTH causes hypercalcaemia through different mechanisms: (1) it enhances the release of calcium from the large reservoir contained in the bones; (2) it enhances active reabsorption of calcium and magnesium from distal tubules and the thick ascending limb; (3) it enhances the absorption of calcium in the intestine by increasing the production of activated vitamin D. PTH also reduces the reabsorption of phosphate from the proximal tubule of the kidney and enhances the uptake of phosphate from intestine and bones into the blood.

PTHrP can also be measured to exclude hypercalcaemia of malignancy, although there is no evidence of any neoplasia in the history. PTHrP is a hormone similar to PTH that is secreted by tumour cells in some neoplastic conditions (lymphoma, anal sac adenocarcinoma). For these reasons, PTH and PTHrP have been measured.

Analyte (units)	Result	Reference Interval
PTH (pg/ml)	**75**	20–65
PTHrP (pmol/l)	<0.1	0.0–0.5

3 What is your suspicion?

High calcium with low phosphate and high PTH are indicative of primary hyperparathyroidism. A small mass in the ventral neck was found during ultrasound examination. Surgical excision was performed. Histopathology was consistent with a parathyroid adenoma.

4 How would you explain the reduced calcium concentration after a few days?

The dog developed hypocalcaemia after surgery to remove the adenoma. This condition is frequently observed because parathyroid adenomas can cause suppression of the other parathyroid gland. The dog was given infusions of calcium gluconate, fed high-calcium diets and given supplemental vitamin D therapy. After 3 days the calcium levels were stable and within normal limits.

FURTHER READING

Skelly B, Mellanby R (2005) Electrolyte imbalances. In: *BSAVA Manual of Canine and Feline Clinical Pathology*, 2nd edn. (eds E Villiers, L Blackwood) British Small Animal Veterinary Association, Gloucester, pp. 113–134.

Stockham SL, Scott MA (2008) *Fundamentals of Veterinary Clinical Pathology*, 2nd edn. Blackwell Publishing, Oxford.

CASE 125

1 How would you describe this anaemia, and what are the possible causes?

There is evidence of a severe anaemia, which is normocytic-normochromic considering that the MCV and MCHC are within normal limits. This is indicative of a poorly regenerative anaemia because most of the RBCs in the circulation are mature (normal cell volume and haemoglobin content) and polychromatophils (high cell volume and low haemoglobin content) are very rare.

Severe normocytic-normochronic anaemia may indicate a pre-regenerative condition, which can occur in the first few days after haemolysis or blood loss because the marrow has not had time to produce reticulocytes. A persistent non-regenerative anaemia indicates a dysfunction of the bone marrow that is not regenerating a replacement population of erythrocytes. This condition may be observed in erythroid hypoplasia, marrow aplasia, red cell aplasia, myelofibrosis, myelitis, myelophthisis and erythroid hyperplasia with maturation arrest.

2 What further investigation would you suggest?

Consider repeating the FBC after 3–4 days to determine if regeneration has become apparent. If the anaemia is still non-regenerative, a bone marrow aspirate is recommended. In this cat a bone marrow aspirate was performed after a couple of days. There is evidence of a marked erythroid hypoplasia/aplasia with normal myelopoiesis and thrombopoiesis. The myeloid:erythroid ratio is 9 (reference interval, 1.2–2.2). This is consistent with pure red cell aplasia (PRCA).

3 Could FeLV infection be related to this?

Experimental infection with FeLV subgroup C virus can induce PRCA; however, this does not appear to be immune mediated and has been attributed to inhibition of early progenitor cells. This condition has also been rarely described in naturally FeLV-infected cats with PRCA.

4 What is your overall interpretation?

The marked erythroid hypoplasia in the bone marrow associated with a severe poorly regenerative anaemia in the peripheral blood is indicative of PRCA, which may have been triggered by/associated with FeLV infection. PRCA is a condition in which marrow suppression is limited to the erythroid lineage. It can be immune mediated, induced by virus or drugs or may be idiopathic.

FURTHER READING

Abkowitz JL (1987) Retrovirus-induced feline pure red cell aplasia. *J Clin Invest* **80**:1056–1063.

Weiss DJ, Wardrop KJ (2010) (eds) *Schalm's Veterinary Hematology*, 6th edn. Blackwell Publishing, Ames.

CASE 126

1 Describe and discuss the haematological abnormalities.

There is a moderate to severe normocytic-hyperchromic anaemia, which is highly regenerative. Regenerative anaemia occurs in the face of recent blood loss or haemolytic destruction of erythrocytes. As no external or internal blood loss was noted, this differential is unlikely. Haemolysis may also lead to an artificially increased MCHC based on the fact that blood haemoglobin is used to calculate the MCHC. Further differentials for an increased MCHC include lipaemia, pigments, severe leucocytosis, Heinz bodies or precipitated immunoglobulins. All of these conditions lead to spectral interferences in haemoglobin detection and therefore a falsely high MCHC.

Causes for haemolysis further include immune-mediated disease, infectious disease (e.g. *Mycoplasma*, *Babesia* or *Ehrlichia* infection), metabolic disease originating from the development of Heinz bodies or eccentrocytes, or inherited disease (e.g. pyruvate kinase [PK] deficiency or phosphofructokinase deficiency). As erythrocytes do not show poikilocytosis on the blood smear and infectious disease is not present, these differentials are unlikely. As this dog is quite young and a Basenji, hereditary PK deficiency should be the primary consideration.

2 Describe the underlying pathophysiology of the most likely cause of this dog's condition.

PK is one of the enzymes of anaerobic glycolysis (Embden–Meyerhof pathway) catalysing the conversion of phosphoenolpyruvate to pyruvate and thus producing ATP. In normal patients, PK is present in the R-isoform. Affected Basenjis display a single base-pair deletion causing a frameshift and truncation of the enzyme, leading to enzyme deficiency. Due to the missing conversion of phosphoenolpyruvate to pyruvate, metabolites prior to this enzymatic step accumulate and erythrocytes become ATP deficient. The erythrocyte membrane becomes defective and RBCs lyse. One of the metabolites accumulating in RBCs is 2,3-diphosphoenolpyruvate (DPG), the important enzyme of the Rapoport–Luebering cycle, also known as DPG shunt. DPG is important for haemoglobin affinity to oxygen. Increased DPG concentrations lead to decreased haemoglobin affinity to oxygen and a shift of the oxygen–haemoglobin curve to the right. As oxygen delivery to tissues is therefore facilitated, affected patients can cope more easily with the developing anaemia.

3 What other diagnostics can you perform to confirm your suspicion of disease?

A definitive diagnosis of PK deficiency can be made by confirming decreased activity of the R-PK isoenzyme. Some assays detect total PK enzyme activity, which is predominantly made up of M_2-type isoenzyme, normally only present in erythroid precursors. In addition to this assay, PCR testing for Basenjis is available, as well as for the West Highland White Terrier and the Beagle. Therefore, affected dogs as well as carriers can be identified.

Patients suffering from the disease may also show laboratory evidence of hepatic failure, as iron overload may cause haemochromatosis and liver cirrhosis. Finally, pancytopaenia may be observed if myelofibrosis develops, which can be confirmed via bone marrow examination (bone marrow core biopsy). The mechanism behind the development of myelofibrosis remains to be determined, unfortunately.

4 What other breeds may have this disease?

Basenjis are the most severely affected breed. Other breeds that may be affected are West Highland White Terriers, Beagles, Miniature Poodles, Cairn Terriers, Dachshunds, Chihuahuas and American Eskimo Toy Dogs. Cats may also suffer from PK deficiency. Breeds affected include Somali, Abyssinian and DSH cats.

FURTHER READING

Kaneko JJ, Harvey JW, Bruss ML (2008) *Clinical Biochemistry of Domestic Animals*, 6th edn. Elsevier, San Diego.

Stockham SL, Scott MA (2008) *Fundamentals of Veterinary Clinical Pathology*, 2nd edn. Blackwell Publishing, Oxford.

Weiss DJ, Wardrop KJ (2010) (eds) *Schalm's Veterinary Hematology*, 6th edn. Blackwell Publishing, Ames.

CASE 127

1 What is the most likely cause for the lymphopaenia?

The most likely cause for the lymphopaenia is stress or excess glucocorticoids.

2 What is the presumptive clinical diagnosis?

The presumptive diagnosis based on the clinical presentation and the biochemical findings is equine metabolic syndrome (EMS, sometimes known as peripheral Cushing's disease) (**Fig. 127.1**).

3 What are the four biochemical findings that indicate this disease most consistently?

The four findings that most consistently indicate EMS are hyperglycaemia, hypertriglyceridaemia, hypercholesterolaemia and hyperinsulinaemia.

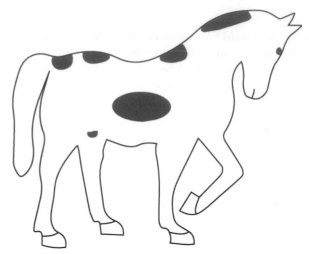

FIG. 127.1 Typical fat deposits found in equine metabolic syndrome. (Courtesy Dr Ernst Leidinger)

4 What calculated measurands can be used in addition to the measured ones?

The calculated measurands that can be used for the evaluation of EMS are:

- Glucose:insulin (G:I) ratio.
- Insulin sensitivity = reciprocal of the square root of insulin (RISQI) = $(\text{insulin})^{-0.5}$.
- Modified insulin:glucose (MIRG) = $800 - 0.30 \times (\text{insulin}-50)^2/(\text{glucose}-30)$.

If the G:I ratio and RISQI are positive, there is no need to calculate the MIRG.

Note: These calculations use conventional units for glucose (mg/dl). Glucose in SI units must be converted to conventional units for these calculations (glucose in mmol/l divided by 0.0555 = glucose in mg/dl).

EMS is likely if RISQI <0.32 (insulin resistance) and MIRG >5.6 and triglycerides >57 mg/dl (>0.644 mmol/l).

Other interpretative guidelines are:

- G:I ratio <4.5 = insulin resistant.
- G:I ratio 4.5–10 = compensated insulin resistance.
- RISQI 0.2–3.2 = compensated insulin resistance.
- RISQI <0.2 = failed compensation, high risk of laminitis.
- MIRG >5.6 = insulin resistant.

The link below is to a calculator that will calculate the RISQI and MIRG and provides some interpretation of the results: http://www.freil.com/~mlf/IR/ir.html (Accessed 1st February 2015).

FURTHER READING

Frank N, Geor RJ, Bailey SR *et al.* (2010) Equine metabolic syndrome. ACVIM consensus paper. *J Vet Intern Med* **24**:467–475.

http://www.ecirhorse.com/index.php/faq (Accessed 1st February 2015).

Kjelgaard-Hansen M, Mikkelsen LF, Kristensen AT *et al.* (2003) Study on biological variability of five acute-phase reactants in dogs. *Comp Clin Path* **12**:69–74.

Walton RM (2012) Subject-based reference values: biological variation, individuality, and reference change values. *J Vet Clin Pathol* **41**:175–181.

CASE 128

1 Is the CRP increase significant based on data on biological variation and reference change value (RCV)?

Based on published data on biological variation (see Appendix 2, p. 264), CRP shows an intra-individual (CV_I) variation of 24.3%, and an optimal analytical variation of 7.2% (CV_A). The RCV is defined as the difference between two serial results in an individual that is statistically significant based on data on biological variation. The formula to calculate the RCV is:

$$RCV = 1.96 \times \sqrt{2 \times \left(CVI^2 + CVA^2\right)} = 70.25\%$$

A difference of 70.25% of the result obtained in July (6.9 mg/l) is 4.9 mg/l. Therefore, the critical difference is located at 6.9 + 4.9 = 11.8 mg/l. As the CRP value in August exceeds the critical difference of 70.25% or 4.9 mg/l at this level, the result indicates a significant change in comparison with the previous result. An early acute-phase reaction may be present. However, as CRP is a major acute-phase protein in dogs, it may rise 10–100-fold in the face of systemic inflammation. As CRP is a sensitive but non-specific parameter and no clinical signs are apparent at the moment, the recommendation given to the practitioner is to closely monitor the patient.

2 What is the index of individuality (IoI) for CRP, and how do you interpret it?

The published IoI for CRP is 0.9 (based on the calculation ($[CV_A^2 + CV_I^2]/CV_G^2]^{1/2}$). While an IoI of <0.6 calculated with this formula inherits a low individuality and subject-based reference intervals can be safely used, an IoI of >1.4 would suggest the use of population-based reference intervals or the use of the RCV. The IoI of CRP is located between 0.6 and 1.4. Therefore, the use of population-based reference intervals is at least questionable. RCV and population-based reference intervals may be used simultaneously to ensure correct interpretation of a patient's result.

FURTHER READING

Fraser CG (2001) *Biological Variation: From Principles to Practice.* AACC Press, Washington.

CASE 129

1 What is your analysis of these results?

There is moderate anaemia that is likely the result of previous red maple leaf toxicosis with methaemoglobin formation and erythrocyte haemolysis. The slight leucocytosis with slight lymphopaenia and monocytosis is consistent with inflammation and/or stress.

The slight to moderate increase in total protein in conjunction with the history of anorexia and not eating and drinking is consistent with dehydration. The degree of anaemia may be worse than indicated since the haematocrit is likely elevated by dehydration. The albumin is within normal limits, but it may be elevated by dehydration and may be decreased if normal hydration status is achieved.

The slight increase in CK is a non-specific finding and may be due to muscle catabolism and/or damage. The slight increase in total bilirubin is likely due to anorexia. Increases up to three times the upper reference limit have been reported with anorexia. Previous haemolysis may also be contributing to the elevation. The hypocalcaemia may be due to decreased intake (anorexia) and is more common with AKI, while hypercalcaemia is more common with chronic renal failure. The moderate increases in urea, creatinine and phosphorus are consistent with a decreased GFR, which may be pre-renal, renal or post-renal. In this horse there is no indication of a post-renal origin. Dehydration (pre-renal) is likely contributing, but a renal cause is considered likely since the USG is <1.020 and reflects a decreased renal concentrating ability in the face of dehydration.

2 What are your differential diagnoses?

The primary concern in this case is AKI, likely due to haemoglobinuric nephrosis and hypovolaemic/hypoxic nephrosis secondary to red maple leaf toxicity. A dehydration (pre-renal) contribution cannot be ruled out and azotaemia would be expected to resolve with fluid therapy if the azotaemia is due to a pre-renal cause alone.

AKI in the horse may result in oliguria, as noted clinically (small amounts of urine produced). The distinction between pre-renal and renal causes of AKI is difficult and pre-renal causes may contribute to the development of renal nephrosis and/or necrosis, which precipitates the primary renal failure.

3 What abnormalities of Na⁺, Cl⁻ and K⁺ would you expect to find?

Hyponatraemia and hypochloraemia are expected. Horses with oliguric or anuric AKI may have variable K⁺ and hyperkalaemia may be present. Horses with polyuric renal failure may have normokalaemia or hypokalaemia.

FOLLOW UP

Fluid therapy was instituted and the urea remained increased at approximately the same level. Creatinine continued to rise over the next 2 days. The lack of improvement in azotaemia with fluid therapy provided further support for AKI. Euthanasia was elected because of the poor prognosis.

FURTHER READING

Alward A, Corriher CA, Barton MH *et al.* (2006) Red maple (*Acer rubrum*) leaf toxicosis in horses: a retrospective study of 32 cases. *J Vet Intern Med* **20**:1197–1201.

Geor RJ (2007) Acute renal failure in horses. *Vet Clin North Am Equine Prac* **23**:577–591.

Schott HC (2007) Chronic renal failure in horses. *Vet Clin North Am Equine Prac* **23**:593–612.

CASE 130

1 What are the granulated cells in the blood smear? What is your diagnosis?

In addition to a few erythrocytes and non-intact neutrophils, several mast cells can be seen. The diagnosis is mastocytaemia.

2 What diseases can lead to this finding on a blood smear?

Mastocytaemia can be caused by neoplastic, inflammatory or infectious diseases. Mast cell tumours in the skin or viscera or mast cell leukaemia may result in mast cells circulating in the blood. Inflammatory disorders may involve various organs (e.g. intestines, lungs, pancreas or skin). Mastocytaemia has been described in parvovirus infection, aspiration pneumonia and pancreatic necrosis. Infectious diseases, such as bacterial peritonitis and sarcoptic mange complicated by pyoderma, may also show increased numbers of mast cells in the blood. Other conditions that may result in mastocytaemia are tissue injuries, immune-mediated haemolytic/regenerative anaemia, renal failure if associated with inflammation and fibrinous pericarditis/pleuritis.

Because of the large variety of diseases potentially accompanied by mastocytaemia, mast cells in a buffy coat smear are not specific for mast cell neoplasia. Therefore, buffy coat examination for mast cells is currently not part of the routine staging of patients with mast cell tumours.

3 Briefly describe the hypersensitivity reaction of which these cells are a part.

Mast cells are an important part of the immediate type hypersensitivity (type 1) reaction, which can be divided into a sensitisation phase and an effector phase. Firstly, allergens (e.g. parasite antigens, insect venoms, bacterial products, viruses, narcotics, chemical agents) exposed to the patient bind to their antigen-specific surface receptor on B cells. B cells then engulf and process the antigen and finally present it on their major histocompatibility complex (MHC)-II molecules, initiating type 1 hypersensitivity reaction by activation of T$_H$2 cells. The function of these cells primarily involves activation of B cells via secretion of IL-4, IL-5, IL-6 and IL-13. Finally, IgE molecules are bound to the mast cell surface FcεRI receptors. The mast cell is sensitised. The effector phase is characterised by cross-linking of these bound IgE molecules, which leads to activation of three different signal cascades, finally culminating in the initiation of a local inflammatory response:

- Secretion of preformed granules (e.g. containing histamine) occurs, increasing local blood flow and vessel permeability.
- Intracellular phospholipase A$_2$ is activated by increased cytoplasmic calcium concentration and phosphorylation by mitogen-activated protein (MAP) kinase, resulting in production of arachidonic acid and finally cyclo-oxygenases and lipoxygenases. Mast cells therefore secrete prostaglandin D$_2$ and the leucotrienes B$_4$, C$_4$ and D$_4$ as well as platelet activating factor, which causes, for example, bronchoconstriction.
- The third signal cascade leads to augmentation of gene transcription factors such as NF-κB through activation of protein kinases. Transcription factors furthermore induce transcription of cytokines (e.g. interleukins of the T$_H$2-type and TNF).

The local inflammatory response is characterised by leucocyte infiltration, increased mucus production and increased blood vessel permeability. Prolonged marked inflammation will result in tissue damage.

4 Where do these cells originate from, and what stimuli lead to their final differentiation?

Mast cells originate from CD34+, c-Kit+ and CD13⁻ precursor cells in the bone marrow. Endothelial as well as epithelial cells and fibroblasts produce the stem cell factor, which leads to differentiation into agranular mononuclear cells. These circulate in the blood and finally migrate into connective tissues where final maturation occurs.

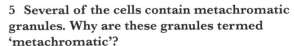

5 Several of the cells contain metachromatic granules. Why are these granules termed 'metachromatic'?

Metachromasia is present if an object (e.g. a mast cell granule) is not stained as anticipated with the dye used. The absorption spectrum of the mast cell granule then varies from the stained surrounding tissue. Mast cell granules are stained purple with methylene blue when they would be expected to stain blue. This phenomenon is called metachromasia.

6 List the three metachromatic dyes.

The three metachromatic dyes are toluidine blue, methylene blue and thionine. Wright's stain and Giemsa stain include metachromatic dyes.

FOLLOW UP

As neither overt clinical signs nor abnormalities in the erythron and leucon were visible, and marked signs of inflammation were not present, several differentials for mastocytaemia could be excluded. The skin tumour was examined using fine needle aspiration and revealed a mast cell tumour as the most likely cause for the haematological finding. Boxers are especially prone to mast cell tumours.

FURTHER READING

McGavin D, Zachary JF (2006) *Pathologic Basis of Veterinary Disease*, 4th edn. Mosby Elsevier, Philadelphia.
Stockham SL, Scott MA (2008) *Fundamentals of Veterinary Clinical Pathology*, 2nd edn. Blackwell Publishing, Oxford.
Weiss DJ, Wardrop KJ (2010) (eds) *Schalm's Veterinary Hematology*, 6th edn. Blackwell Publishing, Ames.

CASE 131

1 How would you explain the presence of rouleaux?

Rouleaux formation is common in some species, especially in horses because they have a negative erythrocyte membrane charge. Increased rouleaux tends also to occur if there is hyperglobulinaemia and hyperfibrinogenaemia, because these can further mask erythrocyte negative surface charge and allow contact of erythrocytes to form the characteristic 'stack of coins' appearance.

2 How would you interpret the anaemia?

There is a slight macrocytic-normochromic anaemia. In horses, regeneration cannot be assessed by polychromasia in the peripheral blood because the bone marrow does not release reticulocytes into the circulation. An increase in MCV may be an indication of a bone marrow response.

In order to assess the regeneration, bone marrow cytology was performed, which showed increased erythropoiesis from the stage of rubriblasts to the stage of reticulocytes. Myeloid cells showed orderly maturatation from myeloblasts to neutrophils. At this point the anaemia was considered to be regenerative. Regenerative anaemia is commonly associated with haemolysis or blood loss.

3 How would you explain the increase in total protein, and what tests would you recommend to further investigate this?

There is a marked hyperproteinaemia with a moderate hypoalbuminaemia and a marked hyperglobulinaemia. Hypoalbuminaemia may be due to decreased synthesis or increased loss. Considering the history of diarrhoea, protein-losing enteropathy is the main differential. This condition should be associated with a concurrent hypoglobulinaemia, which is not observed and is likely to be masked by an increase in globulins for other reasons. Hyperglobulinaemia is commonly observed in association with inflammation and B-lymphoid neoplasia. Serum protein electrophoresis (SPE) may be helpful to further investigate this.

4 Which are the main differential diagnoses?

SPE was performed.

Analyte (units)	Result	Reference Interval
Total globulins (g/l)	**112**	22–40
A:G ratio	**0.1**	0.6–1.5
Alpha-1 globulin (g/l)	0.8	0.6–2.1
Alpha-2 globulin (g/l)	5.4	5.4–7.9
Beta-1 globulin (g/l)	**47.4**	5.7–11.4
Beta-2 globulin (g/l)	**48.5**	1.8–7.2
Gamma globulins (g/l)	8.9	5.7–14.4

Increases in beta globulins alone are infrequent in most species and found in association with active liver disease and suppurative dermatopathies; occasionally the sharp monoclonal spikes of multiple myeloma, Waldenstrom's macroglobulinaemia or lymphoma are seen. Most of these differentials were excluded on the basis of clinical signs (no evidence of dermatopathy, lymphadenopathy or internal or external masses) and laboratory investigations (no increase in liver enzymes, unremarkable abdominal ultrasound, absence of neoplastic cells in the bone marrow).

In the horse, increased levels of beta globulins have been observed in SPE of serum from animals infected with the intestinal parasites *Stronglyus vulgaris* and *Strongyloides westeri*. The peak can appear as a monoclonal gammopathy or a polyclonal gammopathy, as seen in this case, in which an equine-specific immunoglobulin, IgG(T), is produced.

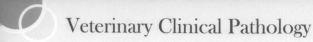

FOLLOW UP
Faecal analysis showed the presence of *S. vulgaris* ova in large numbers.

FURTHER READING
Kaneko JJ, Harvey JW, Bruss ML (2008) *Clinical Biochemistry of Domestic Animals*, 6th edn. Elsevier, London.

Stockham SL, Scott MA (2008) *Fundamentals of Veterinary Clinical Pathology*, 2nd edn, Blackwell Publishing, Oxford.

CASE 132

1 What samples are required to perform UFEE?
A urine specimen and a serum specimen are required. These should be collected at the same time. A diuretic should NOT be used to collect the urine specimen since a diuretic will alter the composition of electrolytes in the urine. The formula for calculation of % clearance for each electrolyte assessed is:

$$\% \text{ clearance-E} = \frac{[E]u}{[E]s} \times \frac{[Cr]s}{[Cr]u}$$

% clearance-E = % clearance of the electrolyte of interest; $[E]u$ = concentration of electrolyte in the urine; $[E]s$ = concentration of electrolyte in the serum; $[Cr]s$ = concentration of creatinine in the serum; $[Cr]u$ = concentration of creatinine in the urine.

2 What electrolytes are assessed?
Electrolytes assessed are sodium (Na), potassium (K), chloride (Cl) and phosphorus (Phos).

3 What are typical reference intervals for UFEE?
Each laboratory will need to establish reference intervals based on results from their instruments/methods. Typical reference intervals for UFEE are:

Electrolyte of Interest	Reference Interval (%)
Sodium	0.02–1.0
Potassium	15–65*
Chloride	0.04–1.6
Phosphorus	0.0–0.5

* Urinary fractional excretion of K will be influenced by diet. This reference interval was developed for horses on grain and grass-hay diet. High-quality alfalfa hay or lush grass hay may result in urinary fractional excretion of K as high as or greater than 150%. Results below 15% have consistently been associated with total body K depletion.

4 In what conditions might UFEE be helpful?
Conditions associated with alteration in UFEE are presented in the following table. Decreased % clearance-Na, increased % clearance-K, decreased % clearance-Cl and decreased % clearance-Phos are not of clinical significance or are precluded by the reference interval.

Alteration in UFEE	Conditions That Should be Considered	Other Expected Findings or Avenues for Investigation
Increased % clearance-Na	Increased dietary Na⁺	History of diet composition and/or supplementation
	Excessive salt block consumption (psychogenic salt eating)	History of rapid salt block consumption and observation of the animal; polyuria common
	Addison's disease (adrenal insufficiency with decreased aldosterone or decreased aldosterone effect)	Concurrent low or low normal serum Na
	Dehydration (hypothesised excretion of Na to normalise serum osmolality; possible altered gastrointestinal Na absorption with dehydration)	High (hypersthenuric) USG, increased serum protein and haematocrit; pre-renal increase in creatinine and urea possible
	Renal tubular insufficiency	Increased urea and creatinine, sub-concentrating or isosthenuric USG, proteinuria and glucosuria in the absence of hyperglycaemia also common
Decreased % clearance-K	Total body depletion of K	Investigate acid–base status and diet. Investigate GI disease that may result in decreased intestinal K absorption. May occur concurrently with myositis and/or laminitis (underlying mechanisms not clear)
Increased % clearance-Cl	Same as for Na	Chloride clearance is expected to show parallel alterations to % clearance-Na
Increased % clearance-Phos	Metabolic/developmental bone disease (secondary nutritional hyperparathyroidism)	Imbalance of calcium:phosphorus ratio in the diet; indicates need for calcium carbonate supplementation
	Renal tubular insufficiency	Increased urea and creatinine, sub-concentrating or isosthenuric USG, proteinuria and glucosuria in the absence of hyperglycaemia also common
	Multifocal recurrent lameness	Mechanism(s) unknown; suggest trial calcium carbonate supplementation should be instituted, regardless of dietary history
	Primary or pseudohyperparathyroidism	Hypercalcaemia with hypophosphataemia. May be difficult to differentiate primary hyperparathyroidism from chronic renal failure with nephrocalcinosis

FURTHER READING

Coffman JR (1981) *Equine Clinical Chemistry and Pathophysiology*. Veterinary Medicine Publishing Company, Bonner Springs.

Lefebvre HP, Dossin O, Trumel C *et al.* (2008) Fractional excretion tests: a critical review of methods and applications in domestic animals. *J Vet Clin Pathol* 37:4–20.

CASE 133

1 Fill in the empty boxes in the Table with the expected findings (prolonged [time], decreased [concentration] or unaffected).

The tests are influenced differently by the various deficiencies in the primary or secondary haemostasis and can thus complement each other in the diagnostic process.

PT is a widely used screening test for the function of the extrinsic pathway. The test is sensitive for deficiencies of factors VII, X, V and II and fibrinogen. Prolonged PT results can have several causes due to reduced production or consumption of functional factors. Disorders where this can occur include liver failure, rodenticide intoxication by vitamin K antagonists, malabsorption, increased globulin levels (i.e. multiple myeloma), DIC and congenital factor deficiency (VII, II or fibrinogen).

aPTT is a screening test of the intrinsic and common pathways. The normal range is strongly reagent and instrument dependent. Prolongation of the results can have several pathogenic mechanisms. It can be due to reduced production or consumption of one factor or a combination of factors. Disorders where this occurs include liver disease, rodenticide intoxication, DIC, malabsorption and congenital factor deficiency (VIII, IX, XI, XII, prekallikrein, high molecular weight kininogen [HMWK], X, V, II and fibrinogen) and congenital deficiency of von Willebrand factor (vWF) due to the reduced half-life of VIII. In addition, prolonged aPTT can be due to inhibitor substances that interfere with fibrin polymerisation, such as heparin, lupus anticoagulant and autoantibodies.

A low platelet count can have several causes. It can be due to decreased or defective platelet production, increased loss or consumption (extensive bleeding, DIC, thrombocytopaenic thrombotic purpura or haemolytic uraemic syndrome), platelet destruction (immune-mediated, non-immune-mediated or complex mechanism or pseudothrombocytopaenia (artefact or spurious).

Buccal mucosal bleeding time (BMBT) evaluates primary haemostasis. It is prolonged in the majority of cases with vWF deficiency and thrombocytopaenia. It has also been reported to be positive in dogs with severe azotaemia and it is usually normal in dogs with coagulation factor deficiencies.

Expected test results in various deficiencies/treatments are as follows:

Condition/Treatment	PT	aPTT	Platelets	BMBT
Thrombocytopaenia	Unaffected	Unaffected	Decreased	Prolonged
DIC	Prolonged	Prolonged	Decreased	Prolonged
Warfarin treatment/ poisoning or vitamin K deficiency	Prolonged	Prolonged	Unaffected	Unaffected
Aspirin treatment	Unaffected	Unaffected	Unaffected	Prolonged
von Willebrand's disease	Unaffected	Prolonged	Unaffected	Prolonged
Haemophilia	Unaffected	Prolonged	Unaffected	Unaffected
Uraemia	Unaffected	Unaffected	Unaffected	Prolonged

FURTHER READING

Lubas G, Caldin M, Wiinberg B *et al.* (2010) Laboratory testing of coagulation disorders. In: *Schalm's Veterinary Hematology*, 6th edn. (eds DJ Weiss, KJ Wardrop) Blackwell Publishing, Ames, pp. 1082–1100.

Russel KE (2006) Platelet kinetics and laboratory evaluation of thrombocytopenia. In: *Schalm's Veterinary Hematology*, 6th edn. (eds DJ Weiss, KJ Wardrop) Blackwell Publishing, Ames, pp. 576–585.

Tarnow I, Kristensen AT (2006) Evaluation of platelet function. In: *Schalm's Veterinary Hematology*, 6th edn. (eds DJ Weiss, KJ Wardrop) Blackwell Publishing, Ames, pp. 1123–1132.

CASE 134

1 What is the likely complication?

Shock, likely sepsis and DIC.

2 Interpret the TEG results.

The TEG tracing is very hypercoagulable as indicated by the low K time, high angle and high MA. The reaction time (R) is the time of latency (i.e. from the time blood is placed in the TEG analyser until initial fibrin formation), measured as an increase in amplitude of 2 mm; it is primarily related to plasma clotting factors and inhibitor activity. The clotting time (K) is the time to clot formation, measured from the end of R until an amplitude of 20 mm is reached; it is a measure of the time it takes from initial clot formation until a predetermined clot strength is reached, and is primarily related to clotting factors, fibrinogen and platelets. The angle (α) represents the rapidity of fibrin build-up and cross-linking, and is mainly dependent on the concentrations of platelets, fibrinogen and clotting factors. The maximum amplitude (MA) is a direct function of the fibrin and platelet bonding, which represents the ultimate strength of the fibrin clot. About 80% of MA is dependent on platelet number and function. Theoretically, all of the TEG parameters are influenced by abnormal haemostasis;

R and K values are increased and α and MA values are decreased in hypocoagulable states, and opposite changes are observed in hypercoagulable states.

3 Explain the pathogenesis of the complication seen in this patient.

In-vivo activation of coagulation is triggered by binding of factor VIIa to exposed tissue factor (TF), which is constitutively expressed on the adventitial cells and pericytes surrounding the blood vessels. Thus, tissue injury that disrupts the endothelial lining of the vessels is normally needed to activate coagulation. However, in inflammatory or pathological states, monocytes, endothelium and perhaps even platelets can be stimulated to express TF. TF binding of factors VIIa and Xa in turn initiates intracellular signal transduction pathways, which induce production of the transcription factors necessary for the synthesis of adhesion proteins, proinflammatory cytokines and growth factors. The activation of coagulation through endothelial damage, tissue damage or platelet/erythrocyte damage ultimately leads to increased thrombin formation. Thrombin cleaves fibrinopeptides A and B from fibrinogen, which is thus transformed to active fibrin monomers. Initially, the effect of thrombin is limited by endogenous anticoagulants, such as antithrombin or protein C. However, with massive activation of thrombin, the endogenous anticoagulants are quickly consumed and the ensuing systemic activation of thrombin leads to widespread fibrin polymerisation, with subsequent micro- and macrovascular thrombosis, which impedes blood flow and ultimately leads to ischaemia with further tissue and/ or organ damage.

CASE 135

1 How would you interpret this anaemia?

There is evidence of a moderate macrocytic-normochromic anaemia with marked evidence of regeneration on blood film examination (marked polychromasia, presence of NRBCs). This condition is commonly observed in dogs with blood loss or ongoing haemolysis and it reflects a bone marrow response to RBC loss/destruction. In view of the presence of spherocytes, autoagglutination and the absence of clinical evidence of blood loss, a haemolytic disorder is considered to be the main differential. The presence of autoagglutination and a positive saline agglutination test is consistent with immune-mediated haemolytic anaemia (IMHA). This condition may be primary (idiopathic autoimmune disease) or secondary (infectious disease, inflammation, neoplastic condition, or drug reaction). Clinical examination and history (no evidence of inflammatory sites or neoplasia or previous treatment) and negative serology (*Ehrlichia, Borrelia,*

Mycoplasma) excluded common causes of secondary conditions, making a primary IMHA the main differential.

2 How would you interpret the mild leucocytosis observed?

The mild leucocytosis plus mild neutrophilia and lymphopaenia are likely to be due to a stress response, which causes changes in leucocyte kinetics secondary to endogenous glucorticoid secretion. The slight increase in glucose is also considered to be stress related. This type of leucogram often accompanies IMHA and a left shift may be seen in some cases.

3 How would you explain the low calcium, and what additional tests would you suggest?

There is a marked hypocalcaemia, which may be due to several causes. The main differentials are decreased calcium mobilisation from bone or decreased absorption from the intestine, or increased urinary excretion of calcium. The absence of renal disease (normal creatinine and urea) makes the latter condition unlikely. Considering the concurrent increase in phosphate, decreased parathyroid hormone (PTH) activity was suspected. PTH is secreted by parathyroid glands and stimulates calcium resorption from bone and increases absorption in the intestine. It also causes increased urinary excretion of phosphate. A decrease in PTH secretion is a common cause of hypocalcaemia and hyperphosphataemia.

4 Give a possible explanation for this case.

There is evidence of a primary hypoparathyroidism and a concurrent primary IMHA. These pathological conditions may be unrelated, although a common generalised immune-mediated disorder has already been described and may be a possible explanation.

FOLLOW UP

PTH analysis was performed.

Analyte (units)	Result	Reference Interval
PTH (pg/ml)	**<10**	20–65

The PTH is below the reference interval. This is consistent with primary hypoparathyroidism, which is commonly associated with parathyroid damage secondary to trauma, surgery, neoplasia or inflammation. An immune-mediated cause is another possible differential.

FURTHER READING

Russell NJ, Bond KA, Robertson ID *et al.* (2006) Primary hypoparathyroidism in dogs: a retrospective study in 17 cases. *Aus Vet J* **84**:285–290.

Stockham SL, Scott MA (2008) *Fundamentals of Veterinary Clinical Pathology*, 2nd edn, Blackwell Publishing, Oxford.

CASE 136

1 How do you interpret the finding visible in Fig. 136.1?

Autoantibodies in IMHA frequently lead to the formation of agglutinates, even in blood placed in a tube containing anticoagulants (i.e. EDTA). The presence or absence of agglutination can easily be confirmed by placing one drop of blood on a glass slide. The non-homogenous, spotted (clumped) arrangement of erythrocytes is consistent with autoagglutination. In addition, icteric plasma is present, which may result from pre-hepatic, hepatic or post-hepatic disease. Haemolysis is a likely cause of increased bilirubin. An important differential finding for the agglutinates present on the slide is rouleaux formation, which may occur in the face of hyperproteinaemia and may mimic the formation of agglutinates on the slide.

2 Which additional test should be performed to confirm the finding?

A saline dilution test (diluted 1 part blood:4 parts saline) would be expected to result in resolution of rouleaux, but true agglutination will persist with saline dilution (**Fig. 136.2**). The presence of autoantibodies can also be confirmed by performing a Coombs test. However, the presence of autoagglutination invalidates the Coombs test and is sufficient for a determination of a likely immune-mediated basis for the anaemia.

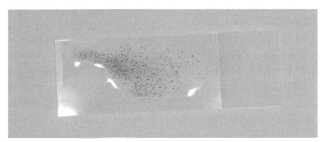

FIG. 136.2 Blood placed on a glass slide and washed with saline.

FURTHER READING

Weiss DJ, Wardrop KJ (2010) *Schalm's Veterinary Hematology*, 6th edn, Blackwell Publishing, Ames.

CASE 137

1 What abnormalities would you expect to find in blood work results if this dog has a coagulopathy secondary to angiostrongylosis (lungworm)?

Haematology, coagulation profile and biochemistry:

- Non-regenerative or regenerative anaemia. Red cell morphology may include aniso- and poikilocytosis because of DIC secondary to the infection.

- Leucocytosis consisting of neutrophilia, monocytosis, eosinophilia and occasionally basophilia caused by the verminous infection.
- Thrombocytopaenia, prolonged aPTT and/or PT, increased fibrinogen and increased D-dimer, all likely a result of DIC. Platelet count may be severely decreased if immune-mediated thrombocytopaenia is also present. BMBT may be prolonged because of a decrease in vWF but in some cases aggravated by thrombocytopaenia.
- Hypoproteinaemia if clinical manifestations of bleeding are present. In most cases hyperglobulinaemia and low fructosamine are present.

Urinalysis findings: usually no abnormal findings, occasionally proteinuria secondary to glomerulonephropathy.

2 What findings would you expect in a faecal examination, and what type of faecal testing is usually necessary to diagnose angiostrongylosis?

Larvae in direct smear may be present, although usually a Baermann test is necessary to confirm the presence of *Angiostrongylus* larvae.

3 What is the prognosis for the coagulopathy in angiostrongylosis?

Prognosis is usually good with aggressive treatment with early detection; if untreated, the prognosis is poor.

CASE 138

1 What is your interpretation of these findings?

The laboratory findings and clinical signs are due to marked thrombocytopaenia.

2 What is the relationship between the laboratory and clinical findings?

The finding of petechiae is consistent with thrombocytopaenia. Some animals will not have clinical signs of bleeding until the platelet count is $<5 \times 10^9/l$, while others will bleed when the platelet count is $<50 \times 10^9/l$.

3 What other clinical findings are commonly observed with this laboratory abnormality?

Other clinical findings that may occur with marked thrombocytopaenia include epistaxis, haematuria, melaena or haematochezia, oozing from the gums or sites of venipuncture, or ecchymoses.

4 Why is evaluation of the peripheral blood film critical?

Evaluation of the peripheral blood film is critical to rule out platelet clumping, which may result in a reduced automated platelet count, and to confirm the thrombocytopaenia by platelet estimate.

5 What is the significance of the few large form platelets seen in the peripheral blood film?

The few large form platelets suggest increased platelet turnover with increased platelet production.

6 What are your differential diagnoses?

Differential diagnoses for thrombocytopaenia include decreased bone marrow production, increased consumption and/or sequestration, and breed-specific conditions. Conditions to be considered include idiopathic immune-mediated thrombocytopaenia, tick-borne disease (*Ehrlichia canis, Anaplasma platys*), DIC, neoplasia, deep vein thrombosis and severe haemorrhage or thrombocytopaenia/macroplatelet syndrome in Cavalier King Charles Spaniels (although in this breed the platelet count is not usually dramatically decreased).

7 What is the most likely clinical diagnosis, and why?

Because of the marked degree of thrombocytopaenia, the most likely clinical diagnosis is idiopathic immune-mediated thrombocytopaenia. Other differentials do not tend to result in such profound thrombocytopaenia, but cannot be completely ruled out without further investigations.

FOLLOW UP

Serological results for tick-borne diseases were negative. There was no indication of other diseases on physical examination. The dog responded well to immunosuppressive corticosteroid therapy.

CASE 139

1 Describe the erythrocytes and make a diagnosis.

The erythrocytes display a moderate anisocytosis and slight poikilocytosis and few echinocytes; rare acanthocytes and shistocytes (not pictured) are present. Several protrusions are visible on the RBC membrane, which are highly suspicious for Heinz bodies, resulting from denatured haemoglobin. As more than 5% Heinz bodies are considered abnormal, Heinz body haemolytic anaemia is the most likely cause for the decreased haematocrit. In general, this type of anaemia is regenerative, as no bone marrow disease is present.

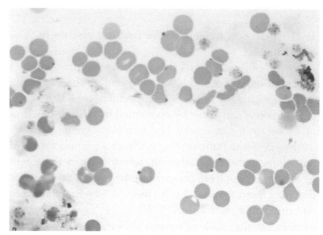

FIG. 139.2 Blood smear from a 7-year-old diabetic cat. New methylene blue, ×100 (oil).

The absence of polychromasia may indicate an early stage of disease.

2 How can you confirm your finding?

New methylene blue stain is used to definitively identify Heinz bodies, which are then visible as refractile structures on the RBC surface. An example of this stain is shown (Fig. 139.2).

3 Briefly describe the pathophysiological changes leading to this condition, including possible causes.

Heinz bodies are consistent with oxidative stress. Various causes have been described including ingestion of onions and garlic as well as administration of certain drugs (e.g. acetaminophen/paracetamol, vitamin K). In cats, diabetes, hyperthyroidism and lymphoma have also been reported as possible causes for Heinz body-induced haemolytic anaemia.

In physiological conditions, the pentose phosphate pathway (also known as the hexose monophosphate pathway) metabolises glucose-6-phosphate to 6-phosphoglycerate and ribulose-5-phosphate, thus generating two NADPHs. NADPH is essential to maintain glutathione in a reduced state. Reduced glutathione works as a free radical acceptor (e.g. from reactive oxygen species). It is therefore of central importance in the protection of RBCs from oxidative injury.

If the amount of oxidants overwhelms the antioxidative protective mechanisms of the RBCs, oxidation of Fe^{2+} to Fe^{3+} and therefore methaemoglobin formation takes place. Further oxidation of reactive sulphydryl groups of methaemoglobin, as well as interaction with oxidised glutathione, leads to irreversible formation of disulphide bonds between the globin chains of the haeme protein. A conformational change of the globin chain subsequently produces haemichromes, which bind to the anion exchange transporter band 3 of the RBC membrane. Thus clusters of copolymers form, precipitate and accumulate as denatured globin molecules. These denatured globin molecules are the Heinz bodies.

FURTHER READING

Kaneko JJ, Harvey JW, Bruss ML (2008) *Clinical Biochemistry of Domestic Animals*, 6th edn. Elsevier, London.

Stockham SL, Scott MA (2008) *Fundamentals of Veterinary Clinical Pathology*, 2nd edn, Blackwell Publishing, Oxford.

Weiss DJ, Wardrop KJ (2010) *Schalm's Veterinary Hematology*, 6th edn. Blackwell Publishing, Ames.

CASE 140

1 What is a sigma metric, and how is it calculated?

A sigma metric is a numeric value that characterises a method's performance in terms of the number of standard deviations or sigmas that fit within the tolerance limit or quality requirement of a test. For analytic processes, the sigma metric is calculated as:

$$\text{Sigma} = [(\%TE_a - \%bias)/\%CV]$$

TE_a = quality requirement for the individual test; CV = coefficient of variation for the individual test.

2 What is the relationship between the sigma metric and application of statistical quality control (QC)?

The higher the sigma metric, the more likely you are to be able to apply a simple QC rule with a low number of QC materials (n = 2–3), a high probability of error detection (P_{ed}) and a low probability of false rejection (P_{fr}).

A 3–4 sigma process often requires 'maximum' QC with a multi QC rule and a high number of QC material results (n = 4–6), and even then P_{ed} may be low. Highly skilled and experienced analysts with experience of analytical methods and instrument systems and a background in analytical quality management should be employed in order to help ensure production of accurate and reliable results.

For a laboratory test with a 4–5 sigma metric, a multi-rule with 2–3 QC materials is often needed to achieve a high P_{ed} and low P_{fr}. Skilled and experienced analysts trained in statistical QC and comfortable in dealing with method performance evaluation and data analysis should be employed in order to help ensure production of accurate and reliable results.

For laboratory tests with ≥5 sigma performance, a simple rule with 2–3 QC materials is usually adequate to provide a high P_{ed} and low P_{fr}. Because of this, less emphasis is placed on the need for skilled analysts to run these tests.

3 Why is knowing the sigma metric for a test important?

Knowledge of the sigma metric provides information about the performance capability associated with a process or a laboratory test. Greater than or equal to 6 sigma metric is considered to reflect 'world class' performance, while a 3 sigma metric is considered to be the minimum performance for a commercial test application. Knowledge of a sigma metric for a test at one or more levels of clinical significance is important since it:

- Allows comparison of tests across various instrument and reagent systems.
- Helps determine likely QC needs.
- Helps determine those tests that may require the most skilled and experienced analysts, those tests that may be in need of performance improvement and those tests for which alternatives should be considered.

FURTHER READING

Westgard JO (2001) *Six Sigma Quality Design and Control: Desirable Precision and Requisite QC for Laboratory Measurement Processes*. Westgard QC Inc., Madison.

CASE 141

1 Discuss the laboratory findings and their significance.

At the time of the first blood sample, CK would be at or near its peak (2–6 hours after damage) but AST would not have peaked (12–24 hours). At the time of the second sample, CK would be past its peak and AST around its peak. The near-peak values reached for each enzyme suggest only slight to moderate muscle damage, and the fact that CK is falling at 24 hours suggests a single incident rather than continuing damage. Overall, the findings are consistent with rhabdomyolysis.

The FE-K is low, suggesting depletion of potassium, which is known to be a predisposing factor to tying up in some cases. FE-Na is normal so sodium deficiency is unlikely to be contributing. Just measuring serum electrolytes rather than FE gives a lot less information, as they are usually normal in such cases.

Calcium was measured as hypocalcaemia is a differential diagnosis here, but it was normal (ionised rather than total Ca would have been better).

2 What would be differential diagnoses for increased FE-Na and FE-K in this horse?

Increased FE-Na: excessive dietary intake, dehydration, renal tubular insufficiency. Increased FE-K: renal disease.

CASE 142

1 Describe and discuss the significant haematological and biochemistry findings as well as the urinalysis.

There is a severe non-regenerative normocytic-normochromic anaemia, which is most likely caused by reduced renal erythropoietin synthesis because of chronic renal failure. Decreased hepcidin elimination by the kidney may also be a factor, resulting in decreased iron availability. A borderline monocytosis is of no clinical significance.

Biochemistry results show a severe azotaemia and hyperphosphataemia, which are suggestive of reduced GFR owing to pre-renal, renal and/or post-renal causes. Non-regenerative anaemia and isosthenuria suggest impaired tubulo-interstitial function and therefore primary renal disease. This is also supported by the presence of renal epithelial cells in the urine. Marked glucosuria in the absence of hyperglycaemia suggests defective renal resorption of glucose associated with damaged or abnormal proximal tubules.

Pyuria, haematuria and bacteriuria suggest infection of the lower or upper urinary tract. Ascending infection of the urinary tract is a likely cause of renal failure in this patient and urine culture and antibiotic sensitivity testing should be performed. Given the age of the dog, congenital renal disease should also be considered; however, histological examination of renal tissue would be necessary to further define the cause of the kidney disease.

Hypoalbuminaemia is moderate and probably represents urinary loss. Albumin is also a negative acute-phase protein and chronic inflammatory processes induce decreased hepatic albumin synthesis. The increased UPCR ratio points towards renal loss; however, as there is an active sediment, the elevation may also be due to haematuria and inflammation of the lower urinary tract. Thus, the UPCR should be re-assessed after treatment of the urinary tract infection.

Marked hypocalcaemia may be induced by three processes. High phosphate plasma concentrations result in formation of $CaHPO_4$ complexes with ionised calcium. Moreover, the high Ca^{2+} multiplied by PO_4^{2-} may cause metastatic calcification of tissues (including the kidney) and thus subsequent hypocalcaemia. Additionally, the increased renal phosphate excretion may be accompanied by excretion of cations including Ca^{2+}.

Slight hypochloraemia without concurrent hyponatraemia is likely due to metabolic acidosis with an increased anion gap caused by the severe hyperphosphataemia and azotaemia. Phosphate is an anion and therefore has the ability to act as an acid. Therefore, increased excretion of another anion (chloride) is an attempt to maintain electrical neutrality.

Vomiting may cause hypochloraemia by loss of a chloride-rich fluid; however, in this case hyponatraemia would also be expected.

The slight increases in ALT and GLDH suggest slight hepatocellular damage.

2 What diagnosis can be made based on the clinical and laboratory findings, and what is the prognosis for this patient?

The findings are consistent with a diagnosis of chronic renal failure and infection of the urogenital tract. The presence of anaemia is indicative of a poor prognosis.

Note: The differentiation between AKI and chronic renal failure is not always as clear as in this case. The poor body condition and anaemia point towards chronic renal failure; in many cases the differentiation can only be made based on the response to treatment and the results of follow-up examinations.

FOLLOW UP

This dog developed anuria and was euthanised because of the poor prognosis. Postmortem examination was performed and the histopathological examination was consistent with renal dysplasia.

CASE 143

1 Is a congenital coagulation factor deficiency likely in this case?

A congenital factor deficiency will not result in prolongation of the BMBT. Evaluation of secondary haemostasis by PT and aPTT analyses is needed to determine if a congenital factor deficiency is likely. Clinical signs associated with secondary haemostasis are often observed when a coagulation factor deficiency is present and include haematoma formation and bleeding into body cavities, including the joints. There is no indication of this type of bleeding in this dog.

2 What types of conditions can result in a prolonged BMBT?

Conditions that result in prolonged BMBT include thrombocytopaenia of any cause, platelet function defects (inherited or acquired) or problems involving the vascular wall or endothelium, such as vasculitis. Inherited platelet function defects include vWD, Basset Hound thrombopathia, platelet-dense storage pool defects in Cocker Spaniels, thrombasthenia of Otterhounds and Great Pyrenees, thrombopathia of Spitz dogs and cyclic haematopoiesis in Grey Collies (also causes thrombocytopaenia).

Drugs that have been associated with decreased platelet function include anaesthetic agents (halothane), phenothiazines, antibiotics (penicillins, sulphas, gentamicin), heparin antihistamines, anti-inflammatory drugs (aspirin, ketoprofen, ibuprofen, indomethacin, phenylbutazone) and calcium channel blockers (verapamil, diltiazem).

Tetracyclines, gentamicin and sulpha drugs impair platelet function *in vitro* but the clinical relevance is not known. Acepromazine, diazepam, ketamine, propofol and halothane impair platelet aggregation, while barbiturates and isoflurane do not. H1 and H2 blockers impair platelet aggregation. H2 blockers are frequently given to thrombocytopaenic animals with gastrointestinal haemorrhage because ulceration cannot be ruled out. Famotidine has less of an effect on platelets than either cimetidine or ranitidine.

Causes of thrombocytopathias that may lead to hyperresponsiveness or prothrombotic states include diabetes mellitus, HAC, nephrotic syndrome, hormone therapy, neoplasms and infectious aetiologies such as feline infectious peritonitis, and heartworm disease.

3 Does a BMBT within normal limits rule out the possibility of von Willebrand's disease in a dog?

A BMBT within normal limits does not rule out the possibility of von Willebrand's disease (vWD) in a dog. There may be some animals with vWD who have a BMBT that is within normal limits. If vWD is suspected or elective surgery on a Doberman Pinscher is to be performed, evaluation of von Willebrand's factor levels should be considered in order to definitively determine if vWD is present. A genetic test for vWD in Doberman Pinschers is available and can be used to determine a clear, carrier or affected status in bitches to be used for breeding. The BMBT is a general screening test. It can be done patient-side and provide a rapid result prior to elective surgery.

FURTHER READING

Jergens AE, Turrentine MA, Kraus KH *et al.* (1987) Buccal mucosal bleeding times of healthy dogs and of dogs in various pathologic states, including thrombocytopenia, uremia and von Willebrand's disease. *Am J Vet Res* **48**:1337–1342.

CASE 144

1 Describe the abnormalities and potential associations, and provide an interpretation.

There is a lymphopaenia consistent with stress/steroids or viral disease.

A moderate hypokalaemia can occur with vomiting/diarrhoea, increased renal loss, diuretic therapy or hyperaldosteronism. Slight hypernatraemia might be due to haemoconcentration, but there is no evidence of hyperalbuminaemia or increase in red cell parameters that would provide additional support for dehydration. There is a moderate to severe hepatocellular injury and necrosis with moderate cholestasis as indicated by increased ALT, GLDH and ALP enzyme activity. Marginal non-specific hyperbilirubinaemia and increased bile acids are consistent with hepatic dysfunction. Markedly increased CK and possibly part of the ALT increase are suggestive of severe muscle injury. Marginal hyperglycaemia is insignificant or stress related. TT4 is within the lower half of the reference interval, consistent with optimal treatment of hyperthyroidism.

Interpretation: hypokalaemic myopathy; moderate to severe hepatopathy.

2 Interpret the follow-up test result and discuss how you would distinguish between primary and secondary causes of this increase.

Markedly increased aldosterone is consistent with feline hyperaldosteronism. To distinguish between primary and secondary hyperaldosteronism it is necessary to perform ultrasonography to evaluate the adrenal glands, possibly test renin concentration and evaluate the liver (for potential cirrhosis) and heart and renal function.

Primary hyperaldosteronism:

- Adrenal neoplasia:
  - ❏ Plasma or serum aldosterone may range from 2 to 30 times the upper limit of the reference interval.
  - ❏ If due to adrenal neoplasia, an enlarged gland (9 mm to >30 mm) is usually identified on abdominal imaging.
  - ❏ Once other causes of hyperaldosteronism are excluded, analysis of plasma renin activity is not necessary.
- Adrenal hyperplasia:
  - ❏ Aldosterone increases are generally lower compared with primary adrenal neoplastic hyperaldosteronism.
  - ❏ Adrenal glands are often unremarkable on ultrasonography.

In this case it is important to prove that the hyperaldosteronism is primary and not secondary. This requires measurement of plasma or serum aldosterone (PA) and plasma renin activity (PRA) and calculation of the PA/PRA ratio:

- Aldosterone – high normal to slightly above the reference interval.

- Renin activity – below or within the lower part of the reference interval.
- Plasma aldosterone (pmol/l) to plasma renin activity (fmol/litre/second) is high and may range from 4.3 to 41.5. Normal reference interval is from 0.3 to 3.8 pmol/l.

Secondary hyperaldosteronism occurs when aldosterone production is increased in response to activation of the renin–angiotensin–aldosterone system, which can occur with congestive heart failure, severe hepatic dysfunction or renal failure. In contrast to primary hyperaldosteronism, the renin concentration will be increased in addition to the changes in aldosterone concentration. Further tests could include liver biopsy (first check coagulation), ECG, urea and creatinine levels, and USG.

3 Give advice regarding the special laboratory tests that may be performed during work up of this condition.
Aldosterone: plasma or serum; reasonably robust hormone (stable at 4°C for 5 days). Plasma renin activity: plasma; special handling requirements, which may include rapid freezing and transportation on dry ice; contact the laboratory prior to testing to establish their specific requirements; interpretation is difficult as enzymatic testing is dependent on testing conditions, which are not standardised; renin activity in humans may be affected by several drugs and the possibility exists that this may also be the case in cats, but further investigation is required.

FURTHER READING
Chiaramonte D, Greco DS (2007) Feline adrenal disorders. *Clin Tech Small Anim Pract* **22**:26–31.
Gunn-Moore D (2005) Feline endocrinopathies. *Vet Clin North Am Small Anim Pract* **35**:171–210.
Schulman RL (2010) Feline primary hyperaldosteronism. *Vet Clin North Am Small Anim Pract* **40**:353–359.
Shiel R, Mooney C (2007) Diagnosis and management of primary hyperaldosteronism in cats. *In Practice* **29**:194–201.
Yu S, Morris JG (1998) Plasma aldosterone concentration in cats. *Vet J* **155**:63–68.

CASE 145

1 What are the round structures besides the erythrocytes represented in the smear?
Erythroid loops, which are often in annular forms but are sometimes disrupted and appear as thin, linear, occasionally convoluted, pale blue bands. Erythroid loops are observed in blood smears prepared

immediately after a viper bite and 24 and 48 hours after envenomation.

2 What is the most probable pathogenic mechanism of formation?
Although no ultrastructural studies were done to clarify the pathogenesis, the structures suggested erythrocyte membrane fragmentation, with loss of haemoglobin, and probably formation of remnants of membrane resulting from intravascular haemolysis.

3 What other cells are associated with these structures?
Echinocytes, spherocytes and erythrocyte ghosts; the phospholipase A2 of the viper venom is responsible both for the morphological changes and the intravascular haemolysis.

FURTHER READING
Masserdotti C (2009) Unusual erythroid loops in canine blood smears after viper-bite envenomation. *J Vet Clin Pathol* **38**:321–325.

CASE 146

1 What number of RBCs is usually needed to see gross discolouration of the urine?
Normal urine samples may contain up to approximately 5 RBCs/hpf (×40) or approximately 5,000 RBCs/ml (range may extend up to 10,000 RBCs/ml). Microscopic haematuria (not visible grossly) may include from 10–2,500 RBCs/hpf or 10,000–2,500,000 RBCs/ml. This may correspond to dipstick findings of trace to +++ RBCs. Gross (macroscopic) haematuria corresponds to >2,500,000 to 5,000,000 RBCs/ml or 2,500–5,000 RBCs/hpf (usually designated as too numerous to count).

2 Why is cloudy urine within expected limits in the horse?
Cloudy or turbid urine is expected in the horse owing to the presence of mucus and expected finding of calcium carbonate and/or calcium oxalate dihydrate crystalluria.

3 Why might additional knowledge about when during urination the haemorrhage is observed be of benefit?
If haematuria occurs throughout urination, the origin may be from the kidneys, ureters and/or urinary bladder. If haematuria occurs at the start of urination, this is likely to reflect origin from the distal urethra. If haematuria occurs at the end of urination, this is most likely to be from the proximal urethra or bladder neck.

4 What are the differential diagnoses for discoloured urine in the horse, and what clinical and/or pathological findings may be helpful in their differentiation?

Differential diagnoses for discoloured urine in the horse and clinical and/or pathological findings that may be helpful in their differentiation are:

- Myoglobinuria. Serum clear (not discoloured), increased CK/AST, clinical signs of muscle pain, urine electrophoresis may help differentiate myglobinuria from haemoglobinuria.
- Haemoglobinuria. Serum ± haemolytic (haemolysed if intravascular haemolysis; RBC ghosts in urine may occur if RBCs have lysed, releasing haemoglobin) ± anaemia (may be present with significant intravascular haemolysis and/or urinary tract haemorrhage of any cause). Intravascular haemolysis may be associated with babesiosis, trypansomiasis or immune-mediated haemolytic anaemia (idiopathic, paraneoplastic or drug induced).
- Oxidised urine caratenoid or other pigments. May occur with exposure of urine to the environment; often apparent in patches of urination in snow or in environment where easily seen by the owner following, but not during, urination.
- Haematuria. May occur with coagulopathy (hepatic insufficiency, DIC, haemophilia) or with urolithiasis, drug toxicity, urinary tract infection, neoplasia, exercise-induced haematuria, proximal urethral tears or renal haemorrhage.
- Coagulopathy. Assess for underlying disease or congenital condition (haemophilia). Evaluate coagulation profile (PT, aPTT, platelet count, peripheral blood film); biochemistry, urinalysis and cytology may help determine if underlying disease is present. Determine if drugs that may interfere with coagulation have been administered.
- Urolithiasis. Rectal palpation, ultrasound and/or urinary tract endoscopy may be helpful for diagnosis.
- Drug/toxicity. Evaluate history, environment and possible access or exposure to drugs or toxins.
- Neoplasia. Evaluate various body systems and organs.
- Urinary tract infection. Examine urine sediment; quantitative urine culture.
- Exercise-induced haematuria. Usually microscopic, occasional gross haematuria. Urinary endoscopy may be helpful to determine if mucosal erosions or ulcerations are present. Diagnosis of exclusion (other possible causes should be excluded). Correlate with periods of exercise.
- Proximal urethral tears. Haemorrhage usually at end of urination and bright red blood. Reported in Quarter horses, Paints and Quarter horse-crosses. Video-endoscopy may be required for demonstration of urethral tears.
- Renal haemorrhage. Usually sudden onset of gross haematuria, often with passage of blood clots in the urine. May be due to renal adenocarcinoma or renal arteriovenous fistulas or be idiopathic. May involve one or both kidneys. May see blood clots emerging from the ureters on endoscopy. May be idiopathic (no primary cause identified, most commonly reported in Arabians).

FURTHER READING
Morgan R (2011) Discoloured urine in the adult horse. How can clinical pathology and imaging help my diagnosis? *Compan Animal* **16:**4–7.

CASE 147

1 What is the most likely diagnosis?

The results of the biochemistry profile indicate that marked hypercalcaemia is present. Considering the absence of azotaemia or isosthenuria, kidney disease seems unlikely in this case. As hyperglobulinaemia is present, a neoplastic aetiology (i.e. lymphoma, multiple myeloma) has to be considered in the differential diagnosis. Primary hyperparathyroidism and vitamin D toxicosis are also possible. Considering the slight increase in PTH in the presence of marked hypercalcaemia, primary hyperparathyroidism is the most likely diagnosis.

2 What are the most frequent clinical signs associated with this diagnosis?

The clinical signs present in this case of hyperparathyroidism are related to the hypercalcaemia. They often include polyuria/polydipsia, decreased activity, gastrointestinal signs (anorexia, vomiting) or neurological signs (mental dullness, coma). Urinary tract signs related to the presence of urinary calculi, metastatic mineralisation of the kidney or urinary infection are possible.

3 What are the causes for this diagnosis?

Primary hyperparathyroidism is caused by the autonomous and excessive secretion of PTH by parathyroid chief cells. This leads to hypercalcaemia and a loss of the negative-feedback control. Pathological findings are adenomas involving one or both glands, carcinomas or adenomatous hyperplasia.

FURTHER READING
Ettinger S. Feldman E (2000) *Textbook of Veterinary Internal Medicine*, 6th edn. Elsevier Saunders, St. Louis.

Stockham SL, Scott MA (2008) *Fundamentals of Veterinary Clinical Pathology*, 2nd edn. Blackwell Publishing, Oxford.

CASE 148

1 There is a discrepancy between the spun PCV performed initially and the haematocrit performed in the clinic. Summarise the pre-analytical, analytical or post-analytical reasons that may influence the result of the microhaematocrit method (spun PCV).

Possible factors influencing the microhaematocrit method include:

- Inadequate mixing of blood. May lead either to a falsely high or a falsely low PCV. Therefore, adequate sample mixing should be assured prior to the measurement.
- Inadequate volume of blood in the EDTA tube. Leads to a falsely low PCV because EDTA is a salt that leads to water loss of the RBCs and makes them shrink. Therefore, the erythrocytes become smaller and the PCV gets lower. This would also be expected to result in an abnormality in the automated haematological evaluation.
- Inadequate centrifugation. Plasma remains between the RBCs, producing a falsely high PCV.
- Misreading of the PCV. Untrained people may have problems correctly identifying the result. It is important to ensure that people performing the measurement know how to do it.

2 Does sample ageing influence the spun PCV?

Yes, sample ageing might influence the PCV. If the sample is delayed in transport for more than a few hours, erythrocytes may get swollen. Therefore, the PCV may be falsely high.

FOLLOW UP

The technician who performed the PCV was contacted after the mismatch had been noted. After discussing the various possibilities of a falsely low PCV, she admitted that the sample had not been mixed prior to assessing it. Therefore, many RBCs sedimented in the tube and could not be included in the measurement.

FURTHER READING

Stockham SL, Scott MA (2008) *Fundamentals of Veterinary Clinical Pathology*, 2nd edn. Blackwell Publishing, Oxford.

CASE 149

1 What is the most likely explanation for the laboratory abnormalities?

The leucogram shows a mild neutrophilia, which probably reflects an inflammatory process. However, the concurrent lymphopaenia, eosinopaenia and mild hyperglycaemia suggest a concurrent stress component. There is also a mild thrombocytopaenia. This could be due to increased consumption (e.g. DIC) or increased destruction. Decreased production due to a bone marrow disorder appears less likely given the absence of other cytopaenias. Measurement of the coagulation times and D-dimers would be recommended to investigate further this finding.

There is a marked azotaemia with increased phosphate. This reflects a decreased GFR. Given that the urea and creatinine are similarly increased, an intrinsic kidney disease is considered more likely. However, a pre-renal component due to dehydration or hypovolaemia cannot be excluded. Urinalysis would be required to further assess the renal function.

A urine sample was collected via cystocentesis and the USG measured 1.020. Given the marked azotaemia, this urine is considered suboptimally concentrated, thus confirming an intrinsic renal disease. Nevertheless, the renal tubules still maintain a residual concentrating ability (the urine is not isosthenuric). A urine sediment examination was also performed and was inactive.

Sodium and chloride are low and this could be due to increased loss (e.g. renal loss, third-space loss, GI sequestration/loss). In proportion, chloride is lower than sodium. This can be estimated by calculating the distance of the electrolytes concentration from the mean value of the reference interval. For example:

- Sodium: reference interval, $139 - 154$ mmol/l; mean value = $(139 + 154)/2 = 146.5$. The sodium concentration of this patient is 137 mmol/l. Therefore, sodium is 9.5 units below the mean concentration value: $146.5 - 137 = 9.5$.
- Chloride: reference interval, $105 - 122$ mmol/l; mean value = $(105 + 122)/2 = 113.5$. The chloride concentration of this patient is 98 mmol/l. Therefore, chloride is 15.5 units below the mean concentration value: $113.5 - 98 = 15.5$.

Physiologically, sodium and chloride should change in parallel. In this case, this discrepancy could be due to additional chloride loss via vomiting or as a result of an underlying acid–base disorder. Evaluation of arterial blood gas results and/or TCO_2 (biochemistry) should be considered.

There is evidence of a hepatocellular injury with signs of biliary obstruction. This cholestasis could either be hepatic, post-hepatic or a combination of the two forms. The CK increase indicates muscular injury.

In summary, the combination of increased liver enzyme activity, azotaemia, electrolyte imbalances and mild hyperbilirubinaemia is more commonly observed in animals affected by leptospirosis. In this dog other differential diagnoses would include pancreatitis or, potentially, pyometra (entire female).

2 What further test would you perform to confirm your diagnosis?

To confirm a diagnosis of leptospirosis, serological titres (MAT test) and blood/urine PCR could be performed. The test used should be chosen depending on the suspected timing of the infection. During the first 10 days of infection, the organism numbers are highest in blood and the antibody titres are low. In this case, the test of choice would be blood PCR. After that, the organism is more numerous in urine and therefore this should be tested by PCR.

Serology (MAT test) is usually negative in the first week of illness as it takes time for the immune system to establish an antibody response. To avoid a false negative, the test should not be performed earlier than 3–4 weeks from the infection (acute titres). Repeating the test after 1 or 2 weeks is also recommended to demonstrate seroconversion. A 4-fold change in titre supports a recent infection.

To rule in/out a pancreatitis, amylase, lipase and cPLI could be measured.

3 What is the pathophysiology behind the biochemistry changes?

Leptospira organisms penetrate abraded skin lesions or mucous membranes and readily replicate in the blood stream. These microorganisms colonise the kidney, where they actively replicate in the renal tubular epithelial cells, causing acute nephritis. In cases of chronic disease, an interstitial nephritis can also occur. This causes renal azotaemia, low USG and proteinuria. In the kidney, the bacteria can also release endotoxins, which may have an effect on the Na/K-ATPase pumps in the nephrons, thus causing electrolyte loss. Electrolyte imbalances may also be a consequence of gastroenteric losses.

In the liver, the leptospiral microorganisms can cause centrilobular necrosis, subcellular damage and biliary obstruction. Increased ALP and total bilirubin are more common than an increase in ALT activity. CK activity can be increased in infected dogs and this is believed to be caused by myositis.

Leucocytosis and thrombocytopaenia are relatively common. Leucocytosis is often associated with an inflammatory response. Thrombocytopaenia is seen in approximately 58% of cases and is probably caused by DIC.

FURTHER READING

Ettinger SJ, Feldmann EC (2005) *Textbook of Veterinary Internal Medicine*, 6th edn. Elsevier Saunders, St. Louis.

Sykes JE, Hartmann K, Lunn KF *et al.* (2010) 2010 ACVIM Small animal consensus statement on leptospirosis: diagnosis, epidemiology, treatment and prevention. *J Vet Intern Med* 25:1–13.

CASE 150

1 Summarise and interpret the abnormalities in these laboratory results.

Microcytosis with occasional cells demonstrating hypochromasia in the absence of anaemia is unlikely to be associated with iron deficiency, but serum iron levels would be useful to rule this out. Microcytosis in a young dog may suggest a portosystemic shunt (PSS).

The leucogram suggests stress. Plasma protein is decreased, but this may be age appropriate considering that this is an adult reference interval. Serum proteins would help evaluate further. There is a slight hyperglycaemia, which may be associated with stress, but a serum fructosamine would help to confirm this. Slight hyperglycaemia may also be post prandial.

Decreased urea may also be associated with decreased synthesis by the liver, which may also be the case with the lowered cholesterol and albumin.

Slight increases in calcium, phosphate and ALP are likely age appropriate, as this is a young growing animal and an ALP increase may be seen with growing bones. The calcium, however, is high considering the lowered albumin (40% of total calcium is albumin bound). An ionised calcium was found to be in the upper reference interval.

Mild increases in hepatocellular parameters suggest slight hepatocellular damage. The marked increase in paired bile acids confirms a defect in liver function. Normal bilirubin indicates no overt cholestasis. Decreased albumin (along with decreased urea and cholesterol) suggests decreased intake, decreased production (liver disease?) or increased loss. The urine dipstick is negative for proteinuria. Slight ALT increase alone may be non-specific and can be due to primary liver change, gut or even heart disease. If there is no evidence of cholestasis, a bile acid would help rule out liver malfunction (bile acids increased as noted above).

There is a reproducible lowered USG with no evidence of active sediment. Urinary tract infection cannot be ruled out on dilute urine and therefore a culture is required. The lowered USG secondary to the PU/PD is most likely due to a washout effect because of the lowered urea, which reduces the medullary interstitial concentration gradient. The presence of biurate crystalluria is commonly seen in cases of PSS because of excessive excretion of ammonia and uric acid in urine.

In summary, the marked increases in bile acids along with the slight liver changes, decreased albumin, urea, cholesterol, presence of the biurate crystalluria and history are suggestive of a liver insufficiency. In a puppy, PSS is likely.

2 Discuss any additional tests you could perform in order to confirm or exclude the possible diagnosis.

Additional tests include a liver Doppler ultrasound. Liver biopsy would help confirm an extrahepatic shunt, which is the most common type seen in small-breed dogs such as the Miniature Schnauzer and Yorkshire Terrier. Note that a full coagulation profile is required prior to biopsy in individuals that have decreased liver function, as these animals may also have a coagulopathy due to decreased production of coagulation factors. Other modalities include transcolonic portal scintigraphy.

A recent study has shown that dogs with a PSS have an impaired ability to eliminate manganese, resulting in increased concentrations in the peripheral blood. Quoted whole blood (EDTA) manganese concentrations of >1,100 nmol/l are highly suggestive of PSS when associated with the appropriate clinical and supportive laboratory findings.

FURTHER READING

Gow, AG, Marques AIC, Yool DA *et al.* (2010) Whole blood manganese concentrations in dogs with congenital portosystemic shunts. *J Vet Intern Med* **24**:90–96.

Winkler JT, Bohling MW, Tillson DM *et al.* (2003) Portosystemic shunts: diagnosis, prognosis, and treatment of 64 cases (1993–2001). *J Am Anim Hosp Assoc* **39**:169–185.

CASE 151

1 How would you classify the anaemia?

Non-regenerative, normocytic-normochromic anaemia.

2 What is your diagnosis, based on the haematology and the blood smear?

Babesia infection, presumably *B. canis*. Two piriform *Babesia* organisms are visible in a RBC.

3 Where on the blood smear would you look for the organisms causing the anaemia?

Babesia organisms are easiest to detect at the edges of the smear (**Fig. 151.2**, short arrows); the feathered edge should be avoided. Alternatively, a smear with a concentration line can be made; *Babesia* accumulate in the concentration line (long arrows).

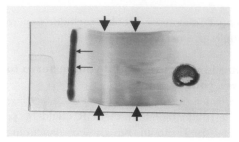

FIG. 151.2 Blood smear with concentration line (see text). (Courtesy Dr Georges Kirtz)

4 Would a serology test (immunoflourescence) or a PCR be useful for further confirmation?

The finding of the organisms is consistent with babesiosis; there is no further test needed for confirmation. *Babesia* serology only indicates seroconversion and antibodies are not found at an early stage of the disease. PCR could be performed but usually takes too long. The aim of the *Babesia* diagnosis is to detect the organisms on a blood smear.

5 What is the most frequent change in the FBC in this infection?

The most frequent finding in babesiosis is a moderate to marked thrombocytopaenia, which is caused by immune-mediated destruction of the platelets. The anaemia as seen in this case is often not prominent. The leucogram may show a leucocytosis or a leucopaenia, often accompanied by reactive lymphocytes.

6 What does the biochemistry profile indicate?

Urea and creatinine indicate renal disease, which can be from damage to the glomeruli by haemoglobin; however, AKI cannot be excluded in this case. Increased globulins are suggestive of an infectious or inflammatory disease. Albumin below the reference interval may be interpreted in the light of renal disease (renal albumin loss). On the other hand, albumin is a negative acute-phase protein; a decrease is seen in infectious or inflammatory disease.

Note: The clinical presentation may differ with *Babesia* species. In Europe, different subspecies of *B. canis* exist that differ in pathogenicity.

FURTHER READING

Leutenegger CM, Pusterla N, Wicki R *et al.* (2002) New molecular tools in the diagnosis of tick-borne diseases. *Schweiz Archiv Tierheilkd* **144**:395–404.

Zygner W, Gojska O, Rapacka G *et al.* (2007) Hematological changes during the course of canine babesiosis caused by large *Babesia* in domestic dogs in Warsaw (Poland). *Vet Parasitol* **145**:146–151.

CASE 152

1 Identify and list the abnormalities and explain their associations.

Mild normocytic-normochromic, non-regenerative anaemia, possibly due to chronic disease. Mild stress leucogram. The borderline elevation in MCHC is unlikely to be of clinical significance since the haemoglobin and PCV show good agreement, but the possibility of slight haemolysis as an underlying cause cannot be ruled out.

Marked hyperkalaemia and marked hypocalcaemia, neither of which is compatible with life, are probably erroneous. This combination of severe hyperkalaemia and hypocalcaemia are suggestive of EDTA contamination. Hypercholesterolaemia may be post prandial, associated with hepatopathies or endocrinopathies (including hypothyroidism with this patient's clinical signs).

Low TT4 and normal TSH are most suggestive of euthyroid sick syndrome (non-thyroidal disease) but hypothyroidism cannot be ruled out.

2 What further tests would you recommend?

Repeat biochemistry on a fresh separated serum sample. Testing FT4 by dialysis. If FT4 is within reference interval, this would confirm euthyroid sick syndrome.

3 Discuss the mechanisms by which EDTA contamination of a serum sample produces marked hyperkalaemia and hypocalcaemia.

EDTA is a chelating agent that binds divalent cations such as Ca^{2+}, Mg^{2+} and Zn^{2+}. It acts as an anticoagulant by binding calcium, which is essential in the clotting cascade. Therefore, if EDTA plasma is used to run biochemistry tests, there will be marked erroneously low calcium. Additionally, there will be erroneously increased potassium because EDTA is usually formulated and used as a dipotassium (K_2EDTA) or tripotassium salt.

4 What other parameter will have been affected by the problem in this profile, and explain why a change is not obvious on evaluation of the profile.

ALP measurement will also be affected if EDTA is the anticoagulant for plasma. The mechanism is similar because it is the chelation of cations such as Mg^{2+} and Zn^{2+} that leads to production of erroneous results because they are necessary cofactors for ALP activity measurement.

5 When collecting blood into multiple different types (plain and anticoagulants) of blood vacutainers, in which order should they be collected?

When collecting blood into three different types of vacutainer tubes, the Clinical & Laboratory Standards Institute guidelines (CLSI, 2007) recommend that the anticoagulant-free tube should be filled first, then the sodium citrate tube and finally the EDTA tube.

DISCUSSION

Inappropriate blood collection, where EDTA in the blood tube for haematological testing contaminates the serum tube, can erroneously affect serum calcium, potassium, ALP, iron, zinc sulphate turbidity test, ammonia, vitamin B12, ACTH and coagulation tests (PT/aPTT), all common tests in veterinary laboratories.

The degrees of decrease in Ca^{2+} and Fe^{2+} and increase in K^+ are directly proportional to the amount of EDTA contamination. Ca^{2+}, Fe^{2+} and K^+ are already affected by a relatively small amount of EDTA. ALP is only affected by a large amount of EDTA and then the decrease is dramatic. Occasionally, this phenomenon can happen when some of the EDTA blood is decanted into the serum tube when there is insufficient blood in the serum tube before submitting it to the laboratory. It can also happen inadvertently when blood is collected directly into vacutainers and the EDTA tube is filled before the serum tube and some backflow has occurred; this contaminated blood is then collected into the plain tube. In this instance, backflow is defined as the possible regurgitation of blood from the evacuated blood collection EDTA tube to the needle or vein. This phenomenon is more likely when evacuated blood collection is performed after tourniquet removal and the pressure in the vein has dropped below that in the blood collection tube. During blood collection into a vacutainer, blood flows from the vein into the tube until the pressure in the tube and vein have reached equilibrium. If the pressure in the vein decreases for any reason, blood will flow back into the vein until pressures in the tube and the vein have reached equilibrium. The volume of the remaining air bubble in the filled tube determines the volume of backflow (air is compressible not the fluid).

REFERENCE AND FURTHER READING

Clinical and Laboratory Standards Institute (2007) *Document H3-A6 – Procedures for the Collection of Diagnostic Blood Specimens by Venipuncture: Approved Standard*, 6th edn. Clinical and Laboratory Standards Institute, Wayne.

Imafuku Y, Meguro S, Kanno K *et al.* (2002) The effect of EDTA contaminated sera on laboratory data. *Clinica Chimica Acta* 325:105–111.

Katz L, Johnson DL, Neufeld PD *et al.* (1975) Evacuated blood-collection tubes: the backflow hazard. *Can Med Assoc J* 113:208–213.

Panteghini M, Bais R (2008) Enzymes In: *Tietz Fundamentals of Clinical Chemistry*. (eds CA Burtis, ER Ashwood, DE Bruns) Saunders Elsevier, St. Louis, p. 326.

Veterinary Clinical Pathology

Young DS, Bermes EW, Haverstick DM (2008) Specimen collection and other preanalytical variables. In: *Tietz Fundamentals of Clinical Chemistry*. (eds CA Burtis, ER Ashwood, DE Bruns) Saunders Elsevier, St. Louis, p. 48.

CASE 153

1 Discuss the haematological abnormalities.

There is a moderate thrombocytopaenia associated with several macroplatelets. In view of the breed, familial macrothrombocytopaenia of CKCSs is most likely. Nevertheless, other underlying pathologies should be excluded. These include immune-mediated destruction of platelets (usually results in severe thrombocytopaenia), infectious disease (e.g. anaplasmosis), platelet consumption (e.g. DIC), platelet sequestration or decreased platelet production in the bone marrow. These are unlikely in this case given the healthy status and absence of other abnormalities.

2 Describe the underlying pathophysiology.

Macrothrombocytopaenia is a common, autosomally recessive hereditary disorder in CKCSs. Between 30 and 50% of the UK and USA populations of CKCSs are thought to have this inherited condition. An underlying missense mutation in this disorder affects the gene encoding for β1-tubulin. The mutation replaces an asparagine, leading to a mischarged aspartic acid, which takes part in the binding site for microtubules in the platelet. In the face of impaired binding, the formation of proplatelets as well as their production by megakaryocytes is abnormal, leading to macroplatelets. Normally, affected dogs do not show any clinical signs or bleeding tendencies since the total platelet volume (plateletcrit) is within normal limits. Platelet counts are often low and interval between 30 and 100 × 10⁹/l. However, as platelets are larger in size, the plateletcrit is well within the reference interval despite the lower platelet count. Therefore, in these patients detecting platelets using an impedance method should be avoided. The quantitative buffy coat analysis can be used to detect the plateletcrit. There is a test available for this inherited macrothrombocytopaenia in CKCSs.

REFERENCE AND FURTHER READING

Davis B, Tovio-Kinnucan M, Shuller S *et al.* (2008) Mutation in beta-1-tubulin correlates with macrothromobocytopaenia in Cavalier King Charles Spaniels. *J Vet Intern Med* 22:540–545.

Stockham SL, Scott MA (2008) *Fundamentals of Veterinary Clinical Pathology*, 2nd edn. Blackwell Publishing, Oxford.

Tvedten H, Lilliehöök I, Hillström A *et al.* (2008) Plateletcrit is superior to platelet count for assessing platelet status in Cavalier King Charles Spaniels. *J Vet Clin Pathol* 37:266–271.

Weiss DJ, Wardrop KJ (2010) (eds) *Schalm's Veterinary Hematology*, 6th edn. Blackwell Publishing, Ames.

CASE 154

1 Summarise and interpret the abnormalities in these laboratory results.

There is evidence of haemoconcentration, which may be due to dehydration, but this is not supported by the protein and albumin being within reference intervals. It can also be seen in animals that have poor renal oxygenation, which may occur in cases of chronic heart disease or diffuse chronic lung disease. Slight increases in PCV may also be seen occasionally in cases of HAC. The lowered MCHC is likely artefactual since anaemia is not present and not clinically significant.

The leucogram suggests stress, due to either endogenous or exogenous steroids. The slight increase in glucose may be due to stress, but can also be seen as a transient change in cases of Cushing's disease (endogenous or exogenous steroids), but one cannot rule out diabetes mellitus (DM). A serum fructosamine would be useful to differentiate stress/Cushing's disease (should show transient increases in glucose) from DM (shows persistent increases in glucose). Glucocorticoids are responsible for gluconeogenesis and they antagonise insulin, resulting in decreased uptake and utilisation of glucose.

Hypercholesterolaemia is associated with a variety of endocrine conditions including hypothyroidism (not supported by history of PU/PD), HAC and DM, and it may also be seen in cases of cholestasis due to decreased clearance.

There are slight increases in hepatocellular parameters with a more marked increase in ALP. An increase in ALT and AST can be seen with slight hepatocellular damage, but ALT can also be raised due to increased permeability changes secondary to glucocorticoids. These may also be associated with glycogen storage in the liver resulting in a steroid hepatopathy.

There is no increase in bilirubin, and thus the marked increase in ALP may be due to steroid induction. Increases >1,000 U/l are highly suggestive of cortisol excess in dogs. A slight increase in sodium and a slight decrease in potassium can be associated with HAC.

The lowered USG may be associated with ADH inhibition with excess cortisol, with resultant PU/PD. The 1+ protein may be attributable to the pH (alkaline pH may induce a 1+ false proteinuria), but can also be seen in cases of HAC, and in this case can be seen with haematuria/urinary tract infection, which is suggested by the active sediment and bacteriuria.

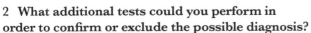
2 What additional tests could you perform in order to confirm or exclude the possible diagnosis?

Further testing would include endocrine testing to rule out/in HAC and serum fructosamine to rule out DM. A urine cortisol:creatinine ratio, an ACTH stimulation test or an LDDST is required to help rule out/in HAC. An increased basal cortisol level is not sufficient evidence of HAC. The results in this dog are shown below:

Analyte (units)	Result	Reference Interval
Fructosamine (μmol/l)	245	<300
Urine cortisol:creatinine ratio	**67**	<15
ACTH stimulation test		
Pre-dexamethasone cortisol (nmol/l)	**190**	28–170
Post-dexamethasone cortisol (nmol/l)	580	<550–607
LDDST		
Pre-dexamethasone cortisol (nmol/l)	**175**	28–170
Post-dexamethasone cortisol (3–4 hour) (nmol/l)	**132**	<40
Post-dexamethasone cortisol (8 hour) (nmol/l)	**127**	<40
HDDST		
Pre-dexamethasone cortisol (nmol/l)	**263**	28–170
Post-dexamethasone cortisol (nmol/l)	**94**	<40
Endogenous ACTH (pmol/l)	**85**	4.4–22.0

SERUM FRUCTOSAMINE

The serum fructosamine result does not support DM.

URINE CORTISOL:CREATININE RATIO

The urine cortisol:creatinine ratio result is suggestive of Cushing's disease if the clinical signs are consistent. This is a useful screening test with a reported 95% sensitivity for canine HAC. It is also useful in cases where HAC is unlikely but needs to be excluded, as a low (normal) result rules out most cases of HAC. However, the test has low specificity (22%), (with many false positives – many causes of polydipsia will give an increased ratio [i.e. DM, diabetes insipidus, pyometra, hypercalcaemia, liver failure]), and thus this test cannot be used to confirm HAC.

Protocol

● Collect a morning urine sample.
● Submit sample with a request for urinary cortisol and creatinine levels.
● It is important to avoid stress.
● Collect urine at home, at least 2 days after the veterinary visit.
● Interpret with care in dogs where the degree of clinical suspicion is not high.

$$ratio = \frac{1,000 \times cortisol\left(nmol/1\right) \times 10^6}{creatinine\left(\mu mol/1\right)}$$

Interpretation

● Values between approximately 10 and 20 are probably normal, but ratios >15 may be due to HAC but could also be due to stress or non-adrenal illness.
● Values of 20 to 50 are suspect if there are supporting clinical signs. This is the 'grey' or equivocal area in which most cases of polydipsia will fall (PU/PD dilutes out creatinine).
● Values >50 are strongly suspect for HAC (but liver disease and diabetes mellitus are likely to be in this area).
● Values >100 are most likely to be due to HAC.

It is thought that the test has similar sensitivity and specificity in cats, but there are few published reports.

ACTH STIMULATION TEST

This result demonstrates a baseline cortisol above the reference interval, but the post-stimulation result is equivocal and may also be due to stress at this level. This result is thus not definitive for HAC.

If there is a high degree of suspicion for HAC, and the result of the ACTH stimulation test is equivocal, then an LDDST should be carried out. If iatrogenic HAC is suspected, the ACTH stimulation test is the test of choice and is also the suggested screening test that can be used to monitor treatment of cushingoid patients with mitotane, ketoconazole or trilostane. The goal with ACTH stimulation is to maximally stimulate the adrenal cortex to see how much cortisol it can make. (**Note:** Anticonvulsant therapy [phenobarbitone and precursors] may cause increase in post-ACTH cortisol results, as well as increased liver enzymes, and some clinical signs that mimic those of HAC, such as PU/PD.)

The ACTH stimulation test is a useful screening test for HAC in dogs but not quite as sensitive as the LDDST (there will be more false negatives with the ACTH stimulation test compared with the LDDST). Data from a number of studies show that 87% of dogs with pituitary tumours and 61% of dogs with adrenal tumours demonstrate an exaggerated response on the ACTH stimulation test. Fourteen percent of dogs with non-adrenal illness give an exaggerated response.

Protocol

Pre- and post-cortisol is analysed 1 hour after injection of synthetic ACTH (0.25 mg IM Cortrosyn) or 2 hours if porcine gel (Cortigel) is used. (**Note:** Each laboratory has its own reference interval.)

LOW-DOSE DEXAMETHASONE SUPPRESSION TEST

The baseline cortisol result is above the reference interval. The dog has not shown suppression at 3 hours to <40 nmol/l or any suppression at 8 hours (<40 nmol/l), which is suggestive of either an adrenal- or pituitary-dependent HAC (see discussion below).

The LDDST tests the integrity of the feedback system by suppression testing using a synthetic glucocorticoid (dexamethasone). In normal animals, ACTH release is suppressed by negative feedback by cortisol. A low dose of dexamethasone acts similarly and suppresses the release of ACTH, which in turn 'turns off' the release of cortisol. HAC causes resistance of the pituitary–adrenal axis to suppression by dexamethasone and the cortisol levels remain high. Dexamethasone is used because it does not interfere with the cortisol assay.

Prednisone contributes 6% and prednisolone 49% to the cortisol measured, and thus animals should be free of these drugs for at least 2–4 weeks prior to testing. Any prolonged topical (including aural or ophthalmic) or systemic steroid therapy can affect ACTH test results. Therapy should be withdrawn (gradually) for a minimum of 2 weeks before testing.

The LDDST is a good screening test for HAC in dogs. It has slightly greater sensitivity than the ACTH stimulation test (i.e. there will be fewer false negatives) but there will be more false positives (it has lower specificity).

Most dogs with adrenal tumours do not suppress at 3 or 8 hours post dexamethasone. This dog's cortisol concentration suppressed at 3 hours but did not remain suppressed at 8 hours. If a dog suppresses at 3 hours, and escapes suppression at 8 hours, it is likely that the dog has pituitary-dependent HAC rather than an adrenal tumour. This 'escape' is due to rapid clearance of the dexamethasone.

The LDDST is of no value for diagnosing HAC, iatrogenic HAC or for monitoring response to treatment. The test can differentiate between pituitary-dependent HAC and adrenal tumours in up to 60% of cases.

In most situations, the LDDST is regarded as the test of choice for diagnosis of HAC in the dog, but not in animals that are already known to have DM and be on insulin therapy.

Protocol (dogs)
Begin test at 0800–0900 hours after withholding food but not water overnight:

- Weigh dog.
- A baseline serum sample (red top tube) is collected and labelled '0 hour'.
- Allow blood to clot at room temperature and then store in refrigerator.
- Inject dexamethasone at 0.01 mg/kg body weight IV. (If the volume is small, it may be helpful to make a 1:10 dilution.)

- Collect further serum samples at 3 or 4 hours and again at 8 hours post injection and label them appropriately.
- Submit blood tubes to the laboratory as soon as possible (cortisol is stable for 40 hours at 4°C).

Interpretation
Combined data from studies show that normal healthy dogs will show suppression at both 4 and 8 hours, and dogs with HAC will not show suppression. (**Note:** Each laboratory has its own reference interval.)

If there is >50% suppression from the baseline and the 8 hour cortisol is <40 nmol/l, this result will exclude 98% of cases of HAC. If clinical signs suggest that HAC is highly likely and the above results are obtained, then the test should be repeated in 4 weeks. (**Note:** Highly stressed animals and some with non-adrenal illness may fail to suppress.) There is poor specificity (high false-positive rate), with reported specificity of 44–73%.

For adrenal tumours, most cases (100%) fail to suppress regardless of criteria, but lack of suppression can also be due to a pituitary-dependent tumour (35–40% of cases). Pituitary-dependent HAC will not suppress and cannot be differentiated from adrenal-dependent disease. It is important to differentiate pituitary-dependent HAC from an adrenal tumour by ultrasound examination and/or by HDDST or an endogenous ACTH assay.

If the degree of suspicion is not high or if the clinical signs are not classic, then it is important to rule out other possibilities such as renal or hepatic disease and DM, because failure to suppress is not specific for HAC. Up to 56% of dogs with chronic stressful illness will not suppress. (**Note:** Bile acid testing will not differentiate liver disease from HAC as both may have increases in bile acids.)

For pituitary-dependent HAC there should be >50% suppression from the baseline 0 hour cortisol level at 3–4 hours or suppression to <40 nmol/l at 3–4 hours post dexamethasone, but there should be escape to >40 nmol/l at 8 hours. (**Note:** Each laboratory has its own reference interval.)

DISCRIMINATORY TESTS
High-dose dexamethasone suppression test
The results of the HDDST do not show suppression to <40 nmol/l at 8 hours, suggesting either an adrenal- or a pituitary-dependent tumour. This test is used to help differentiate if the HAC is pituitary dependent or due to an adrenal tumour. It should be used only after a diagnosis of HAC has been made using either the LDDST or the ACTH stimulation test.

The HDDST has no value in cases of hypoadrenocorticism or iatrogenic HAC. When the concentration of dexamethasone is high enough, it will decrease the release of ACTH from the pituitary microadenoma and the decrease in ACTH will decrease cortisol release.

Protocol

Same as that for the LDDST except the dose of dexamethasone is 0.1 mg/kg body weight and it is only necessary to take baseline 0 hour and 8 hour post-dexamathasone serum samples.

Interpretation

Dogs that suppress (>50% suppression or suppress to <40 nmol/l) at 8 hours have pituitary-dependent HAC (PDH), whereas failure to suppress usually indicates adrenal-dependent HAC (ADH); however, some dogs (15%) with PDH may also fail to suppress. Apparent ADH cases are best further evaluated by ultrasonography of the adrenals or radiology if considering adrenalectomy.

Endogenous ACTH assay

This result in this dog is high, indicating PDH. This test will probably eventually replace the HDDST. There are special sampling requirements (chilled/frozen, no glass tubes):

● ADH (and iatrogenic): ACTH chronically suppressed.
● PDH: ACTH secreted excessively.

Other diagnostic modalities

● Abdominal ultrasound:
  ❏ Dogs with pituitary tumours demonstrate bilateral enlargement of the adrenals due to excess ACTH stimulation of the glands.
  ❏ Dogs with adrenal tumours may show enlargement of a single gland (unilateral) and the gland may also be mineralised. The other normal gland is often suppressed through normal physiological processes, and will generally be smaller.
● Abdominal radiographs. Not useful for visualising normal adrenal glands or bilaterally enlarged glands (pituitary-dependent disease). Mincralisation of the adrenal may be seen with adrenal tumours.
● Other imaging. A CT scan can be useful to verify diagnosis of a pituitary macroadenoma.

FOLLOW UP

A large pituitary macroadenoma was found in this dog.

FURTHER READING

Behrend EN, Kennis R (2010) Atypical Cushing's syndrome in dogs: arguments for and against. *Vet Clin North Am Small Anim Pract* **40**:285–296.

Chastain C, Franklin R, Ganjam V *et al.* (1986) Evaluation of the hypothalamic pituitary-adrenal axis in clinically stressed dogs *J Am Anim Hosp Assoc* **22**:435–442.
Feldman EC, Nelson RW (2004) Canine hyperadrenocorticism. In: *Canine and Feline Endocrinology and Reproduction*, 3rd edn. Saunders, St Louis.
Kooistra HS, Galac S (2010) Recent advances in the diagnosis of Cushing's syndrome in dogs. *Vet Clin North Am Small Anim Pract* **40**:259–207.

CASE 155

1 What does the FBC tell you?

The RBC count is indicative of haemoconcentration or (primary, secondary) polycythaemia. However the clinical findings together with the total protein and serum albumin concentration, as well as the hypernatraemia, make hypertonic dehydration the most likely cause. The mature neutrophilia with a marked lymphopaenia and the monocytosis are consistent with a stress leucogram. The mild thrombocytopaenia would need further evaluation and may, in the case of fever, indicate DIC, but a coagulation profile was not performed in this case.

2 What might the finding of NRBCs indicate?

Peripheral NRBCs can occur with multiple conditions. In heat stroke it has been hypothesised that they are the result of hyperthermic damage of the bone marrow matrix. Their presence in blood is also a negative prognostic factor in this condition.

3 What does the urinalysis indicate?

The low USG and fine granular casts are the strongest indicators of tubular damage; the oxalate crystals are an incidental finding but may be one potential route of calcium loss. A single measurement of the urine pH provides limited information. Together with the azotaemia, AKI is the most likely diagnosis.

Confronted with the findings, the owner admitted that the dog had been locked up in a car on a hot summer day for several hours. The findings described here are consistent with heat stroke.

FURTHER READING

Aroch I, Segev, G, Loeb *et al.* (2009) Peripheral nucleated red blood cells as a prognostic indicator in heat stroke in dogs. *J Vet Intern Med* **23**:544–551.
Bosak JK (2004) Heat stroke in a Great Pyrenees dog. *Can Vet J* **45**:513–515.
Bruchim Y, Klement E, Saragusty J *et al.* (2006) Heat stroke in dogs: a retrospective study of 54 cases (1999–2004) and analysis of risk factors for death. *J Vet Intern Med* **20**:38–46.

A similar case has been described in:

Thrall MA, Baker D, Campell TW (2004) *Clinical Case Presentations for Veterinary Hematology and Clinical Chemistry*. Lippincott, Williams & Wilkins, Philadelphia.

CASE 156

1 What is your assessment of the arterial pH?

The arterial pH is within the reference interval. However, abnormalities of PaO_2, $PaCO_2$ and HCO_3^- indicate an acid–base abnormality is present, regardless of the pH. Normal physiological adaption does not return the pH to normal. Therefore, if the pH is normal, but bicarbonate concentration and $PaCO_2$ are markedly abnormal, there are primary derangements, acting in opposite directions, in both systems.

If the pH is normal and the bicarbonate concentration and $PaCO_2$ are only slightly abnormal, the patient may have an acid–base imbalance in both systems or only in one system. When the bicarbonate concentration and $PaCO_2$ are only slightly abnormal, acid–base analysis does not reliably establish whether only one system or both systems are involved, or which system is involved.

2 What is your assessment of the likely underlying aetiology for this arterial pH?

Because the $PaCO_2$ and HCO_3^- are both moderately decreased, a mixed acid-base disorder is suspected. This may be a metabolic acidosis with respiratory alkalosis. Because the PaO_2 is slightly increased, an extrathoracic respiratory alkalosis is present.

3 Is there appropriate compensation for this condition, and what does it suggest?

The anion gap is within the reference interval, so there is a secretional acidosis.

4 What might be underlying causes for this condition?

Secretional metabolic acidoses occur as a result of excessive bicarbonate loss from the body. Excessive amounts of bicarbonate can be lost in urine, gastrointestinal fluids (pancreatic juice) and saliva (ruminants only). The cellular processes that provide the bicarbonate for the fluid being lost also provide hydrogen protons to the blood. Normally, the bicarbonate in the fluid is reabsorbed from the fluid and there is no net increase in bicarbonate loss. However, during certain diseases, bicarbonate is not reabsorbed from the fluid, resulting in excessive bicarbonate loss and an increase in the hydrogen concentration in the blood. Hence, a secretional metabolic acidosis develops. In order to maintain electroneutrality, the decrease in plasma

bicarbonate concentration must be accompanied by either a concurrent increase in the plasma concentration of another anion or a concurrent decrease in plasma sodium concentration. Several physiological systems, discussed earlier, protect the plasma sodium concentration and prevent it from decreasing dramatically concurrent with the decrease in plasma bicarbonate concentration. Therefore, in order to maintain electroneutrality, the plasma concentration of another anion must increase. Chloride is the only anion of significant concentration in plasma that can be physiologically controlled without causing further acid–base imbalances. At sites of bicarbonate formation and secretion, chloride is transported with H^+ into blood, while HCO_3^- is secreted into the fluid produced (e.g. saliva, pancreatic juice) with Na^+ or K^+. As a result, plasma chloride concentration increases concurrent with and equal to the decrease in plasma bicarbonate concentration. Secretional metabolic acidoses have been called hyperchloraemic metabolic acidoses because plasma chloride concentration increases to offset the decrease in bicarbonate concentration. In some cases of secretional metabolic acidosis, plasma sodium concentration is low and plasma chloride concentration is not increased. As a result, relying on plasma/serum chloride concentration to determine the type of metabolic acidosis can cause misdiagnosis. Secretional metabolic acidoses have also been called normal anion gap acidoses because the anion gap does not change, as the decrease in bicarbonate anions is accompanied by an equal increase in chloride anions. The term secretional metabolic acidosis more accurately reflects the pathophysiological process which is occurring.

Administration of chloride-containing acid (HCl) or administration of large amounts of sodium chloride (dilutional acidosis) can cause hyperchloraemic metabolic acidosis that is not of secretional origin.

There is concurrent respiratory alkalois. Extrathoracic respiratory alkaloses occur as a result of hyperventilation caused by CNS lesions, emotional stress or decreased oxygen carrying capacity of the blood and are associated with normal or slightly increased arterial blood oxygen concentrations. It is easy to understand how hyperventilation resulting in decreased arterial blood CO_2 concentration and normal or increased arterial blood oxygen concentration can result from CNS and emotional conditions. However, development of decreased arterial blood CO_2 concentration with normal or increased arterial blood oxygen concentration caused by decreased blood oxygen carrying capacity may, at first, be confusing. In blood, most oxygen is carried bound to haemoglobin. Oxygen bound to haemoglobin is in equilibrium with oxygen in plasma and provides a reservoir of oxygen. As oxygen diffuses from plasma into tissues, plasma oxygen is replenished from the oxygen reservoir provided by haemoglobin-bound oxygen. Decreased haemoglobin concentration (classic anaemia) or decreased haemoglobin oxygen carrying capacity (cyanide toxicity, nitrate toxicity, carbon monoxide toxicity) decreases the haemoglobin-bound oxygen reservoir. As a result, plasma and functional haemoglobin are normally saturated or slightly supersaturated with oxygen when the blood leaves the lungs. However, plasma and haemoglobin are quickly depleted of oxygen (PaO_2 decreases) after blood enters the tissues because the haemoglobin-bound oxygen reservoir is low. The decrease in PaO_2 stimulates oxygen-sensitive receptors to increase respiratory rate and depth, increasing alveolar ventilation and inducing respiratory alkalosis. Because hyperventilation does not greatly increase the alveolar oxygen concentration, but does markedly decrease the alveolar CO_2 concentration, an extrathoracic respiratory alkalosis develops, while increased oxygen delivery to tissues is minimal.

FURTHER READING

Dibartola SP (2012) *Fluid, Electrolyte and Acid-Base Disorders in Small Animal Practice*, 4th edn. Elsevier Saunders, St. Louis.

CASE 157

1 Based on what is known about biological variation in creatinine in dogs, are two samples adequate to estimate the homeostatic setting point for creatinine within an individual dog (assuming chronic stable renal disease)?

The number of samples required to obtain an estimate within a certain percentage of the true individual homeostatic setting point of the individual can be calculated using a formula based on a simple standard error of the mean estimate:

$$n = [Z \times [CV_A^2 + CV_I^2]^{1/2}/D]^2$$

Z = the number of standard deviations appropriate to the probability and 1.96 is very often used since this is the 95% probability (p <0.05) level; CV_A = the analytical precision at the level of the homeostatic setting point; CV_I = the within-subject biological variation; D = the percentage deviation allowed from the true homeostatic setting point. For creatinine, CV_I = 14.6% (see Appendix 2, p. 264). The chosen D = 10%.

If the within-dog variation (CV_I) for creatinine is 14.6% and the CV_A for a particular laboratory is 1.0%, looking at a situation where we would like to know the mean creatinine within 10% of the 'true value', with 95% probability, the formula is applied as follows:

$$n = [Z \times [CV_A^2 + CV_I^2]^{1/2}/D]^2$$
$$n = [1.96 \times [1.0^2 + 14.6^2]^{1/2}/10]^2$$
$$n = [1.96 \times [1.0 + 213.16]^{1/2}/10]^2$$
$$n = [1.96 \times [214.16]^{1/2}/10]^2$$
$$n = [1.96 \times 14.63/10]^2$$
$$n = [28.68/10]^2$$
$$n = 2.868^2$$
$$n = 8.23$$

Therefore, it will require eight analyses to determine the mean homeostatic setting point of creatinine within 10%, with 95% probability, on an instrument with CV_A of 1.0%. If the instrument has a higher CV_A, such as 5%, this will change the calculation as follows:

$$n = [Z \times [CV_A^2 + CV_I^2]^{1/2}/D]^2$$
$$n = [1.96 \times [5.0^2 + 14.6^2]^{1/2}/10]^2$$
$$n = [1.96 \times [25.0 + 213.16]^{1/2}/10]^2$$
$$n = [1.96 \times [238.16]^{1/2}/10]^2$$
$$n = [1.96 \times 15.432/10]^2$$
$$n = [30.25/10]^2$$
$$n = 3.025^2$$
$$n = 9.15$$

This shows that if the CV_A increases, the number of analyses needed for an accurate estimate will increase. If the percentage deviation from the homeostatic setting point changes, this will also influence the result. If we want to know within 20% rather than 10%, using the above formula it is as follows:

$$n = [Z \times [CV_A^2 + CV_I^2]^{1/2}/D]^2$$
$$n = [1.96 \times [5.0^2 + 14.6^2]^{1/2}/20]^2$$
$$n = [1.96 \times [25.0 + 213.16]^{1/2}/20]^2$$
$$n = [1.96 \times [238.16]^{1/2}/20]^2$$
$$n = [1.96 \times 15.432/20]^2$$
$$n = [30.25/20]^2$$
$$n = 1.513^2$$
$$n = 2.29$$

In this situation, two samples would be adequate to estimate the homeostatic setting point for creatinine in a dog within 20%, with 95% probability.

In conclusion, application of the IRIS recommendations (www.iris-kidney.com) will depend on a number of factors, including the analytical CV, the probability factor, and the stringency of the estimate of creatinine (D) that is desired.

FURTHER READING

Fraser CG (2001) *Biological Variation: From Principles to Practice.* AACC Press, Washington DC.

Veterinary Clinical Pathology

CASE 158

1 What is your assessment of these findings?

The haematological findings indicate the presence of pancytopaenia. The combination of slightly low plasma protein and slightly decreased number of erythrocytes is consistent with the bleeding noted clinically. The anaemia appears to be non-responding – this may be due to recent development without sufficient time to see a response in the peripheral blood, but the presence of a non-responding anaemia with panctyopaenia is suggestive of bone marrow pathology resulting in decreased production of all cell lines (myeloid, erythroid, megakaryocytes/platelets). The marked thrombocytopaenia is consistent with the clinical signs of bleeding from mucous membranes (bleeding from the anus, petechiae, epistaxis, red urine suggesting haematuria).

2 What are your differential diagnoses?

Differential diagnoses include acute septicaemia, aflatoxicosis, sweet clover poisoning or toxicity associated with trichloroethylene-extracted soybean meal, bracken fern toxicity or the haemolytic syndrome of babesiosis.

FOLLOW UP

This cow died. Postmortem investigations did not identify infection or hepatic or renal disease. Evaluation of the pasture shared by the two cows did not reveal the presence of sweet clover. The pasture was bare and bracken fern was present over a large proportion of the pasture. No feeding was provided to supplement that pasture. No ticks were found on the animal and the farmer indicated that periodic pour-on treatment for ticks and lice had been applied. Bracken fern toxicity was diagnosed.

Bracken fern (*Pteridium aquilinum* or *Pteris aquiline*) occurs worldwide and may affect multiple species, and in monogastric animals this is due to thiamine deficiency. Enzootic haematuria with development of bladder tumours (epithelial, fibrous or vascular origin) in cattle may occur with chronic, low-grade ingestion. Haemorrhagic syndrome, as seen in this case, may occur with acute toxicity. This usually requires at least several weeks to months of bracken fern ingestion. Ptaquiloside is thought to be the agent that is toxic to the bone marrow and it may be carcinogenic. In cattle with the acute haemorrhagic presentation, mortality is usually >90% and a very low platelet count is a poor prognostic indicator.

CASE 159

1 What does the ELISA SNAP-Test detect?

The ELISA tests IgG antibodies against the C6 protein of *Borrelia* organisms. This protein is part of the variable major protein-like sequence expression (VlsE) on the outer membrane of the spirochaete. VlsE is one component responsible for the evasion of the immune system of the host, as the sequence is changed rapidly by *Borrelia* clones. The protein is not present while the spirochaete is living in the tick.

2 How do you interpret the result of the ELISA?

This dog is living in an endemic area for *B. burgdorferi* and has been exposed to ticks. He shows a positive *B. burgdorferi*-specific test result and suffers from clinical signs compatible with Lyme borreliosis. Therefore, already three of four criteria are fulfilled to establish the diagnosis Lyme borreliosis. The fourth criterium would be a substantial improvement of clinical signs after appropriate antibiotic therapy (e.g. doxycycline 10 mg/kg PO for 28–30 days). However, after experimental infection of dogs, 15% remain asymptomatic and do not show clinical signs of Lyme disease. Additionally, dogs infected with the organism display antibodies over many years. This dog may have been infected with *B. burgdorferi* long ago and the present finding may be incidental. Therefore, other causes for the lameness (e.g. infectious diseases such as anaplasmosis, which is also transferred by ticks, or injuries such as a ruptured cruciate ligament) should be excluded prior to diagnosing Lyme borreliosis.

3 Might the test be positive owing to previous vaccination?

The test will not be positive because of previous vaccination. Vaccine-specific antibodies are dominantly OspA (outer surface protein A). This protein is rarely expressed in naturally infected dogs. OspA is present in the tick, but after a few hours of blood sucking the protein structure is changed to OspC. This is the key for the spirochaetes to infect the gut of the tick and therefore get into the new host during the feeding times. Cross-reactivity of the C6 test to vaccine-specific OspA has not been reported.

Editors' note: Several ELISA tests exist to test for borreliosis. Knowledge of the test used and the specific antigens detected is important.

FURTHER READING

Gerber B, Haugl K, Eichenberger S *et al.* (2009) Follow-up of Bernese Mountain dogs and other dogs with serologically diagnosed *Borrelia burgdorferi* infection: what happens to seropositive animals? *BMC Vet Res* **5**:8.

Krupka I, Straubinger RK (2010) Lyme borreliosis in dogs and cats: background, diagnosis, treatment and prevention of infections with *Borrelia burgdorferi sensu strict*. *Vet Clin North Am Small Anim Pract* **40**:1103–1119.

Littman MP, Goldstein RE, Labato MA *et al.* (2006) ACVIM Small Animal Consensus Statement on Lyme disease in dogs: diagnosis, treatment, and prevention. *J Vet Intern Med* **20**:422–434.

CASE 160

1 The nurse comes to you with a urine specimen that is testing 2+ positive for leucocyte esterase on dipstick analysis, but no neutrophils are seen in the urine sediment examination. She is concerned that one of these results is in error. What can you tell the nurse regarding this situation in a cat?

Leucocyte esterase is positive in urine from cats that does not contain leucocytes and, therefore, is of no diagnostic value in cats. It can be positive when leucocytes are present in the urine, but because most cats show a positive result when leucocytes are not present, this test is not helpful. The mechanism for the false-positive reaction in cats is not known, but may be due to the presence of non-leucocyte esterases in the urine. Freezing of the urine has been shown to eliminate the false-positive reactions.

2 What if this urine specimen were from a dog?

In dogs, leucocyte esterase dipstick testing is insensitive for detection of leucocytes. Sensitivity of approximately 46% has been reported, with specificity of approximately 93.2%. When the leucocyte esterase-positive results are obtained from the urine of dogs, quantitative urine culture results are frequently also positive. However, false-negative reactions may occur (low sensitivity).

3 What other test pad results available on some dipsticks may be unreliable or of limited use in dogs and/or cats?

Nitrite (reduced form of nitrates) on the dipstick is used to screen for bacteriuria in people, but has been found to be unreliable in dogs and cats. It does not consistently detect significant bacteriuria. The USG pads on dipsticks are also unreliable in dogs and cats, likely because of the greater buffering capacity of feline and canine urine compared with human urine.

Urobilinogen dipstick testing in humans is used to screen for hepatic disease, haemolytic disorders and patency of the bile duct. Urobilinogen is rarely positive in dog and cat specimens and when positive is usually only 1+. This may be due to the fact that urobilinogen is unstable and may be oxidised to urobilin if the urine is acidic or exposed to light following collection. Urobilin will not result in a positive reaction with the dipstick tests used to detect urobilinogen.

4 What urine dipstick tests may be of different significance in the dog and cat?

Urine dipstick analysis for bilirubin may be of differing significance in the dog and the cat. Small quantities of bilirubin are commonly observed in the urine of normal dogs. This may be due to a low renal threshold for bilirubin.

Over 60% of normal male dogs have been reported to have a 1+ or greater Ictotest reaction. When male dogs with normal serum bilirubin values were evaluated, approximately 50% had 1+ or greater Ictotest results and approximately 25% were positive using the Chemstrip test. Conversely, a high percentage of dogs with negative tests for bilirubinuria were found to have increased serum bilirubin concentrations. This has been hypothesised to be the result of an inhibitor of the test reaction. In addition, bilirubin in urine is unstable and may be oxidised to form biliverdin if allowed to stand at room temperature. This will not be detected by diazotisation reactions common on dipsticks for detection of bilirubin. Light also degrades bilirubin. Urine should not be filtered or centrifuged prior to dipstick evaluation for bilirubin since precipitates of calcium carbonate and/or phosphate may absorb bilirubin.

However, bilirubin in the urine of healthy cats is virtually non-existent. If bilirubinuria is detected by dipstick analysis of urine from a cat, evaluation for a variety of conditions is indicated. These include primary hepatic disease, diabetes mellitus, feline infectious peritonitis, haemolysis and FeLV-related disorders.

Bilirubinuria in both dogs and cats is more commonly seen in males compared with females.

FURTHER READING
Osborne CA, Stevens JB (1999) *Urinalysis: A Clinical guide to Compassionate Patient Care.* Bayer Corporation, Shawnee Mission.

CASE 161

1 What test can be used for evaluation for possible cryptorchidism in this horse?

The hCG stimulation test can be used for diagnosis of cryptorchidism in the horse. The protocol is as follows:

- Baseline serum testosterone time 0.
- Administration of 10,000 IU hCG (Chorulon) IV.
- Testosterone (serum) 2 hours post hCG. Cryptorchid stallions will show testosterone significantly elevated from baseline (usually a minimum of twice baseline).

Oestrone sulphate can also be used for diagnosis of cryptorchidism in horses >3 years of age. Oestrone sulphate is not suitable for diagnosis of cryporchidism in donkeys. An hCG stimulation test may be needed if a borderline result is obtained with oestrone sulphate.

2 What recommendations would you make for detection of cryptorchidism in a dog or cat?

An hCG or GnRH test can be used for diagnosis of cryptorchidism or testicular remnants in the dog and cat, according to the following protocols. In the male cat, the presence of penile spines is indicative of the influence of testosterone. A retained testicle/testicular remnant is the most common source for testosterone, but adrenal neoplasia may also result in testosterone production.

Cat: GnRH stimulation test

- Collect baseline serum testosterone sample at time 0.
- Administer 250 µg of GnRH (Cystorelin) IM.
- Collect post-GnRH sample at 60 minutes.
- Cryptorchid/testicular remnant cats will have ≥ twice baseline testosterone levels following GnRH stimulation.

Cat: hCG stimulation test

- Collect baseline serum testosterone sample at time 0.
- Administer 250 IU of hCG.
- Collect post-hCG sample at 4 hours.
- Cryptorchid/testicular remnant cats will have ≥ twice baseline testosterone levels following hCG stimulation.

Dog: GnRH stimulation test

- Collect baseline serum testosterone sample at time 0.
- Administer 25 µg total dose or 2 µg/kg (whichever is the larger dose) IM.
- Collect post-GnRH sample at 60 minutes.
- If the dog is >2 years of age, 'stimulating' the testicular tissue may be of benefit 3 days after GnRH injection, followed by collection of the stimulated sample at 60 minutes following the GnRH injection on the fourth day.
- Cryptorchid/testicular remnant dogs typically show ≥ twice baseline testosterone samples following stimulation.

Dog: hCG stimulation test

- Collect baseline serum testosterone sample at time 0.
- Administer 44 µg/kg hCG IM.
- Collect post-hCG sample at 4 hours.
- Cryptorchid/testicular remnant dogs typically show ≥ twice baseline testosterone samples following stimulation.

CASE 162

1 What are the cells shown (long arrows and arrow heads)?

Two mast cells (long arrows) and three basophils (arrow heads) are shown. Mast cells were counted as atypical cells during the differential count. Mast cells are medium to large 'round cells' that contain fine magenta cytoplasmic granules. Basophils are granulocytic cells that contain fine cytoplasmic lavender granules. The main morphological feature that helps in distinguishing these two cell types is the shape of the nucleus. In fact, while mast cells have round to oval nuclei, basophils have segmented nuclei similar to those observed in neutrophils.

2 What is the significance of this finding, and what further test would you perform?

Mast cells are not usually found in the peripheral blood of healthy animals and their presence always indicates an underlying disease. In dogs, mast cells can occasionally be seen in circulation during severe reactive or inflammatory processes and, therefore, mastocytaemia is not always a reflection of an underlying mast cell tumour (MCT). In cats, the incidence of mastocytaemia is very low and most of the time is associated with an MCT either involving the bone marrow or a visceral organ such as the spleen or the gastrointestinal tract. However, a few cases of feline mastocytaemia have been recently reported associated with other tumours, such as lymphoma and haemangiosarcoma.

In this case, further investigation would include abdominal imaging and bone marrow aspiration. Abdominal ultrasonography revealed an enlarged hypoechoic spleen. Following fine needle aspiration, cytology indicated a splenic MCT. This finding alone would be sufficient to explain the mild mastocytaemia but, given the mild non-regenerative anaemia, a bone marrow aspirate was also performed. This showed a mild focal bone marrow involvement.

3 What are the differential diagnoses for the anaemia?

In this cat, the main differential diagnoses for the non-regenerative anaemia include bone marrow infiltration, chronic blood loss and decreased or ineffective erythropoiesis.

As in dogs, mast cell granules contain vasoactive substances including histamine. These substances may cause gastroenteric ulcerations, leading to anaemia of chronic blood loss. Because of this, red cell morphology (microcytic-hypochromic anaemia) and faecal analysis for occult blood may aid in the diagnosis of this paraneoplastic condition. Ineffective erythropoiesis during neoplasia may be due to a combination of factors including increased red cell precursors, apoptosis or chronic inflammation.

This is a case of a feline splenic MCT with a secondary paraneoplastic anaemia and mild mastocytaemia and basophilia. In cats, MCTs can be classified into three distinct entities: splenic/visceral, intestinal or cutaneous mast cell tumours.

The most common clinical signs in cats with the splenic form of MCT are usually non-specific and include vomiting (especially if gastrointestinal ulcerations are present), weight loss and anorexia. Splenectomy is considered the treatment of choice even if involvement of other organs is found.

FURTHER READING
London C, Thamm D (2013) *Whithrow and MacEwen's Small Animal Clinical Oncology*, 5th edn. Elsevier Saunders, St. Louis, pp. 335–355.
Piviani M, Walton RM, Patel RT (2013) Significance of mastocytemia in cats. *J Vet Clin Pathol* **42**:4–10.

CASE 163

1 What is the significance of: (a) the +++ positive leucocyte reaction; (b) the ++ positive protein reaction; (c) the + positive blood?

(a) The finding of +++ leucocytes (or rather leucocyte esterase) in the absence of leucocytes in the sediment has no significance. This reaction occurs extremely frequently; the cause is not well understood but may be due to various interferents in animal urine.

(b) The cause for the ++ proteinuria is not clear. The urine sample is adequately concentrated and therefore kidney disease is unlikely, but cannot be excluded. Also a pre-renal proteinuria (overload proteinuria) is possible. However, further tests are needed to determine if this is a persistent finding.

(c) The + blood reaction without the finding of RBCs in the sediment is of questionable significance. RBCs could become lysed in urine, but no ghosts (RBC membranes) were reported. The most plausible explanation is a spurious positive reaction caused by the presence of +++ bilirubin. The orange–brown colour of the urine sample is most likely due to bilirubin and not to blood. In the author's experience, a massive bilirubinuria is frequently mixed up with blood in the urine by pet owners.

2 Which crystal is shown in Fig. 163.2?

The crystal is a bilirubin crystal, resembling star-like, plant-like or sometimes also rhomboid structures of orange–yellow colour. Frequently, cells (squamous epithelial cells, transitional cells) are also stained by bilirubin.

3 What is the next step in a cat with this finding?

Because of the higher renal threshold, the finding of bilirubin in the urine of a healthy cat is rare. Therefore, any finding of bilirubin in a cat's urine must not be ignored and should prompt a close screening of the liver by ultrasound and laboratory tests.

FOLLOW UP

In this cat, grossly elevated liver enzymes and a bilirubin concentration of 318.06 µmol/l (reference interval, <10.26 µmol/l) was found. The cat died a few days later and cholangiohepatitis was found on necropsy and histopathology.

FURTHER READING
Holan KM, Kruger JM, Gibbons SN *et al.* (1997) Clinical evaluation of a leukocyte esterase test-strip for detection of feline pyuria. *Vet Clin Pathol* **26**:126–131.
Osborne CA, Stevens JB (1999) *Urinalysis: A Clinical Guide to Compassionate Patient Care.* Bayer Corporation, Shawnee Mission.
Stockham SL, Scott MA (2008) *Fundamentals of Veterinary Clinical Pathology*, 2nd edn. Blackwell Publishing, Oxford, pp. 457–462.

CASE 164

1 Describe and discuss the biochemistry changes.

The pancreatic enzymes amylase and lipase are markedly increased (more than 3-fold), which is indicative of pancreatic acinar cell damage, most likely because of acute pancreatitis. Another cause could be pancreatic neoplasia.

Moderate hypocalcaemia is present, which has been reported in the face of acute pancreatitis. Although the exact pathomechanism is unclear, entry of calcium into damaged membranes or extravasation of protein-bound calcium may be the cause. Traditionally, the formation of calcium soaps by binding of calcium to fatty acids has been considered. Parathyroid damage during surgery of the thyroid gland may contribute.

Slight hyperproteinaemia based on slight hyperalbuminaemia indicates dehydration. Sample desiccation (heating prior to analysis, spinning of tube without a plug, sample sitting on analyser in open cup with delay in testing) may cause hyperproteinaemia and hyperalbuminaemia, but is unlikely with good specimen handling and techniques.

Mild hyperbilirubinaemia is present in pre-hepatic, hepatic or post-hepatic disease. There is no haemolysis or anaemia, which excludes pre-hepatic causes. Slightly increased ALT enzyme activity indicates hepatocellular damage. Therefore, an hepatic cause of hyperbilirubinaemia could be possible. However, the most likely cause is post-hepatic disease, such as obstructive cholestasis, in conjunction with acute pancreatitis. This may be the result of inflammation and/or swelling in the area of the bile duct, resulting in its obstruction. This is further supported by a marked increase in ALP enzyme activity. Its liver isoenzyme is located in hepatobiliary epithelial cells with induction of the enzyme in the face of cholestasis.

Mild hypercholesterolaemia is frequently observed in acute pancreatitis, probably due to altered lipoprotein metabolism because of inflammatory cytokines or obstructive cholestasis.

Diagnosis: acute pancreatitis with obstructive cholestasis and slight hepatocellular damage.

2 What further analyses would you recommend to confirm your diagnosis?

Further analyses to confirm acute pancreatitis are:

- Canine pancreatic lipase immunoreactivity (cPLI) is a sensitive and specific test for pancreatitis in dogs and should be performed in cases suspicious for pancreatitis. In this case, the degree of increase in amylase and lipase is classic for pancreatitis, so assessment of cPLI is unlikely to be needed. It will not help differentiate the underlying cause for pancreatitis (idiopathic, neoplastic, inflammatory, pancreatic abscess, other).
- Canine trypsin-like immunoreactivity (cTLI) detecting trypsinogen, trypsin and trypsin bound to proteinase inhibitors. May be increased in about 40% of patients with pancreatitis. The advantage over assessment of amylase and lipase is only minimal. As with cPLI, it is not needed for the diagnosis in this case.
- Abdominal ultrasonography to diagnose the underlying aetiology, such as pancreatic neoplasia or pancreatic abscess.
- Exploratory laparotomy with pancreatic biopsy may be necessary to make a definitive diagnosis. Disadvantages to consider include an increased risk of anaesthesia for the patient. Additionally, the biopsy may miss the area(s) of abnormality as these are often localised and may or may not be macroscopically apparent.

CASE 165

1 What types of gammopathy can be identified on serum protein electrophoresis using capillary zone electrophoresis?

- Monoclonal gammopathy (**Fig. 165.1**). Production of a single clone of immunoglobulin due to clonal expansion of neoplastic lymphocytes.
- Biclonal gammopathy (**Fig. 165.2**):
  - ❑ Production of two classes of immunoglobulin by two separate B cell clones.
  - ❑ Production of one class of immunoglobulin by a single clone of B cells with different dimerisation patterns.

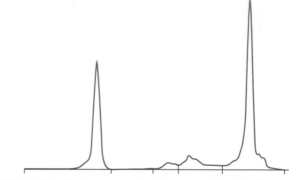

FIG. 165.1 Canine monoclonal gammopathy. Capillary zone electrophoresis.

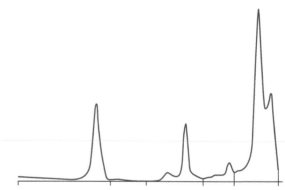

FIG. 165.2 Canine with suspected biclonal gammopathy. Capillary zone electrophoresis.

  - ❑ Production of separate heavy chain isotypes by a single clone of B cells ('isotype switching').
  - ❑ Production of light chains only (described in a cat).
- Polyclonal gammopathy (**Fig. 165.3**). Production of multiple subclasses/classes of immunoglobulins.
- Oligoclonal gammopathy (**Fig. 165.4**):
  - ❑ Polyclonal gammopathy with restricted migration.
  - ❑ Oligoclonal gammopathies may be indistinguishable from a monoclonal gammopathy or as narrow bands, base slightly wider than the albumin band.
  - ❑ Oligoclonal gammopathies may be recognised as tall 'monoclonal-like' peaks superimposed upon a broad 'polyclonal-like' base. This is due to specific B-cell stimulation resulting in secretion of a few restricted classes of immunoglobulins (*E. canis*, feline lymphocytic/plasmacytic gingivitis–stomatitis, possibly some cases of babesiosis).
  - ❑ Same pattern theoretically could be seen with B-cell neoplasia in an animal with concurrent antigenic stimulation.

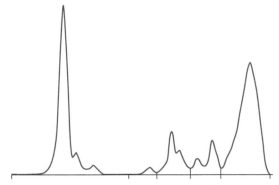

FIG. 165.3 Feline polyclonal gammopathy. Capillary zone electrophoresis.

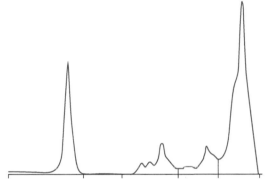

FIG. 165.4 Canine with suspected oligoclonal gammopathy. Capillary zone electrophoresis.

CASE 166

1 How do you interpret the result of the ELISA?
The ELISA detects IgM and IgG antibodies against *B. burgdorferi* and is positive. Although the clinical signs match Lyme disease, dogs frequently show positive serological titres without having the disease. This occurs especially in endemic areas for the spirochaetes. Other causes for the clinical signs should be ruled out prior to diagnosing Lyme borreliosis. Additionally, if this ELISA is not specifically detecting antibodies against the C6 protein of *B. burgdorferi*, false-positive results due to vaccination may occur.

2 How would you proceed with this dog with regard to additional laboratory testing?
A second, confirmatory test has to be performed to exclude a false-positive result due to vaccination. This could be an ELISA detecting the C6 protein or a Western blot. The latter discriminates specific bands for the disease as well as antibodies resulting from vaccination. If the test is still positive, a therapeutic trial with doxycycline (10 mg/kg PO over 30 days) is indicated. If the patient shows substantial

improvement in clinical signs after a few days of therapy, the diagnosis of Lyme borreliosis can be established.

Frequently, co-infections with other tick-borne organisms occur. Therefore, exclusion of other tick-borne diseases, such as anaplasmosis, is warranted since clinical signs may be similar.

Lyme nephritis, a suspected immune-mediated glomerulonephritis, is still a theme under discussion. Nevertheless, exclusion of proteinuria is recommended in a dog with an established diagnosis of Lyme borreliosis to exclude renal disease.

Finally, the owner must be educated that vaccination does not replace adequate tick control. Preventive action against ticks is highly recommended (e.g. permethrin application, amitraz collar) to avoid infection with other diseases transmitted by ticks (e.g. *Anaplasma phagocytophilum*, *Ehrlichia* spp., *Babesia* spp., *Bartonella* spp., *Mycoplasma* spp.).

Editors' note: Several ELISA tests exist for borreliosis, so knowledge about the specific antigens detected and possible need for further confirmatory testing is important.

FURTHER READING

Gerber B, Haugl K, Eichenberger S *et al.* (2009) Follow-up of Bernese Mountain dogs and other dogs with serologically diagnosed *Borrelia burgdorferi* infection: what happens to seropositive animals? *BMC Vet Res* **5**:8.

Krupka I, Straubinger RK (2010) Lyme borreliosis in dogs and cats: background, diagnosis, treatment and prevention of infections with *Borrelia burgdorferi sensu strict*. *Vet Clin North Am Small Anim Pract* **40**:1103–1119.

Littman MP, Goldstein RE, Labato MA *et al.* (2006) ACVIM small animal consensus statement on Lyme disease in dogs: diagnosis, treatment, and prevention. *J Vet Intern Med* **20**: 422–434.

CASE 167

1 How would you classify this anaemia, and what are possible causes?
The anaemia observed at day 1 was normocytic-normochromic with poor evidence of regeneration. Reticulocyte evaluation was recommended to further quantify the regeneration. A reticulocyte count of 52 × 10^9/l confirmed a non-regenerative condition. The main differentials for a non-regenerative, normocytic-normochromic anaemia are a pre-regenerative condition (e.g. acute haemolysis, acute blood loss), anaemia due to insufficient bone marrow production (e.g. bone marrow neoplasia or suppression or damage), or anaemia of chronic disease. The haemolytic appearance of the blood might be spurious due to *in-vitro* haemolysis, although acute haemolysis is a possible differential in this case.

Haematology at day 3 showed a significant regenerative response and confirmed that the anaemia initially observed was pre-regenerative, likely due to acute haemolysis. Acute haemolytic anaemia was diagnosed finally.

2 What RBC morphological abnormalities can be observed in the blood film?

Two schistocytes can be seen in the centre of the film. Schistocytes are erythrocyte fragments with pointed extremities and are commonly the result of the impact of erythrocytes with fibrin strands in the peripheral blood. They are commonly observed in DIC, microangiopathic haemolytic anaemia, iron deficiency anaemia, myelofibrosis, heart failure, glomerulonephritis, dyserythropoiesis and haemangiosarcoma. The combination of haemolytic anaemia and evidence of schistocytes make a microangiopathic haemolytic anaemia the main differential. Microangiopathic haemolytic anaemias are a subgroup of haemolytic anaemias characterised by mechanical damage to RBCs in the circulation, which may be the main cause of the lysis of the cells. DIC and haemolytic–uraemic syndrome (HUS) are a couple of possible causes of this.

3 How would you classify the azotaemia in this patient?

There was evidence of a marked azotaemia, which could be pre-renal (dehydration), renal (kidney dysfunction) or post-renal (urinary obstruction). The evidence of poorly concentrated urine made a renal azotaemia more likely. Considering the acute onset of the clinical signs, this was consistent with AKI.

4 What would be your main differential for a dog with acute onset of haemolytic anaemia, thrombocytopaenia and azotaemia?

The combination of microangiopathic haemolytic anaemia, thrombocytopaenia and AKI is highly suggestive of acute HUS. DIC is less likely as a possible cause of thrombocytopaenia because the coagulation times assessed at a follow-up examination are within reference interval. Leptospirosis is another possible differential for AKI, although serology and PCR were performed and were negative.

HUS is a condition commonly associated with *E. coli serotype 0157* infection, which has been reported to be the main cause of HUS. Toxins produced by this bacteria destroy intestinal epithelial cells and enter the vascular system, inducing specific localised damage to glomerular capillary and renal arteries with formation of thrombi and consequent renal dysfunction and mechanical damage to erythrocytes (microangiopathic haemolytic anaemia). A serological test performed to identify this specific serotype of *E. coli* was positive, confirming the initial suspicion.

The dog was treated with antibiotics, IV fluid therapy and diuretics to induce diuresis. Unfortunately, she remained oliguric and the azotaemia worsened. Peritoneal dialysis was started, although despite multiple dialysis sessions, the azotaemia did not significantly decrease and the dog remained anuric. After 4 days of hospitalisation she was euthanised.

FURTHER READING

Dell'Orco M, Bertazzolo W, Pagliaro L *et al.* (2005) Hemolytic-uremic syndrome in a dog. *J Vet Clin Pathol* 34:264–269.

Douglas JW, Wardrop KJ (2011) *Schalm's Veterinary Hematology*, 6th edn. Wiley-Blackwell, Ames.

Holloway S, Senior D, Roth L *et al.* (1993) Hemolytic uremic syndrome in dogs. *J Vet Intern Med* 7:220–227.

Stockham SL, Scott MA, (2008) *Fundamentals of Veterinary Clinical Pathology*, 2nd edn. Blackwell Publishing, Oxford.

CASE 168

1 What is your assessment of the biochemistry findings at day 15 and day 30 following the institution of treatment?

The findings at days 15 and 30 show resolution of the increased urea, creatinine and phosphorus, indicating resolution of the dehydration. The decline in total protein, albumin and globulins also likely reflects better hydration. However, there is now slight hypoproteinaemia with hypoalbuminaemia that deserves further investigation as to an underlying cause. There is a trend for declining ALP and ALT, which is encouraging, but both remain increased compared with their reference interval.

2 Based on your knowledge of biological variation in the dog, index of individuality and reference change value, what findings do you consider likely to be statistically 'significant' or 'highly significant'?

Information on biological variation for various analytes in dogs is shown in Appendix 2 (p. 264). The CV_A provided will be used as representative of the laboratory in which this patient's data was generated. (**Note:** The CV_A may differ with instruments/methods, so the CV_A will also differ between laboratories and CV_A specific for the laboratory being used should be used for these types of calculations.)

The Table below summarises the index of individuality (IoI) from Appendix 2 (p. 264), the changes in analytes and the reference change values (RCVs) at 95% probability ('significant') and 99% probability ('highly significant') levels for this patient.

Analyte	IoI (from Appendix 2)	Change in Analyte from Day 1 to Day 15 (%)	Change in Analyte from Day 15 to Day 30 (%)	Change in Analyte from Day 1 to Day 30 (%)	RCV (95% probability) 'Significant' (%)	RCV (99% probability) 'Highly Significant' (%)
Creatinine	0.87 (intermediate)	50	16.67	58.3	41.26	54.30
Total protein	1.10 (intermediate)	16.67	4.00	20.00	7.8	10.3
Albumin	1.04 (intermediate)	20	5.00	24.00	8.00	10.52
Glucose	0.37 (low)	5.80	3.08	8.70	28.26	37.19
ALP	3.90 (high)	30.34	13.27	39.59	24.30	31.98
ALT	2.32 (high)	20.00	9.18	27.35	28.31	37.26

The IoI for creatinine and total protein and albumin is intermediate (IoI between 0.6 and 1.4), indicating that the RCV may be of benefit, but not providing the strongest support for its use. The IoI for glucose is low (<0.6), indicating that a population-based 95% reference interval (the traditional reference interval) is likely to be the best standard for making judgements about alterations in this analyte. The IoI for ALP and ALT is high (>1.4), indicating that the RCV is likely to be more useful than the population-based reference interval in making judgements about changes in serial results for these analytes.

Based on the changes documented in this Table, the change in creatinine (decreasing trend) between days 1 and 15 is 'significant' (>41.26%) but does not qualify as a 'highly significant' change (>54.3%). The change between days 1 and 30 qualifies as a 'highly significant' change. The change in hydration status and decline in other analytes reflective of improved GFR (urea, total protein, albumin) provide further support for improved hydration, as noted clinically.

The changes in total protein (decreasing) between days 1 and 15 and between days 1 and 30 are statistically 'highly significant'. This concurs with the use of the population-based reference interval and indicates that further evaluation for an underlying cause for decreasing total protein should be investigated. Hepatic dysfunction could be investigated by a bile acid stimulation test. Urinalysis should be considered to determine if urinary tract loss of protein may be contributing. Likewise, the changes in albumin are similar in degree and significance to those of the total protein.

The changes in glucose do not meet levels of statistical significance but are reassuring when the population-based reference interval is applied, since there is normalisation of the glucose level.

The changes in ALP (decreasing) achieve 'significant' levels between days 1 and 15 and 'highly significant' levels between days 1 and 30. This suggests that there is some resolution of the cholestatic component, either spontaneously or because of the treatment that was instituted. However, the changes in ALT (decreasing) are not statistically 'significant' or 'highly significant'. Although the trend is encouraging, the variation in ALT could be due to biological variation within this individual and may not reflect a true improvement in the hepatocellular condition.

3 Do you feel that these results are also of clinical significance? If so, why?

Correlation with other evaluations and tests helps provide support for the clinical significance of the changes in laboratory data. However, since the total protein and albumin are now low and the ALT has failed to show improvement considered to be statistically 'significant' or 'highly significant' based on information about biological variation of these analytes in the dog, further investigation should be considered. Use of the RCV helps provide quantitative evidence for evaluation of laboratory findings and their interpretation.

4 What additional testing would you recommend?

It is possible that there may be continued improvement with time and continued monitoring is an option since the patient's clinical condition is good. Alternatively, further investigations may include radiographic and ultrasound evaluations of the liver, a bile acid stimulation test to determine if hepatic dysfunction may be the cause of declining albumin, and urinalysis to determine if there is urinary protein loss. Ultimately, liver biopsies may be required to determine the most definitive diagnosis with regard to the liver condition. Prior to liver biopsy, evaluation of a coagulation profile (including platelet count, aPTT and PT) is recommended.

FURTHER READING

Fraser CG (2001) *Biological Variation: From Principles to Practice*. AACC Press, Washington DC.

Walton RM (2012) Subject-based reference values: biological variation, individuality, and reference change values. *J Vet Clin Pathol* **41**:175–181.

CASE 169

1 What is your assessment of these findings?

The haematological findings are consistent with a moderate responding anaemia. There is slight leucocytosis and neutrophilia without lymphopaenia, suggesting inflammation.

The slight hyperbilirubinaemia in the absence of other bio-chemistry abnormalities is suggestive of a pre-hepatic origin for the haemolysis. The microagglutination noted in the blood film suggests that an immune-mediated basis for the anaemia is likely.

2 What is the most likely clinical diagnosis?
The most likely clinical diagnosis is haemolytic anaemia, possibly immune-mediated haemolytic anaemia.

3 What are the differential diagnoses, and what other tests should be considered in this case?
Haemolytic anaemia in cattle may occur secondary to bacterial, viral or protozoal infections, drug exposure, liver disease, toxic plant exposure and/or neoplasia. Evaluation to determine if infection is present (rule out common problems such as mastitis, pneumonia, metritis, traumatic reticulopericarditis with infection, internal abscess) is recommended. A Coombs test should be considered to determine if the anaemia has an immune-mediated basis.

FOLLOW UP
A Coombs test was positive in this cow. No evidence of infection, neoplasia or toxic plant exposure was found in subsequent evaluations. A clinical diagnosis of idiopathic immune-mediated haemolytic anaemia was made.

FURTHER READING
Dixon PM, Matthews AG, Brown R et al. (1978) Bovine autoimmune-hemolytic anemia. Vet Rec 103:155–157.
Nassiri SM, Saeedeh D, Khazralinia P (2011) Bovine immune-mediated haemolytic anemia: 13 cases (November 2008–August 2009). J Vet Clin Pathol 40:459–466.

CASE 170

1 What is your assessment of these results?
The hyperglycaemia is likely to be due to stress associated with the seizure and/or transport to the veterinary clinic. This does not completely rule out transient hypoglycaemia as an underlying cause for the seizure, but given the normal behaviour and nursing prior to the seizure, hypoglycaemia appears unlikely.

The moderate increase in CK is likely due to muscle damage sustained during the seizure. The marked hypo-calcaemia with hyperphosphataemia is highly suggestive of hypoparathyroidism. There is no history of marked exercise, lack of nursing (decreased dietary intake), hypoalbu-minaemia or severe renal or liver disease that would account for hypocalcaemia. There is no indication of hypomagne-saemia that may result in secondary hypoparathyroidism (required for release of PTH from the parathyroid gland).

2 What additional tests would be needed to confirm the likely diagnosis in this case?
Additional tests to confirm a diagnosis of hypoparathyroidism include ionised calcium assay, fractional excretion of electrolytes and PTH assay. You would expect the ionised calcium to be decreased, the fractional excretion of calcium to be increased and the PTH to be low/undetectable.

3 What are the pathophysiological bases for the observed abnormalities?
The pathophysiological mechanisms underlying these abnormalities includes decreased calcium mobilisation from bone due to absence of PTH activation of osteoclasts. The absence of PTH results in increased renal excretion of calcium. Calcium excretion is increased because of decreased tubular reabsorption and phosphate reabsorption in the proximal tubule is increased, thus causing hyperphosphataemia. PTH stimulates the enzyme 1-a-hydrolase, which catalyses the activation of 1,25-hydroxy-vitamin D (calcitriol), which normally facilitates intestinal absorption of calcium. In the absence of sufficient calcitriol, hypocalcaemia is further accentuated.

FOLLOW UP
The ionised calcium in this foal was found to be decreased. She failed to respond to calcium and vitamin D3 supplementation and was euthanised 1 week later.

The syndrome of neonatal hypoparathyroidism in foals has been reported to be either permanent or transient. Some foals may recover with calcium and vitamin D3 supplementation. The underlying basis is hypothesised to be due to dysgenesis or hypoplasia if permanent, or idiopathic if transient. When detected, a guarded prognosis is warranted, with continued monitoring of the clinical and laboratory findings following treatment.

FURTHER READING
Schwarz B, van den Hoven R (2011) Seizures in an Arabian foal due to suspected prolonged transient neonatal hypoparathyroidism. Equine Vet Educ 24:225–232.
Torobio RE (2011) (ed) Endocrine diseases. Vet Clin North Am Equine Pract 27.

CASE 171

1 What is the pink inclusion in the cytoplasm of the erythrocyte?
The pink inclusion visible in the erythrocyte is a distemper virus inclusion. These bodies are composed of aggregates of viral nucleocapsids. They form within nucleated cells during maturation of erythroid precursors in the bone

marrow and persist in circulating RBCs; they can be also detected in the cytoplasm of leucocytes within blood smears.

2 How long would you expect inclusions to be observed in blood smears?

Distemper virus inclusions are detectable in circulating RBCs during the viraemic stage of infection. Their number is unpredictable and the lack of detectable inclusion bodies does not rule out distemper infection.

3 How can the disease be confirmed?

PCR on a blood sample is usually mandatory. Since distemper virus is an RNA virus, a reverse transcriptase PCR must be used.

FOLLOW UP

A reverse transcriptase PCR for distemper virus was positive.

FURTHER READING

Kubo T, Kagawa Y, Taniyama H *et al.* (2007) Distribution of inclusion bodies in tissues from 100 dogs infected with canine distemper virus. *J Vet Med Sci* **69**:527–529.

CASE 172

1 Discuss which panel of laboratory markers you would recommend.

Acute-phase proteins (APPs) are the markers of choice to exclude inflammation with high sensitivity. A panel of APPs may be of benefit. This should include a major APP, which is defined as a protein showing a marked (>10-fold) and rapid increase in concentration after an insult. Secondly, a moderate APP should be included. Moderate APPs rise less (1–10-fold) and more slowly. Additionally, their concentration also declines more slowly. Finally, a negative APP that declines in the presence of an acute-phase reaction should be part of the panel.

In horses, SAA is a major APP, showing a rapid, up to 10-fold increase after an insult. It increases after colic or other inflammatory causes as well as in the face of bacterial infections. Moderate APPs known to react in horses are fibrinogen and haptoglobin. Fibrinogen is historically used as a marker for inflammatory disease in horses, although it reacts quite slowly. It increases over 24–72 hours after an insult. Fibrinogen is still widely used, especially as the heat precipitation detection method is quick. The other moderate APP, haptoglobin, rises 1–10-fold following surgery, but also in the face of non-infectious causes such as arthritis and carbohydrate-induced laminitis. Albumin may be used as a negative APP.

2 What actions does serum amyloid A (SAA) contribute to an inflammatory reaction?

SAA is produced in the hepatocytes as well as in extrahepatic locations such as the mammary gland and the joints. SAA directly interferes with the inflammatory reaction. It downregulates the inflammatory response, as it inhibits lymphocyte proliferation and myeloperoxidase release. It also favours inflammation, as it enhances the recruitment of inflammatory cells to the site of injury. In extrahepatic tissues, SAA serves as a local protector.

FURTHER READING

Cray C, Zaias J, Altman NH (2009) Acute phase response in animals: a review. *Comp Med* **59**:517–526.
Crisman MV, Scarratt WK, Zimmerman KL (2008) Blood proteins and inflammation in the horse. *Vet Clin North Am Equine Pract* **24**:285–297.

CASE 173

1 What is your interpretation of the profile results, and what are the possible aetiologies?

Increased ALT at this level suggests a hepatocellular insult with leakage of the cytosolic enzyme. Possible causes include inflammatory, toxic, neoplastic or traumatic disease. Concurrent hyperbilirubinaemia and increased bile acids are consistent with cholestasis. Causes include post-hepatic disease (pancreatitis, pancreatic neoplasia and choleliths) or intrahepatic disease (cholangiohepatitis, neoplasia, chronic hepatitis). The increase in ALT activity typically associated with chronic hepatitis is less than noted here, but profile changes cannot reliably be used to discriminate between different hepatic pathologies. In this case, cholestasis secondary to pancreatitis is unlikely given the cPLI result.

2 How might you investigate further?

Ultrasound examination of the biliary tree and gallbladder and assessment of the hepatic size may allow differentiation between post-hepatic and hepatic disease and identification of any localised hepatic or pancreatic masses, but ultimately, diagnosis relies on biopsy. Histological examination usually allows classification of the pathological process but may not be able to determine the aetiology.

FOLLOW UP

Hepatic biopsy revealed a moderate, periportal inflammatory cell infiltrate including neutrophils with small numbers of lymphocytes and plasma cells. The hepatocytes displayed an increased mitotic rate with periportal bile duct proliferation and fibrosis, with foci of bridging fibrosis between the portal tracts. Plugs of bile were identified in the biliary canaliculi. Prussian Blue staining revealed large amounts of iron-positive pigment throughout the liver in Kupffer cells and, occasionally, in hepatocyte cytoplasm. The histological diagnosis of cholangiohepatitis was made but the underlying cause was not evident. Fresh material (bile or hepatic parenchyma) was not collected for culture, although in hindsight this would have been useful. The underlying cause of the cholangiohepatitis was not identified. Possible predisposing factors include biliary obstruction, impaired hepatic perfusion and compromised immune function. The presence of increased Kupffer cell iron deposits has been noted in association with inflammatory and chronic hepatopathies (Fuentealba *et al.*, 1997; Schultheiss *et al.*, 2002).

The dog was treated with symptomatic therapy, fluid therapy and a combination of amoxicillin/clavulanic acid and metronidazole. She made an uneventful recovery.

REFERENCES

Fuentealba C, Guest S, Haywood S *et al.* (1997) Chronic hepatitis: a retrospective study in 34 dogs. *Can Vet J* **38**:365–373.

Schultheiss PC, Bedwell CL, Hamar DW *et al.* (2002) Canine liver iron, copper and zinc concentrations and association with histological lesions. *J Vet Diagn Invest* **14**:396–402.

CASE 174

1 How do you interpret the negative result of the rapid in-house test?

This dog originates from a country where *E. canis* is endemic and it carried ticks. If it is the brown dog tick *Rhipicephalus sanguineus*, the risk is pretty high that he is infected. A negative result from the rapid in-house test does not exclude acute infection, as antibodies need time to develop and may not be detected until day 21 post infection. A false-negative result of the test is unlikely, as the ELISA in-house tests usually have a high sensitivity with very few false-negative results. However, a false-negative result cannot be fully excluded.

2 How would you proceed with the patient?

To definitively rule out *Ehrlichia* infection, paired samples at least 1–2 weeks apart should be analysed. Alternatively, one EDTA sample may be submitted for PCR analysis, which is able to detect *Rickettsia* organisms (4 days post infection). Finally, a haematological examination may be useful. Typical abnormalities associated with *E. canis* infection may be neutropaenia and thrombocytopaenia. *Ehrlichia* morulae are diagnostic for infection and occur early in the infection, but may be few or not detected on blood film evaluation.

FOLLOW UP

PCR was performed and the result was positive. Therefore very early infection with *E. canis* organism was diagnosed.

FURTHER READING

Harrus S, Waner T (2011) Diagnosis of canine monocytotropic ehrlichiosis (*Ehrlichia canis*): an overview. *Vet J* **187**:292–296.

Neer MT, Breitschwerdt EB, Greene RT *et al.* (2002) Consensus satement on ehrlichial disease of small animals from the Infectious Disease Study Group of the ACVIM. *J Vet Intern Med* **16**:309–315.

CASE 175

1 Would there be any benefit in analysing the two patient samples in duplicate in order to estimate the homeostatic setting point for creatinine in an individual dog with chronic stable renal disease?

The dispersion of a result obtained by a single or multiple analyses of one or more samples is calculated from the formula:

$$\text{Dispersion} = Z \times [(CV_A^2/n_A) + (CV_I^2/n_S)]^{1/2}$$

Z = the number of standard deviations appropriate to the probability selected – 1.96 for 95% ($p < 0.05$); CV_A = the precision at the level of the result; n_A = the number of replicate assays or measurements; CV_I = the within-subject biological variation = 14.6% for creatinine in the dog; n_S = the number of patient samples.

Therefore, if we take two samples from a dog with chronic stable renal disease and analyse each of these once and have a CV_A of 2.9%, the dispersion of the result is as follows:

$$
\begin{aligned}
\text{Dispersion} &= Z \times [(CV_A^2/n_A) + (CV_I^2/n_S)]^{1/2} \\
&= 1.96 \times [2.9^2/1 + 14.6^2/2]^{1/2} \\
&= 1.96 \times [8.41/1 + 213.16/2]^{1/2} \\
&= 1.96 \times [8.41 + 106.58]^{1/2} \\
&= 1.96 \,[114.99]^{1/2} \\
&= 1.96 \,[10.723] = 21.02\%
\end{aligned}
$$

So, at a mean creatinine of 150 µmol/l, the dispersion around this mean = 150 ± 21.02% = 150 ± 31.53 = 118.47–181.53. This is a wide range of results and could result in a change in the category of disease based on the recommended cut-offs in the dog.

If we take two samples from a dog with chronic stable renal disease and analyze each of these in duplicate and have a CV_A of 2.9%, the dispersion of the result is as follows:

$$\begin{aligned}
\text{Dispersion} &= Z \times [(CV_A{}^2/n_A) + (CV_I{}^2/n_S)]^{1/2}\\
&= 1.96 \times [2.9^2/2 + 14.6^2/2]^{1/2}\\
&= 1.96 \times [8.41/2 + 213.16/2]^{1/2}\\
&= 1.96 \times [4.205 + 106.58]^{1/2}\\
&= 1.96\,[110.785]^{1/2}\\
&= 1.96\,[10.525] = 20.63\%
\end{aligned}$$

So, at a mean of 150 µmol/l, the dispersion of the result around the mean would be 150 mmol/l ± 20.63% = 150 ± 30.95 = 119.05–180.95. This represents a marginal improvement compared to a single analysis.

If we take three samples from a dog with chronic stable renal disease and analyse each of these once and have a $CV_A = 2.9\%$, then the dispersion is:

$$\begin{aligned}
\text{Dispersion} &= Z \times [(CV_A{}^2/n_A) + (CV_I{}^2/n_S)]^{1/2}\\
&= 1.96 \times [2.9^2/1 + 14.6^2/3]^{1/2}\\
&= 1.96 \times [8.41/2 + 213.16/3]^{1/2}\\
&= 1.96 \times [4.205 + 71.05]^{1/2}\\
&= 1.96\,[75.258]^{1/2}\\
&= 1.96\,[8.675] = 17.00\%.
\end{aligned}$$

So, at a mean of 150 µmol/l, the dispersion of the result around the mean would be 150 mmol/l ± 17% = 150 ± 25.50 = 124.5–175.50. This would represent an improvement and less risk of misclassification of chronic renal disease, based on the recommended cut-off values. However, this still covers a wide range of creatinine results.

Note: Use of cut-offs recommended by the IRIS may be further compromised by a lack of traceability and standardisation of calibration of assays for creatinine analysis. An argument can be made that standardisation of calibration and traceability are needed in order to use cut-off values that are not instrument and method specific.

FURTHER READING

Dispersion Calculator and Critical Number of Test Samples. http://www.westgard.com/dispersion-calculator-and-critical-number-of-test-samples.htm (Accessed 17th November 2014)

Fraser CG (2001) *Biological Variation: From Principles to Practice.* AACC Press, Washington DC.

International Renal Interest Society. Staging of Chronic Renal Disease. http://www.iris-kidney.com/_downloads/N378.008%20IRIS%20Website%20Staging%20of%20CKD%20PDF.PDF (Accessed 17th November 2014)

CASE 176

1 Describe the haematological abnormalities. What do you see on the blood smear? State the underlying pathophysiological mechanism.

Results of the haematological examination are unremarkable except for an increased reticulocyte count. In the absence of anaemia, this may be due to excitement or recent exercise, but could also indicate increased RBC turnover. As the haematocrit is within the reference interval but the reticulocytes are increased, continuous haemorrhage or haemolysis of low volume may be present.

The blood smear shows slight polychromasia and slight anisocytosis, as well as slight to moderate poikilocytosis based on the presence of some acanthocytes and rare shistocytes. Causes for acanthocytes are not fully understood, but changes in the membrane composition of erythrocytes are likely. Therefore, an increased cholesterol:phospholipid ratio is present in the RBC membrane. The increased amount of cholesterol in the erythrocyte membrane causes protrusion of the outer part of the RBC membrane, with visible irregular outlines of the cells. Causes may include metabolic disease such as hepatic or renal disease. In addition to the metabolic changes, fragmentation of the RBCs is another possible cause. Haemangiosarcoma is a frequently mentioned cause for acanthocytes.

Abdominal neoplasia (e.g. haemangiosarcoma) with an oozing haemorrhage should be considered after taking into account the possible increased RBC turnover.

2 How would you proceed with this patient?
Abdominal ultrasound to rule out hepatic or splenic neoplasia should be the first step to consider.

FOLLOW UP
Abdominal ultrasound confirmed the presence of splenic neoplasia. Laparotomy was performed and the spleen removed. Histopathology revealed haemangiosarcoma.

FURTHER READING

Stockham SL, Scott MA (2008) *Fundamentals of Veterinary Clinical Pathology*, 2nd edn. Blackwell Publishing, Oxford.

Weiss DJ, Wardrop KJ (2010) *Schalm's Veterinary Hematology*, 6th edn. Blackwell Publishing, Ames.

CASE 177

1 Summarise and interpret the abnormalities in these laboratory results.

There is a slight non-regenerative anaemia, which may be attributable to an anaemia of chronic disease. The anaemia is likely more severe than is apparent, considering the degree of dehydration as evidenced by the increased plasma protein and albumin.

There is a slight leucocytosis with a mild non-specific neutrophilia and monocytosis, which may suggest mild inflammation. There is a lymphocytosis and eosinophilia (opposite of stress leucogram, which is usually seen in a sick dog). Extremely ill animals (under severe stress) would normally be expected to have lymphopaenia and eosinopaenia. The fact that they do not show this is diagnostically significant. This is most often associated with Addison's disease (hypoadrenocorticism). Other differentials for lymphocytosis include antigenic stimulation, physiological lymphocytosis or infectious diseases such as ehrlichiosis. There is a slight eosinophilia, which may also be associated with hypersensitivity, allergic disease or parasitic disease.

Increased plasma protein may be associated with dehydration as evidenced by the elevation of serum proteins/albumin.

The Na:K ratio is close to 15:1, which at this level is most likely to be associated with hypoadrenocorticism. This is not a feature of all cases, especially those with predominantly glucocorticoid deficiency. Other differentials that may also cause increased potassium and decreased Na:K ratio include certain breeds that may have increased K^+ in their RBCs, such as the Japanese Akita, Shiba Inu and Shar Pei. There may be shift of K^+ from within the RBC to the serum if there is prolonged exposure of the serum to the clot (lack of prompt serum separation). Sometimes, elevated K^+ may be the result of release from platelets (especially if thrombocytosis is present) and can occur with tissue damage or lysis of tumour cells during chemotherapy. Uroabdomen, chylothorax, salmonellosis, *Trichuris* (whip worm), severe metabolic acidosis and congestive heart failure can also be associated with low ratios. Oliguric or anuric renal disease may also be associated with hyponatraemia and hyperkalaemia. The response to ACTH stimulation would help to distinguish these diseases.

Primary hypoadrenocorticism is associated with decreased aldosterone which, under normal circumstances, acts at the nephron, where it stimulates sodium and chloride reabsorption from the proximal renal tubule and sodium absorption with exchange for potassium in the distal tubule. Aldosterone secretion is influenced by the renin–angiotensin system and plasma potassium level. Decreased aldosterone production causes a decrease in the exchange of potassium for sodium and water conservation in the distal renal tubule, with resulting potassium retention. The reduced cortisol interferes with the efficiency of the potassium pump, allowing potassium to pass from the cells into the extracellular fluid (ECF).

The initial decrease in ECF volume due to aldosterone is mild and theoretically this can be countered by thirst and ADH secretion, but plasma Na^+ tends to decrease. If the water loss is not replaced, then the resultant dehydration can mask the decrease in sodium level. This dehydration can also mask underlying anaemia and in this case makes the anaemia more profound.

K^+ is moderately elevated but is in excess of that expected attributable to acid–base shifts alone.

There is a moderate azotaemia present with a USG of 1.022. This suggests renal disease but as the sodium and chloride are low, the kidneys may not be able to concentrate the urine owing to sodium loss and renal medullary washout. Pre-renal azotaemia is seen in 80% of cases of Addison's disease. Aldosterone deficiency causes impaired sodium retention, resulting in hypovolaemia, hypotension and reduced renal perfusion.

Increased phosphate is usually due to decreased renal clearance.

There is a slight to moderate hypercalcaemia, which may be in part due to an apparent hypercalcaemia as the albumin is increased and 40% of total calcium is albumin bound. Renal disease may also cause a hypercalcaemia. Increased calcium resorption from the gastrointestinal tract is thought to occur in cases of hypoadrenocorticism. Elevation of calcium can also be associated with humoral hypercalcaemia of malignancy, cholecalciferol toxicity and granulomatous disease.

A lowered TCO_2 suggests a metabolic acidosis with increased anion gap, the latter due to the presence of unmeasured anions. Uraemic and lactic acids are most likely and may be associated with decreased tissue perfusion secondary to the hypotension and from decreased renal tubular excretion of H^+ secondary to aldosterone deficiency.

Except for the inadequate urine-concentrating ability (see discussion on azotaemia above), the urinalysis is unremarkable.

2 What additional tests could you perform in order to confirm or exclude the possible diagnosis?

A single low basal cortisol level (<55 nmol/l) can be used as supporting evidence of hypoadrenocorticism. An ACTH stimulation test would verify the diagnosis.

FOLLOW UP

The ACTH stimulation test results in this patient were: pre-stimulation serum cortisol, <10 nmol/l; post-stimulation serum cortisol, <10 nmol/l. Dogs with hypoadrenocorticism should show: baseline (pre-stimulation) cortisol levels <45 nmol/l; post-ACTH cortisol levels <55 nmol/l. The lack of stimulation with the ACTH stimulation test in combination with the hyponatraemia/hypochloraemia and hyperkalaemia confirms a diagnosis of hypoadrenocorticism. Dogs with hypoadrenocorticism commonly have decreased basal serum cortisol concentrations, which do not increase or increase only slightly after ACTH stimulation.

SUMMARY
Hyponatraemia, hypokalaemia and a Na:K ratio of 16.5:1, along with a lack of a stress leucogram (lymphopaenia) in a sick dog is highly suggestive of hypoadrenocorticism. An inadequate response to ACTH stimulation confirms this disease. The azotaemia, with evidence of inadequate urine-concentrating ability, suggests primary renal disease, but is more likely due to a combination of pre-renal azotaemia and decreased renal concentrating ability secondary to mineralocorticoid (aldosterone) deficiency and medullary washout.

FURTHER READING
Feldman EC, Nelson RW (2004) *Canine and Feline Endocrinology and Reproduction*, 3rd edn. Saunders, St. Louis.
Greco DS (2007) Hypoadrenocorticism in small animals. *Clin Tech Small Anim Pract* 22:32–35.
Lennon EM, Boyle TE, Hutchins RG *et al.* (2007) Use of basal serum or plasma cortisol concentrations to rule out a diagnosis of hypoadrenocorticism in dogs: 123 cases (2000–2005). *J Am Vet Med Assoc* 231:413–416.
Rose BD (1994) *Clinical Physiology of Acid-Base and Electrolyte Disorders*. McGraw-Hill, New York, pp. 164–173.
Roth L, Tyler RD (1999) Evaluation of low sodium:potassium ratios in dogs. *J Vet Diagn Invest* 11:60–64.

CASE 178

1 What can you do to determine the underlying cause for this lower than desirable level of performance capability?

You could investigate the cause for a less than desirable performance by using a quality goal index (QGI), which is determined by the following formula:

$$QGI = Bias/1.5\ CV$$

The QGI ratio is based on the relative extent to which both bias and precision meet the quality goals of $1.5(TE_a/6)$ for bias and $TE_a/6$ for precision (CV).

This is interpreted as follows:

QGI	Problem
<0.8	Imprecision
0.8–1.2	Imprecision and inaccuracy
>1.2	Inaccuracy

Further investigation to improve performance in precision and/or accuracy, depending on the results of the QGI, may be of benefit in determining if performance can be improved in order to achieve a sigma metric of ≥6, indicative of 'world class performance'.

FURTHER READING
Dr David Parry. *Quality goal index: its use in benchmarking and improving sigma quality performance of automated analytic tests.* Guest essay. http://www.westgard.com/guest34.htm (Accessed 17th November 2014).

CASE 179

1 Discuss the laboratory findings and their significance.

There is a slight, normocytic, marginally hypochromic anaemia. Although the erythrocytes, haemoglobin and spun PCV are only just below the reference intervals, in a fit Thoroughbred gelding they should be at least in the middle if not at the high end. The anaemia is suspicious for anaemia of inflammatory disease (AID). This results from decreased iron availability (increased uptake of iron by macrophages, local binding of iron by apolactoferrin released by neutrophils, decreased iron absorption from the gut) and can occasionally lead on to the microcytic, hypochromic anaemia expected in iron deficiency. Iron sequestration has an antibacterial effect. Erythrocyte survival is also decreased in AID (premature removal by macrophages due to erythrocyte surface alterations), as is erythropoiesis (cytokines [e.g. IL-1, TNF-alpha], decreased erythropoietin production). Decreased serum TIBC and increased serum ferritin can be used, if necessary, to distinguish AID from iron deficiency anaemia where TIBC is high and serum ferritin low. The latter is a good indicator of total body iron stores.

A mild leucopaenia with neutropaenia and lymphopaenia are also common in low-grade chronic inflammation and suggest increased consumption and/or decreased production.

2 What is your interpretation, and what are your recommendations?

Overall, the results point towards a chronic inflammatory condition or a post-viral syndrome. Serum amyloid A (SAA) is a major acute-phase protein in horses and may be used to rule in/out systemic inflammatory disease. As most of these chronic inflammatory conditions and post-viral syndromes are of respiratory origin in this type of horse, bronchoalveolar lavage is indicated. However, as TIBC and serum ferritin have not been done, iron deficiency due to chronic haemorrhage cannot be completely ruled out. Chronic blood loss in the equine athlete may occur with chronic parasitism, a bleeding gastrointestinal ulcer or repeated exercise-induced pulmonary haemorrhage, although the magnitude of haemorrhage usually associated with these conditions and the regenerative capacity of the bone marrow suggest that the latter two conditions are less likely.

CASE 180

1 What is your assessment of these findings?
The slight microcytic-normochromic anaemia is likely associated with chronic disease (based on biochemistry findings [see below]). The slight leucocytosis with neutrophilia and monocytosis without lymphopaenia suggest inflammation with necrosis.

The increased pre- and post-prandial bile acids support the presence of hepatic dysfunction. This is further supported by the slight increase in ALT and ALP and the slight decrease in albumin.

The slightly low total calcium is likely the result of the decreased albumin with decreased protein binding. The pattern of low albumin with increased globulins is typical of hepatic disease and is likely due to decreased hepatic clearance of endotoxins and/or other factors that may result in increased inflammatory and/or immune globulins. The low protein C level provides further support for decreased hepatic synthetic function and decreased hepatoportal blood flow.

2 What does the protein C result support as a likely underlying cause?
The low protein C suggests that a portosystemic shunt is the most likely cause. Low protein C levels help differentiate portosystemic vascular anomalies from microvascular dysplasia (most have protein C >70%), but can be seen with other causes of severe hepatic disease and hepatic failure.

3 What other biochemistry alterations are common with this suspected condition?
Other biochemistry alterations that are common with portosystemic shunt include hypocholesterolaemia, hypoglycaemia, low urea and creatinine and hypoalbuminaemia. The degree of decrease in these analytes tends to be greater with portosystemic shunts compared with microvascular dysplasia.

4 What might you expect to see on urinalysis?
Ammonium biurate crystalluria and/or hyposthenuric USG are common findings on urinalysis from dogs with portosystemic shunts.

FURTHER READING
Toulza O, Center SA, Brooks MB *et al.* (2006) Evaluation of protein C activity for detection of hepatobiliary disease and portosystemic shunting in dogs. *J Am Vet Med Assoc* **229:** 1761–1771.

CASE 181

1 How would you distinguish relative from absolute erythrocytosis?
Relative erythrocytosis is characterised by an increased haematocrit with a normal total RBC mass resulting from a decrease in plasma volume. This condition is commonly due to dehydration caused by external losses of body fluids. It is commonly associated with clinical evidence of dehydration and an increase in serum total protein and urea. An increase in total RBC mass defines the absolute polycythaemia.

In this dog the increase in haematocrit is accompanied by a concurrent increase in RBCs, there is no clinical evidence of dehydration and the biochemistry is unremarkable. These findings are suggestive of absolute erythrocytosis.

2 How would you distinguish primary from secondary absolute erythrocytosis?
Absolute erythrocytosis is further divided into primary or secondary erythrocytosis, and the latter is further classified as physiologically appropriate or inappropriate. Primary polycythaemia is a rare myeloproliferative disorder described in dogs and cats and is commonly diagnosed by exclusion of other possible causes of erythrocytosis. Secondary polycythaemia may be appropriate if this is a consequence of persistent hypoxia, as observed in congenital heart defects, lung diseases and haemoglobin dysfunctions. Secondary inappropriate polycythaemia refers to disease processes leading to increased serum erythropoietin (EPO), such as EPO-producing neoplasia.

3 What further investigations would you suggest, and what is your suspicion?
Arterial blood gases are useful for detecting hypoxia. In the case of appropriate secondary erythrocytosis, partial pressure of oxygen is expected to be low. Measurement of EPO may also be helpful. EPO is commonly low or normal in primary erythrocytosis and is usually increased in secondary erythrocytosis, in particular in animals with EPO-secreting tumours (renal carcinoma, renal lymphoma).

In this dog, the absence of signs of hypoxia (normal partial pressure of oxygen, no heart or lung diseases) and the presence of a renal mass detected on ultrasound makes an inappropriate secondary erythrocytosis the main differential (**Fig. 181.1**).

FOLLOW UP
Inappropriate secondary erythrocytosis was confirmed by EPO results, which were significantly above the reference interval.

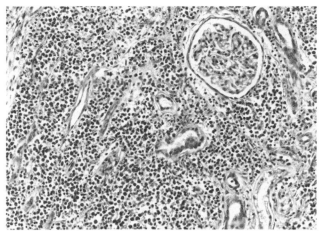

FIG. 181.1 Histological section of renal mass. Renal lymphoma, glomerular structure (top right) and a monomorphic infiltrate of lymphoid cells in the cortical area. ×40.

Analyte (units)	Result	Reference Interval
Erythropoietin (mU/ml) (RIA)	**64**	8.4–28

Postmortem examination revealed the presence of a renal lymphoma, which is likely to be the cause of the erythrocytosis caused by inappropriate EPO production.

FURTHER READING
Stockham SL, Scott MA (2008) *Fundamentals of Veterinary Clinical Pathology*, 2nd edn. Blackwell Publishing, Oxford.
Weiss DJ, Wardrop KJ (2011) *Schalm's Veterinary Hematology*, 6th edn. Wiley-Blackwell, Ames.

CASE 182

1 What laboratory test would you recommend?
A submaximal exercise test may be of benefit. This test is good at detecting subclinical rhabdomyolysis without risk of overexertion. If muscle stiffness is noted during exercise, the exercise should be terminated. This test is conducted prior to and following regular moderate exercise (routine exercise session of approximately 15 minutes duration that includes walking, trotting and cantering/galloping).

Protocol

● Collect pre-exercise serum specimen for CK and AST determinations:
  ❑ Expect CK to be within reference interval (intervals may differ slightly amongst laboratories, 150–300 U/l).
  ❑ Expect AST to be within reference interval (intervals may differ slightly amongst laboratories, 250–350 U/l).

● Collect post-exercise (regular moderate exercise) specimen for CK and AST determination at 2–4 hours post exercise:
  ❑ Should not see more than a doubling of resting CK levels.
  ❑ Should see little or no change in AST.
● Collect serum specimen 24 hours post exercise for CK and AST determinations.

2 How do you interpret your recommended test?
There should be a return of CK to baseline levels. Expect no more than a 50% increase in AST. There should be no observable clinical signs of stiffness or muscle pain.

If the above criteria are not fulfilled, the results of the test are abnormal and support a muscle problem. A normal test does not rule out the possibility of tying up, but a positive test provides support for it.

FURTHER READING
Robinson NE, Sprayberry KE (2009) *Current Therapy in Equine Medicine*, 6th edn. Saunders Elsevier, St. Louis.

CASE 183

1 What cells can be seen in Fig. 183.1?
The cells are transitional epithelial cells arranged in sheets. These cells – often arranged in clumps – are a typical finding if urine samples are collected by catheterisation. They have been traumatically exfoliated by the tip of the catheter. This method is not the diagnostic procedure of first choice if a sample for sediment evaluation is needed.

2 Is there evidence of neoplasia?
There is no cytological evidence of a transitional cell carcinoma. The slight nuclear abnormalities and the slight anisocytosis are commonly found in transitional epithelial cells.

3 What is the pinkish structure in Fig. 183.2?
The pinkish structure is a budding yeast (*Candida* was isolated on culture). This is a very uncommon finding in urine and might be the result of faecal contamination of the catheter. In some animals with a history of antibiotic treatment, immunosuppression or diabetes mellitus, there may be true urinary fungal infection. Correlation with the results of fungal culture on a cystocentesis specimen is recommended if yeast are found on urine sediment evaluation.

CASE 184

1 What tests would you recommend for this patient?
An FBC and peripheral blood film morphological evaluation would be helpful in determining if additional abnormalities

other than the severe anaemia are present. A jaundiced foal agglutination test is a rapid test that may be helpful in determining if neonatal isoerythrolysis is present.

2 What is your interpretation of these tests?

The procedure and interpretation for the jaundiced foal agglutination test are as follows:

Protocol

- Set up seven clear tubes, each with 1 ml of saline. Label consecutively as 1:2, 1:4, 1:8, 1:16, 1:32, 1:64 and BLANK.
- Make serial dilutions of the mare's plasma or colostrum by adding 1 ml to tube 1 and mixing with pipette and then removing 1 ml from this tube into the next tube, mix and remove 1 ml to the third tube, and so on. Discard 1 ml from the sixth tube (labelled 1:64).
- Add one drop of the foal's whole EDTA blood to each of the seven tubes and mix by agitation or gentle rocking.
- Centrifuge tubes for 2–3 minutes at speeds suitable for separation of plasma/serum.
- Pour or pipette off supernatant from each tube, taking care not to disturb the erythrocytes in the bottom of the tube. Observe the status of the red cell button.

Interpretation

- Complete agglutination causes cells to remain firmly packed in a button at the bottom of the tube, and they will not move when the tube is tilted. Negative samples show free movement of cells when the tube is tilted.
- Positive reactions are taken to be >1:16 dilution (i.e. if the 1:1 or higher dilutions form firmly fixed buttons, the foal is likely a neonatal isoerythrolysis case). The results are less certain with colostrum, with more false positives.

Suspected neonatal isoerythrolysis cases based on this test can be confirmed by blood typing of the sire and dam.

FURTHER READING

Paradis MR (2006) *Equine Neonatal Medicine: A Case-Based Approach.* Elsevier Saunders, Philadelphia.

CASE 185

1 How do you explain the positive result of the ELISA in-house test and the negative result of the PCR?

There are four main reasons that may explain the present results. First, in-house rapid tests are screening tests. The major characteristic of a screening test is a high diagnostic sensitivity, which implies few false-negative results, so animals that are free of the disease are correctly identified. There may be some false-positive results, so a confirmatory test has to follow a screening test. The confirmatory test should have a higher specificity (i.e. comprises less false-positive results) and, therefore, excludes patients wrongly identified as diseased by the ELISA test. From the analytical point of view, a false-positive ELISA result is expected with a high sensitivity screening procedure.

Second, another analytical reason may be a false-negative PCR result. This may take place if an inadequate sample is submitted, there is unsuccessful extraction of the organism or inherent technical problems occur. An inadequate sample may be from the wrong location (e.g. blood, when the organism is sequestered in an internal organ and not circulating in the blood) or if the sample is incorrectly preserved or handled, resulting in degradation of the organism.

Third, rapid in-house tests are not able to only identify *E. canis*, but also show cross-reactivity to other *Ehrlichia* spp. (e.g. *Ehrlichia chaffeensis*). However, although cross-reactivity has to be kept in mind when interpreting test results, it is unlikely in this case as *E. chaffeensis* does not occur in Spain.

The fourth and possibly most likely explanation is that antibodies may persist for several months to years after infection of the dog is cleared and antigen is neither present nor detectable. This finding has been observed in patients treated against rickettsiosis. In patients originating from endemic areas of the disease, such as Spain, it is more likely that dogs have previously been infected. Therefore, antibodies may be detectable but antigen not detected.

2 Which organism transmits *Ehrlichia* spp., and what other infectious agents may it carry?

E. canis is transmitted by the brown dog tick *Rhipicephalus sanguineus*. This vector may also carry *Hepatozoon canis* and *Babesia canis vogeli*. Clinical signs may be complicated if a patient is infected by multiple organisms.

FURTHER READING

Harrus S, Waner T (2011) Diagnosis of canine monocytotropic ehrlichiosis (*Ehrlichia canis*): an overview. *Vet J* **187**:292–296.

Neer MT, Breitschwerdt EB, Greene RT *et al.* (2002) Consensus statement on ehrlichial disease of small animals from the Infectious Disease Study Group of the ACVIM. *J Vet Intern Med* **16**:309–315.

CASE 186

1 How would you interpret the changes in liver enzymes?

The biochemistry showed a mild to moderate increase in GLDH and AST, indicating hepatocellular damage.

The mild increase in AST could also reflect muscle damage, considering the concurrent increase in CK. The increase in ALP and GGT was supportive of cholestasis. Urea, glucose, protein and bile acids were within normal limits and did not suggest liver dysfunction. A diagnosis of cholestatic hepatopathy was made.

2 According to the history, what are your main differentials?
The biochemistry results were supportive of a cholangio-hepatopathy. The evidence of hepatomegaly and distended bile ducts on abdominal ultrasound confirmed this, although these findings were considered to be non-specific and did not add any additional information to the diagnosis. The presence of characteristic skin lesions raised the suspicion of photosensitisation, a condition usually associated with primary liver disease or secondary to ingestion of certain plants.

3 What further investigations would you suggest?
Histopathology is the test of choice in order to further investigate the liver problem. A liver biopsy was performed and multiple samples collected. The clinical history and clinical findings, in association with the histological evidence of megalocytosis of hepatocyes, fibrosis, and bile duct hyperplasia, were considered pathognomonic for ragwort poisoning.

The toxic compound of the plant (pyrrolizidine alkaloid) is metabolised by the liver into pyrrole. This acts on the hepatocytes, preventing cell division (with resulting megalocytosis) and then causing cellular death (with subsequent fibrosis). If the damage is extended, there may be evidence of liver dysfunction and also neurological signs secondary to insufficient ammonia excretion. The evidence of specific skin lesions (peeling in white areas such as a facial blaze and sock) is considered another important feature of ragwort poisoning and was observed in this case. Reduced metabolisation of chlorophyll (normally present in all green plants) may cause an accumulation in the body (mainly in the skin), activation by sunlight, with a consequent release of inflammatory mediators, and tissue damage. Dermatitis (mud fever, dew poisoning or pastern dermatitis) may occur.

Identification of ragwort (Senecio jacobaea) in the pasture confirmed the diagnosis. The absence of liver dysfunction (bile acid assay is within reference interval) and the gradual improvement suggested the poisoning was not too severe and that the prognosis for recovery is good.

CASE 187

1 What condition do you suspect may be present based on the clinical findings and/or the severe anaemia?
In a hunting dog with this presentation and severe, apparently non-responding anaemia, which may be due to acute development (too early to see a bone marrow response in the peripheral blood), phosphofructokinase (PFK) deficiency is the primary consideration. This condition is an autosomal recessive disease that has been reported in Cocker Spaniels, English Springer Spaniels, Whippets, German Spaniels (Wachtelhunds) and in mixed-breed dogs with some ancestor in common with these breeds.

2 What is the pathophysiology underlying the suspected condition?
This disease is a result of a missense mutation affecting energy metabolic pathways in skeletal muscle and within erythrocytes. The deficiency causes a reduction in erythrocyte 2,3-diphosphoglycerate, resulting in increased affinity of haemoglobin for oxygen binding and a higher erythrocyte pH. The erythrocytes exhibit increased fragility under alkalotic situations of increased exercise, excitement, extreme temperature and barking. Muscles suffer from exertional myopathy.

Episodes of discoloured urine are attributed to intravascular haemolysis with haemoglobinuria and bilirubinuria. Poor performance in the hunting field or in field trials is attributed to exertional myopathy, with muscle cramping and sometimes complete refusal to move.

3 Are there any potential differential diagnoses, and what tests would you run to determine if these are likely?
Other potential differentials include babesiosis (intravascular haemolysis); PCR would help determine if this is present. Immune-mediated haemolytic anaemia (IMHA) (idiopathic or secondary to drugs or neoplasia) should be considered, but the absence of spherocytes, the presence of intravascular haemolysis (not common with IMHA), the results of other examinations and the young age in this particular patient suggest this possibility is unlikely. A Coombs test would provide support for IMHA if positive, but a negative test does not rule it out.

Hunting dog hypoglycaemia may contribute to poor performance despite an initial enthusiastic response. Evaluation of a serum or plasma glucose result taken post exercise at a time of demonstration of clinical signs would help rule this out. Evaluation of CK may also be helpful since increased CK (and subsequent increase in AST) would be expected with PFK deficiency. There is a genetic test available for PFK deficiency. In this case the patient was found to be affected (homozygous) for the trait.

FURTHER READING
Skibild E, Dahlgard K, Rajpurohit Y et al. (2001) Haemolytic anaemia and exercise intolerance due to phosphofructokinase deficiency in related Springer Spaniels. J Small Anim Pract 42:298–300.

CASE 188

1 How would you classify the anaemia?

Non-regenerative, macrocytic anaemia. The macrocytosis cannot be explained by the regeneration; it is possible that the patient has an innate macrocytosis. Alternatively, platelet clumps may have been recorded as erythrocytes or there may be erythrocyte swelling if this is an aged specimen.

2 What is your diagnosis based on the haematology and serology results and the blood smear?

Anaplasma phagocytophilum infection (anaplasmosis, formerly canine granulocytic ehrlichiosis). Two morulae, consisting of elementary bodies in a neutrophil, are visible. This finding is consistent with anaplasmosis; no further test is needed for confirmation.

3 Why are antibodies to the organism causing this anaemia not detectable here?

Seroconversion (with IgM antibodies) starts briefly after the occurrence of morulae in the blood; therefore, it is too early at this stage to expect IgG antibodies.

4 What is the most frequent change in the FBC in this infection?

The most frequent finding is a moderate to marked thrombocytopaenia, which is caused by immune-mediated destruction of the platelets. The anaemia as seen in this case is often not prominent. The leucogram may show a leucocytosis or a leucopaenia.

FURTHER READING

Carrade DD, Foley JE, Borjesson DL *et al.* (2009) Canine granulocytic anaplasmosis: a review. *J Vet Intern Med* 23: 1129–1141.

Kirtz G, Czettel B, Thum D *et al.* (2007) *Anaplasma phagocytophilum* in einer österreichischen Hundepopulation: eine Prävalenzstudie (2001–2006) [*Anaplasma phagocytophilum* in an Austrian population of dogs: a study of seroprevalency (2001–2006)]. *Kleintierpraxis* **52**:562–568.

CASE 189

1 What are the QGIs associated with each of these test/instrument combinations and the interpretations of the most likely reason for the <6 sigma performance?

Test	Instrument	QGI	Interpretation of Problem
A	1	0.61	Imprecision
A	2	1.56	Inaccuracy
B	1	1.0	Both inaccuracy and imprecision
B	2	0.67	Imprecision

2 What can be done to help improve inaccuracy and/or imprecision for a particular test?

Inaccuracy may be improved by more frequent calibration or inclusion of a 'correction factor' to reduce or eliminate bias. If reference intervals are established for each analyser separately, this may provide a basis for interpretation that takes into account the bias present with the individual instrument. Careful attention to the method of bias estimation should be considered. Evaluation of certified standards or comparison with a 'gold standard' method should be considered to determine whether the bias estimate is a true reflection of the accuracy of the method/instrument used.

Imprecision may be harder to improve since there is a degree of imprecision inherent in each instrument/method. Sometimes, imprecision may be improved by increased attention to routine maintenance and instrument cleaning or by changing reagents or calibrators.

CASE 190

1 What are the main differential diagnoses for the hyponatraemia?

There is a significant hyponatraemia and hypochloraemia and sodium and chloride have decreased proportionately. Hyponatraemia occurs when the ratio between the 'total body sodium' ($tbNa^+$) and the 'total body water' (tbH_2O) is decreased. Hyponatraemia can be seen in hypo-, normo- or hypervolaemia. The most common causes of hyponatraemia are:

- Loss of sodium greater than the loss of water:
  - Gastrointestinal losses of sodium (vomiting, diarrhoea, gastrointestinal sequestration) followed by increased water intake but without replacement of Na^+ in the diet (such as with anorexic animals that continue to drink).
  - Renal losses (hypoadrenocorticism, prolonged diuresis, intrinsic renal disease).
  - Third-space losses (pleural or abdominal cavities).
- Water retention:
  - Oedematous disorders: congestive heart failure, nephrotic syndrome, hepatic cirrhosis.
  - Non-oedematous conditions: syndrome of inappropriate ADH secretion (SIADH), psychogenic polydipsia (PP).

2 What is the diagnostic approach to these changes?

Hyponatraemia, in most cases, is associated with plasma hypo-osmolality. Therefore, the first diagnostic step for this patient was to measure the plasma osmolality: this was 270 mOsmol/kg [290–315 mOsmol/l].

Once the plasma osmolality is known, this should be interpreted in the context of the volaemic status of the animal. The patient's volaemic status can be estimated based on the results of the physical examination, the PCV, the total protein concentration and the blood pressure, all in conjunction with the clinical history.

If the plasma hypo-osmolality is associated with hypovolaemia, the main differential diagnoses for the hyponatraemia include gastrointestinal loss, third-space loss and hypoadrenocorticism.

On the other hand, if the patient is normovolaemic or hypervolaemic, the following conditions should be considered: severe liver disease, congestive heart failure and nephrotic syndrome, which are usually associated with oedema and/or effusions; PP and SIADH, which are not accompanied by oedema or ascites.

The blood pressure of this patient was 130 mmHg (normovolaemic/slightly hypervolaemic). This, the absence of gastrointestinal clinical signs and a negative ACTH stimulation test ruled out the possibility of increased loss of sodium.

Liver disease, cardiovascular disease and nephrotic syndrome were also excluded following extensive imaging studies and by the blood and urine results. The remaining differential diagnoses were SIADH and PP. Given the normal measured water intake, SIADH was considered more likely.

SIADH is a condition characterised by an excessive secretion of ADH in the absence of either osmotic or non-osmotic stimuli. This is essentially the opposite of diabetes insipidus. As a consequence, the ingested water is retained, causing increasing of the tbH_2O and secondary hyponatraemia. The plasma volume is usually modestly expanded and oedema or effusion do not occur. The volume expansion stimulates the renin–angiotensin–aldosterone system, resulting in reduced tubular absorption of sodium and leading to natriuresis. The main diagnostic features of SIADH are:

- Hyponatraemia with modest volume expansion but without oedema.
- Plasma hypo-osmolality.
- Urine osmolality greater than that appropriate for the plasma osmolality (>100 mOsm/kg).
- Natriuresis despite the plasma hyponatraemia (>20 mmol/l in humans).

The clinical signs are the result of water intoxication and patients are often presented for neurological complaints. As in this case, diagnosis is made by excluding other causes of hyponatraemia and meeting the diagnostic criteria listed above. In this patient, the diagnosis of SIADH was further supported by the increased fractional excretion of sodium (42 mmol/l) and the inappropriately high urine osmolality (230 mOsmol/l; [100–200 mOsmol/l]).

SIADH is a rare condition in dogs. In the veterinary literature, single case reports have been published. SIADH has been found in association with filarial infestation, amoebic granulomatous meningoencephalitis (GME), undifferentiated carcinoma and a neoplasm in the hypothalamic region. A few cases of idiopathic SIADH have also been described.

FURTHER READING

DiBartola SP (2006) Disorders of sodium and water: hypernatremia and hyponatremia. In: *Fluid, Electrolyte, and Acid-Base Disorders in Small Animal Practice*, 3rd edn. Saunders Elsevier, St. Louis, pp. 47–79.

Feldman EC, Nelson R (2004) Water metabolism and diabetes insipidus. In: *Canine and Feline Endocrinology and Reproduction*, 3rd edn. Saunders, St. Louis, pp. 2–44.

Stockham SL, Scott MA (2008) *Fundamentals of Veterinary Clinical Pathology*, 2nd edn. Blackwell Publishing, Oxford, pp. 495–557.

CASE 191

1 What is your analysis of these findings?

The slight increase in MCV may be due to cellular swelling with ageing of a sample that has come through the post. It is unlikely to be of significance in the absence of other abnormalities of the erythron. The slight leucopaenia and neutropaenia is likely due to the increased demand for leucocytes associated with the diarrhoea. The moderate lymphopaenia may be due to inflammation, immunosuppression and/or stress.

The moderate decrease in albumin with low normal total protein and slight hyperglobulinaemia and decreased A:G ratio is likely secondary to protein-losing enteropathy (PLE) associated with the diarrhoea. The serum protein electrophoretic pattern (low albumin with mild increase in alpha-2 and beta-1 fractions) suggests an acute inflammatory response. Hypoalbuminaemia may be multifactorial in this patient: primary and/or secondary to negative acute-phase response and/or PLE. Other contributions may include protein-losing nephropathy (not ruled out in this case) and decreased hepatic production (should be considered in light of the increase in bile acids). The slight increase in GLDH indicates hepatocellular insult. This may be secondary to poor blood flow to the liver associated with the gastrointestinal condition and/or a primary hepatic insult such as endotoxin showering from the GI tract.

The slight increase in CK may be due to muscle damage associated with recumbency (if the animal is weak or debilitated) and/or muscle catabolism.

Veterinary Clinical Pathology

The low phosphorus is suggestive of gastroenteritis with decreased intestinal absorption and the hypocalcaemia is likely the result of decreased albumin and therefore of protein-bound calcium. Decreased intake/absorption could also contribute to both these electrolyte abnormalities.

2 What additional testing may be of benefit in this case?

Additional testing that may be of benefit includes:

- Faecal culture for *Salmonella* and other pathogens.
- Faecal parasite evaluation.
- Rectal cytology (looking for inflammation).
- Serum amyloid A (if further confirmation of inflammation and acute-phase reaction is desired).
- Urinalysis (rule out possible urinary tract loss of protein).
- Repeat evaluation of serum biochemistry and FBC with blood film evaluation to determine trends in laboratory results that help with the prognosis.

CASE 192

1 Considering the breed, what is the most likely diagnosis in this patient?

Miniature Schnauzers may have idiopathic hyperlipidaemia. The exact genetics, however, are still unknown.

2 What differential diagnoses should you consider?

Several differential diagnoses have to be taken into account when hyperlipidaemia is detected. Besides physiological post-prandial increases, secondary hyperlipidaemia has to be considered. This includes endocrinological diseases such as hypothyroidism, diabetes mellitus and HAC. Furthermore, cholestatic disorders, pancreatitis and the nephrotic syndrome may cause increases in cholesterol and/or triglycerides.

Increases in hepatocellular enzymes indicate hepatocellular damage as well as potential cholestasis.

3 Which disease is often associated with hyperlipidaemia, also in Miniature Schnauzers?

Acute pancreatitis is frequently observed in association with hyperlipidaemia. It has not been determined whether hyperlipidaemia is the primary cause of the pancreatitis or a consequence, although a causal relationship is suspected. The pathophysiological mechanism is not fully understood. Possibly, diminished insulin concentration impairs lipoprotein lipase activity. Secondly, cytokines may be involved in changes in the lipoprotein metabolism, leading to increased VLDL concentrations.

FURTHER READING

Stockham SL, Scott MA (2008) *Fundamentals of Veterinary Clinical Pathology*, 2nd edn. Blackwell Publishing, Oxford.

CASE 193

1 What is your assessment of these results?

The mild leucocytosis based on a slight neutrophilia with toxic changes, associated with left shift and lymphopaenia, is suggestive of acute inflammation. The intracellular morulae observed within neutrophils are consistent with canine granulocytotropic rickettsial infection. Since *Anaplasma phagocytophilum* and *Ehrlichia ewingii* are microscopically indistinguishable organisms that infect neutrophils, both should be considered as differentials in this dog.

The increased C-reactive protein supports the presence of an active inflammatory process. The slight hyperglycaemia is most likely the consequence of excitement or fright. Steroid-associated hyperglycaemia due to stress may be another explanation for this finding. The increased ALP associated with the mild hyperbilirubinaemia reflects cholestasis, most likely without hepatocellular damage since the liver enzymes are not increased. Endogenous cortisol production due to stress may also contribute to ALP increase.

2 What are the bases for the aetiology and pathogenesis for the present case?

Anaplasmosis and ehrlichiosis are both tick-borne diseases. *Amblyomma americanum* has been reported as the primary vector for *E. ewingii*, while different species of tick from the genus *Ixodes* are the main vectors of *A. phagocytophilum*. Transmission of *A. phagocytophilum* by direct contact with blood or respiratory secretions has also been reported in humans. Moreover, experimental studies have demonstrated transplacental infection in cows.

A minimum feeding time of 24–48 hours is required for *Ixodes* spp. ticks to transmit *A. phagocytophilum*. Disease incubation after a tick bite is 1–2 weeks for this pathogen. The time required from tick attachment to *E. ewingii* transmission in unknown, but clinical signs of infection are observed by 18–28 days.

A. phagocytophilum and *E. ewingii* are small gram-negative, obligate intracellular bacteria that invade granulocytes, forming membrane-bound, intracytoplasmic colonies of organisms known as morulae. Within cells both pathogens can delay neutrophil apoptosis, providing additional time for their replication.

Although the pathogenesis of the clinical findings remains poorly understood for *E. ewingii*, proposed mechanisms for both pathogens may include cytokine myelosuppression, autoantibodies, infection of haematopoietic precursors and blood cell consumption, especially of platelets.

Indeed, thrombocytopaenia is a clinically pathological abnormality described for both diseases, especially with *E. ewingii*, although platelet counts within the reference interval do not rule out the diagnosis. Occasionally, slight anaemia has also been reported.

3 What additional tests would be needed to confirm the likely diagnosis in this case?

The ELISA-based rapid in-house tests are good screening assays to differentiate the present granulocytotropic rickettsial infection. There is no serological cross-reactivity between the response to *E. ewingii* and *A. phagocytophilum*. In contrast, cross-reactivity exists in the response to *E. ewingii* and *E. canis* and some strains of *E. chaffeensis*, and between *A. phagocytophilum* and *A. platys*.

In general, PCR is a more sensitive diagnostic tool than searching for circulating morulae and provides reliable species-specific confirmation. PCR allows for a specific diagnosis, whereas serological testing can reflect only prior exposure and potentially there may be cross-reactivity to closely related rickettsiae. Another advantage of the molecular diagnostic technique is early detection. In *A. phagocytophilum*-infected dogs, positive PCR results may be obtained 6–8 days earlier than the first appearance of morulae in peripheral blood. In contrast, seroconversion occurs 2–5 days after the first appearance of morulae in peripheral blood. Then, antibody titres to *A. phagocytophilum* may remain detectable for at least 8–24 months.

Because all *Ehrlichia* spp. (ruling out *E. canis*, which requires a longer course of antibacterial therapy) and *Anaplasma* spp. infections are responsive to treatment with tetracyclines, differentiating between infections with these organisms is usually of zoonotic concern for the owner or of academic importance more than it is of clinical relevance to the ill dog.

FOLLOW UP

Molecular analyses were performed on EDTA-anticoagulated peripheral blood. A fragment of the 16S ribosomal RNA gene was amplified from total blood DNA, using forward and reverse *Anaplasmataceae*-specific primers. The sequence obtained was identical to other *A. phagocytophilum* 16S rRNA sequences reported in GenBank.

FURTHER READING

Cocayne CG, Cohn LA (2012) *Ehrlichia ewingii* infection (canine granulocytotropic ehrlichiosis). In: *Infectious Diseases of the Dog and Cat*. (ed CE Greene) Saunders, Philadelphia, pp. 241–244.

Diniz PP, Breitschwerdt EB (2012) *Anaplasma phagocytophilum* infection (canine granulocytotropic anaplasmosis). In: *Infectious Diseases of the Dog and Cat*. (ed CE Greene) Saunders, Philadelphia, pp. 244–256.

Little SE (2010) Ehrlichiosis and anaplasmosis in dogs and cats. *Vet Clin North Am Small Anim Pract* **40**:1121–1140.

CASE 194

1 What is your interpretation of these findings? Can you localise the bleeding problem to a specific part of the coagulation cascade?

The history, clinical signs and point of care result of only a prolonged aPTT with normal PT and platelet count is consistent with a generalised bleeding disorder affecting the intrinsic system.

2 What additional haemostatic tests are indicated?

Additional relevant testing includes testing for haemophilia A (FVIII) or B (FIX), the most common congenital coagulation disorders.

FURTHER READING

Lubas G, Caldin M, Wiinberg B *et al*. (2010) Laboratory testing of coagulation disorders. In: *Schalm's Veterinary Hematology*, 6th edn. (eds DJ Weiss, KJ Wardrop) Blackwell Publishing, Ames, pp. 1082–1100.

CASE 195

1 Which acute-phase proteins (APPs) would you examine to assess the health status of cattle?

The most sensitive APPs in cattle are serum amyloid A (SAA) and haptoglobin. Both are considered to be major APPs and rise in the face of mastitis, metritis, peritonitis and endocarditis. The kinetics of both proteins vary. SAA rises earlier and declines more rapidly than haptoglobin. It has also been observed that both of these APPs rise after parturition. Despite that, post-partum metritis could be suspected by markedly increased haptoglobin concentrations. Additionally, increased haptoglobin concentrations 2 months after calving appear to be associated with an increased intergestational interval.

Moderate APPs in cattle are α-1-acid glycoprotein, ceruloplasmin and fibrinogen. However, the detection of ceruloplasmin has received less attention in the last decade and α-1-acid glycoprotein is considered the main moderate APP in cattle.

Extrahepatic SAA produced in the mammary gland (MAA), as well as haptoglobin measured in milk, are known to rise when mastitis is present. Detection of both proteins in milk may be used as an early indication of subclinical mastitis. MAA has proved to be more accurate than the California mastitis test.

2 What actions does ceruloplasmin perform?

Ceruloplasmin transports copper and scavenges free radicals known to create oxidative stress in the cow. As copper plays a favourable role in wound healing and the formation of collagen, ceruloplasmin plays a supporting role in tissue remodelling after injury.

FURTHER READING

Chan JPW, Chang CoC, Hsu WL *et al.* (2010) Association of increased serum acute-phase protein concentrations with reproductive performance in dairy cows with postpartum metritis. *J Vet Clin Pathol* **39**:72–78.

Cray C, Zaias J, Altman NH (2009) Acute phase response in animals: a review. *Comp Med* **59**:517–526.

Eckersall PD, Bell R (2010) Review. Acute phase proteins: biomarkers of infection and inflammation in veterinary medicine. *Vet J* **185**:23–27.

Safi S, Khoshvaghti A, Jafarzadeh SR *et al.* (2009) Acute phase proteins in the diagnosis of bovine subclinical mastitis. *Vet Clin Pathol* **38**:471–476.

CASE 196

1 For foal number 1, what are your main differential diagnoses? What other tests may be helpful for differentiating these diagnoses?

The main differential diagnoses are ruptured urinary bladder and diarrhoea with electrolyte loss. Concurrent hyperkalaemia and hypochloraemia would be expected with both conditions, but often ruptured urinary bladder results in abdominal distension with fluid retention. The creatinine in the abdominal fluid is more than twice the serum creatinine in most cases. There may or may not be pollakuria and/or stranguria and straining to urinate may be misinterpreted as straining to defaecate. Ultrasound evaluation of the abdomen may be successful in demonstrating urinary bladder rupture. If new methylene blue dye is injected by catheter into the urinary bladder, it will show up in the abdominal fluid within 15 minutes if a rupture is present.

Observation of the diarrhoea will be helpful in determining if it is the underlying cause of the reported clinical signs, but the possibility of concurrent diarrhoea and urinary bladder rupture should not be ignored. Neutrophilic leucocytosis is common with both conditions, although there may be variations in leucocyte response depending on the rapidity of development and the underlying cause. Failure of passive transfer of maternal antibody and sepsis may predispose to urinary bladder rupture, so evaluations to determine if these are present are indicated.

2 For foal number 2, is the slightly low calcium likely to be the cause of the clinical signs? Why or why not?

Total serum calcium of 2.0 mmol/l is not sufficiently low to result in the described clinical signs. Usually, clinical signs due to hypocalcaemia will not develop until total serum calcium is <1.75 mmol/l and ionised calcium is <0.7 mmol/l. The possibility of slightly low serum calcium due to hypoproteinaemia with decreased protein binding should be considered.

3 For foal number 3, what are your differential diagnoses? What other laboratory findings would provide support for these diagnoses?

Hyperammonaemia may occur with intestinal disease, presumably due to overgrowth of urease-producing bacteria and/or increased absorption of ammonia because of intestinal inflammation. More commonly it is associated with hepatic disease. This has been reported with iron toxicity, *Rhodococcus equi* infection and portosystemic shunt. Evaluation of serum AST, GLDH, ALP, GGT and bile acids should help determine if hepatic disease is likely. Interpretation of intestinal hyperammonaemia relies on elimination of hepatic causes and observation of signs of diarrhoea or intestinal upset.

FURTHER READING

Axon JE, Palmer JE (2008) Clinical pathology of the foal. *Vet Clin North Am Equine Pract* **24**:357–385.

Divers TJ, Warner A, Vaala WE *et al.* (1983) Toxic hepatic failure in newborn foals. *J Am Vet Med Assoc* **183**:1407–1413.

Hillyer MH, Holt PE, Barr FJ *et al.* (1993) Clinical signs and radiographic diagnosis of a portosystemic shunt in a foal. *Vet Rec* 132:457–460.

Johnson AL, Gilsenan WF, Palmer JE (2012) Metabolic encephalopathies in foals: pay attention to the biochemistry panel! *Equine Vet Educ* **24**:233–235.

CASE 197

1 What are the most important morphological features of the blood smear?

There are small coccoid bacteria arranged singly or in short rows in epimembranary position on the RBCs, consistent with *Mycoplasma haemocanis*. No platelets or platelet clumps are visible in the background, confirming the low automated platelet count.

2 What is the most probable pathogenesis of the disease diagnosed in this dog?

Haemotrophic mycoplasmosis usually occurs with 'stress' and can be secondary to other primary diseases such as intestinal parasitism or infectious disease; splenectomised dogs are predisposed to develop the disease; the infection leads to immune-mediated haemolytic anaemia. Moderate anaemia is also present in this case but erythrocytes are normocytic-normochromic indicating a non-regenerative anaemia at present. The cause may be acute disease prior to visible regeneration.

3 How can the diagnosis be confirmed?

PCR and electron microscopy are the best way to confirm the diagnosis.

FOLLOW UP

Mycoplasma spp. infection was confirmed by PCR.

FURTHER READING

Hulme-Moir KL, Barker EN, Stonelake A *et al.* (2010) Use of real-time quantitative polymerase chain reaction to monitor antibiotic therapy in a dog with naturally acquired *Mycoplasma haemocanis* infection. *J Vet Diagn Invest* **22:** 582–587.

Roura X, Peters IR, Altet L *et al.* (2010) Prevalence of hemotropic mycoplasmas in healthy and unhealthy cats and dogs in Spain. *J Vet Diagn Invest* **22:**270–274.

CASE 198

1 What is your assessment of these findings?

The increased refractometer total protein and fibrinogen may be due to dehydration associated with the anorexia for 4 days. The increased urea and creatinine may also be due to dehydration (pre-renal), but further assessment following rehydration and treatment will be needed to determine if concurrent renal disease may be present. The clinical signs suggest that a post-renal cause of the increase in urea and creatinine is unlikely. The slight increase in CK may be due to muscle damage associated with the falling.

The abnormalities of the CSF are the most striking and consistent with a neutrophilic pleocytosis and inflammatory condition involving the CNS, and this is consistent with the clinical signs. The marked decrease in CSF glucose suggests metabolism of glucose, often associated with infection, despite the absence of infectious agents in the CSF.

2 What are the most likely clinical diagnoses/ differential diagnoses?

Primary concerns include brain abscess or purulent meningitis/meningoencephalitis associated with late dehorning and inadequate attention to the dehorning sites.

Editors' note: This case illustrates the fact that haematological findings may be without abnormality when there is a localised site of ongoing active inflammation. The absence of haematological abnormality does not rule out the possibility of inflammation.

FOLLOW UP

Radiography of the head (**Fig. 198.2**) showed area of lucency consistent with osteomyelitis over the poll. Euthanasia was elected and at postmortem examination an abscess was found in this area, with erosion of bone.

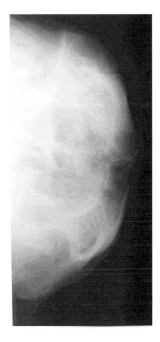

FIG. 198.2 Radiograph of the head. Poll at right, ear at the bottom. Note the areas of radiolucency consistent with osteomyelitis at the poll.

CASE 199

1 What are the structures in the cytoplasm of the erythrocytes?

Babesia canis organisms are visible in the erythrocytes. Babesial parasites vary in size from large (2.5–5.0 μm) to small (1.0–2.5 μm). The large protozoal organism shows a tear drop-shaped profile, with weakly eosinophilic cytoplasm and an eccentric small nucleus, and commonly appears in pairs or in groups of four. Three species of large (*B. canis, B. vogeli, B. rossi*) and three species of small (*B. gibsoni, B. conradae, B. microti*-like) *Babesia* have been identified in the dog, although more than 100 species are recognised to infect domestic and wild animals.

2 What is the most probable pathogenesis of the disease diagnosed in this dog?

These protozoa are transmitted by tick bite, transplacentally or by blood transfusion and can be secondary to some other primary disease, such as infectious disease. Babesiosis may cause both intravascular and extravascular haemolysis. Mechanisms of haemolysis include damage by protozoal proteases, immune-mediated destruction of erythrocytes and oxidative damage, followed by haemoglobinuria.

3 What other examination can be useful in the management of this disease?

Quantitation of serum antibodies by ELISA is useful in evaluation of the immune response of the dog; determination and monitoring of the renal and urinary parameters are useful in follow up. PCR is necessary for detecting infection in animals with very low-grade parasitaemia.

FURTHER READING

Harvey JW (2012) *Babesia* species. In: *Veterinary Hematology: A Diagnostic Guide and Color Atlas.* (ed. JW Harvey) Saunders Elsevier, St. Louis, pp. 82–85.

CASE 200

1 What is your assessment of these findings?

The slight increase in RBC count and haematocrit suggests dehydration. The total protein may be increased by dehydration, suggesting it is lower than the results represented here, although a fall to below reference interval with rehydration is unlikely. The fibrinogen is increased compared with the reference interval but does not suggest an increase when compared with the total protein (fibrinogen does not exceed 10% of total protein). There is a slight leucocytosis with mature neutrophilia and left shift indicated by an increase in band cells; these findings support the presence of an acute inflammatory condition.

2 What is/are your diagnosis/differential diagnoses?

Based on the clinical signs, pneumonia is a primary concern, but other causes of acute inflammation cannot be ruled out. Further physical examination may help to localise the likely site of inflammation.

Appendices

1 Conversion Factors

To convert from SI units to old/conventional units, divide by the conversion factor.

	SI Units	Conversion Factor	Old/Conventional Units
Haematology			
PCV	l/l	0.01	%
RBCs	$\times 10^{12}$/l	1	$\times 10^6$/µl
Erythrocytes	$\times 10^9$/l	1	$\times 10^3$/µl
Nucleated cell count	$\times 10^9$/l	1	$\times 10^3$/µl
Eosinophils	$\times 10^9$/l	1	$\times 10^3$/µl
Fibrinogen	g/l	100	mg/dl
MCV	fl	n/a	fl
MCH	pg	n/a	pg
MCHC	g/l	10	g/dl
Biochemistry			
ALP	U/l	1	IU/l
ALT	U/l	1	U/l
ACTH	pmol/ml	0.22	pg/ml
Albumin	g/l	10	g/dl
Ammonia (NH_4)	µmol/l	0.587	µg/dl
Amylase	U/l	1	U/l
AST	U/l	1	U/l
Bilirubin	µmol/l	17.1	mg/dl
Calcium	mmol/l	0.2495	mg/dl
Carbon dioxide	mmol/l	1	mEq/l
Chloride	mmol/l	1	mEq/l
Cholesterol	mmol/l	0.0259	mg/dl
Copper	µmmol/l	0.157	µg/dl
Cortisol	nmol/l	27.59	µg/dl

	SI Units	Conversion Factor	Old/Conventional Units
Creatine kinase (CK)	U/l	1	IU/l
Creatinine	µmol/l	88.4	mg/dl
GGT	U/l	1	U/l
GLDH	U/l	1	U/l
Globulin	g/l	10	g/dl
Glucose	mmol/l	0.0555	mg/dl
Iron, binding	µmol/l	0.179	µg/dl
Iron, total	µmol/l	0.179	µg/dl
Lipase	U/l	1	IU/l
	U/l		Cherry-Crandall U
Magnesium	mmol/l	0.4114	U/l
Osmolality	mmol/l	1	Osm/kg
Phosphorus	mmol/l	0.323	mg/dl
Potassium	mmol/l	1	mEq/l
Protein, total	g/l	10	g/dl
SDH	U/l	1	IU/l
Selenium	µmol/l	0.1266	µg/dl
Sodium	mmol/l	1	mEq/l
Triglycerides	mmol/l	0.0113	mg/dl
Triiodothyronine (T3)	nmol/l	0.0154	µg/dl
Thyroxine (T4)	nmol/l	12.5	µg/dl
Urea nitrogen	mmol/l	0.357	mg/dl
Uric acid	mmol/l	59.48	mg/dl
Vitamin E	µmol/l	2.322	mg/ml

2 Biological Variation

Recommendations for analytical coefficient of variation (CV), bias and total error (TE) based on biological variation of various biochemical and haematological analytes in dogs. The index of individuality is calculated using the 'inverse' formula, so a high index of individuality corresponds to a high degree of individual variation.

	Information From the Literature			Traditional Quality Specifications Based on Biological Variation²									Alternative TE Based on Biological Variation³			Index of Individuality (II)⁴ (Category⁵)	RCV or Critical Difference⁶	RCV or Critical Difference⁷
Measurand	CV_G = Between Dog¹	CV_I = Within Dog¹	CV_A¹	CV Opt	CV Des	CV Min	Bias Opt	Bias Des	Bias Min	TE Opt	TE Des	TE Min	Alt TE Opt	Alt TE Des	Alt TE Min		95% Probability 'Significant'	99% Probability 'Highly Significant'
RBC	4.4	5.4	2.8	1.35	2.70	4.05	0.87	1.74	2.61	3.10	6.20	9.29	2.23	4.46	6.68	0.73 (Intermed)	16.86%	29.67%
Hct	5.2	6.4	1.1	1.6	3.20	4.80	1.03	2.06	3.09	3.67	7.34	11.01	2.64	5.28	7.92	0.80 (Intermed)	18.00%	23.69%
Hgb	4.7	5.9	2.9	1.48	2.95	4.43	0.94	1.89	2.83	3.38	6.76	10.14	2.44	4.87	7.31	0.72 (Intermed)	18.22%	23.98%
WBC	12.3	12.1	3.7	3.03	6.05	9.08	2.16	4.31	6.47	7.16	14.29	21.45	5.00	9.98	14.98	0.97 (Intermed)	35.18%	46.16%
ALT	23.7	9.7	3.2	2.43	4.85	7.28	3.20	6.40	9.60	7.21	14.40	21.61	4.01	8.00	12.01	2.32 (High)	28.31%	37.26%
AST	10.9	11.4	3.3	2.85	5.70	8.55	1.97	3.94	5.91	6.67	13.35	20.02	4.70	9.41	14.11	0.92 (Intermed)	32.90%	43.30%
ALP	34.2	8.6	1.7	2.15	4.30	6.45	4.41	8.82	13.22	7.96	15.92	23.86	3.55	7.10	10.64	3.90 (High)	24.30%	31.98%
Alb	3.0	2.4	1.6	0.60	1.20	1.80	0.46	0.93	1.39	1.45	2.91	4.36	0.99	1.98	2.97	1.04 (Intermed)	8.00%	10.52%
TP	3.1	2.6	1.1	0.65	1.30	1.95	0.51	1.01	1.52	1.58	3.16	4.74	1.07	2.15	3.22	1.10 (Intermed)	7.82%	10.30%
Creatinine	12.9	14.6	2.9	3.65	7.30	10.95	2.44	4.88	7.31	8.46	16.93	25.38	6.02	12.05	18.07	0.87 (Intermed)	41.26%	54.30%
Cholesterol	15.1	7.3	3.0	1.83	3.65	5.48	2.10	4.19	6.29	5.12	10.22	15.33	3.02	6.02	9.04	1.91 (High)	21.88%	28.79%
Glucose	3.8	9.5	3.7	2.38	4.75	7.13	1.28	2.56	3.84	5.21	10.40	15.60	3.93	7.84	11.76	0.37 (Low)	28.26%	37.19%
Fructosamine	4.2	11.1	2.8	2.78	5.55	8.33	1.48	2.97	4.45	6.07	12.13	18.20	4.59	9.16	13.75	0.37 (Low)	31.73%	41.76%
Potassium	3.6	3.3	0.1	0.83	1.65	2.48	0.61	1.22	1.83	2.07	3.94	5.92	1.37	2.72	4.09	1.09 (Intermed)	9.15%	12.05%
Total T4	17.2	17.0	4.0	4.25	8.50	12.75	3.02	6.05	9.07	10.03	20.08	30.11	7.01	14.03	21.04	0.99 (Intermed)	40.41%	63.71%
cTSH	43.6	13.6	8.8	3.40	6.80	10.20	5.71	11.42	17.13	11.32	22.64	33.96	5.61	11.22	16.83	2.69 (High)	44.91%	59.01%
Iron	17.2	17.8	0.7	4.45	8.90	13.35	3.09	6.19	9.28	10.43	20.88	31.31	7.34	14.69	22.03	0.97 (Intermed)	49.37%	64.99%
Fibrinogen	19.0	17.1	2.8	4.28	8.56	12.84	3.20	6.39	9.59	10.26	20.51	30.78	7.06	14.12	21.19	1.10 (Intermed)	48.03%	63.21%
C-reactive protein	29.3	24.3	7.2	6.08	12.16	18.24	4.76	9.52	14.27	14.79	29.58	44.37	10.03	20.06	30.10	1.16 (Intermed)	70.25%	92.46%
α-1-AGP	67.0	9.6	8.1	2.40	4.80	7.20	8.46	16.92	25.38	12.42	24.84	37.26	3.96	7.92	11.88	5.33 (High)	34.82%	45.82%
Haptoglobin	20.2	17.0	4.9	4.25	8.50	12.75	3.30	6.60	9.90	10.31	20.63	30.94	7.01	14.03	21.04	1.14 (Intermed)	49.04%	64.54%

RCV = reference change value.

CV Opt = recommended optimal analytical CV based on $CV_A \leq 0.25CV_I$

CV Des = recommended desirable analytical CV based on $CV_A \leq 0.5 CV_I$

CV Min = recommended minimally acceptable analytical CV based on $CV_A \leq 0.75 CV_I$

Bias Opt = recommended optimal Bias based on B $\leq 0.125(CV_I^2 + CV_G^2)^{1/2}$

Bias Des = recommended desirable Bias based on B $\leq 0.250 (CV_I^2 + CV_G^2)^{1/2}$

Bias Min = recommended minimally acceptable Bias based on B $\leq 0.375(CV_I^2 + CV_G^2)^{1/2}$

TE Opt = recommended optimal TE based on $TE_A \leq 1.65(0.25CV_I) + 0.125(CV_I^2 + CV_G^2)^{1/2}$

TE Des = recommended desirable TE based on $TE_A \leq 1.65 (0.50CV_I) + 0.250 (CV_I^2 + CV_G^2)^{1/2}$

TE Min = recommended minimally acceptable TE based on $TE_A \leq 1.65 (0.75CV_I) + 0.375(CV_I^2 + CV_G^2)^{1/2}$

Alt TE Opt = recommended optimal TE based on $TE_A \leq 1.65$ (CV Opt). (Calculation from Oosterhuis, WP (2011) Gross overestimation of total error based on biologic variation. Letter to the Editor. *Clin Chem* **57**:1334–1336.)

Alt TE Des = recommended desirable TE based on $TE_A \leq 1.65$ (CV Des) (Calculation from Oosterhuis, WP (2011) Gross overestimation of total error based on biologic variation. Letter to the Editor. *Clin Chem* **57**:1334–1336.)

Alt TE min = recommended desirable TE based on $TE_A \leq 1.65$ (CV Min) (Calculation from Oosterhuis, WP (2011) Gross overestimation of total error based on biologic variation. Letter to the Editor. *Clin Chem* **57**:1334–1336.)

Superscript designations

1. Jensen AL, Kjelgaard-Hansen M (2006) Method comparison in the clinical laboratory. *Vet Clin Pathol* **35**:276–86.

2. Calculation formulas from:

Fraser CG, Petersen PH, Libeer JC et al. (1997) Proposals for setting generally applicable quality goals solely based on biology. *Ann Clin Biochem* **34**:8–12.

Fraser CG (2001) Quality specifications. In: *Biological Variation: From Principles to Practice*. AACC Press, Washington DC, pp. 29–66.

Sciacovelli L, Secchiero S, Zardo L et al. (2001) External quality assessment schemes: need for recognized requirements. *Clinica Chimica Acta* 309:183–199.

3. Calculation formula using CV Opt, CV Des and CV Min from Oosterhuis WP (2011) Gross overestimation of total error based on biologic variation. Letter to the Editor. *Clin Chem* **57**:1334–1336.

4. Index of Individuality (II) = CV_G/square root of $(CV_I^2 + CV_A^2)$. Interpretation: >1.7 = high II; RCV likely to provide better determination of significant difference in sequential analyses; use of 95% population-based reference interval may hamper diagnostic sensitivity. <0.7 = low II; use of 95% population-based reference interval is valid. Between 0.7 and 1.7, RCV may be of benefit in determining significant difference in sequential analyses. **Note:** The II will change with assays having a CV_A different from that presented in this table. See Fraser CG (2001) Quality specifications. In: *Biological Variation: From Principles to Practice*. AACC Press, Washington DC, pp. 29–66.

5. Categories of II: high (>1.7); intermediate (Intermed) (0.7–1.7); low (<0.7).

6. RCV = $1.96 \times \sqrt{2 \times \left(CV_I^2 + CV_A^2\right)}$ = 95% probability = 'significant' change. Calculated using CV_A^1 provided in this table from information in the literature.

From: Fraser CG (2001) *Biological Variation: From Principles to Practice*. AACC Press, Washington DC. See also: Walton RM (2012) Subject-based reference values: biologic variation, individuality, and reference change values. *Vet Clin Pathol* **41**:175–181.

7. RCV = $2.58 \times \sqrt{2 \times \left(CV_I^2 + CV_A^2\right)}$ = 99% probability = 'highly significant' change. Calculated using CV_A^1 provided in this table from information in the literature.

From: Fraser CG (2001) *Biological Variation: From Principles to Practice*. AACC Press, Washington DC. See also: Walton RM (2012) Subject-based reference values: biologic variation, individuality, and reference change values. *Vet Clin Pathol* **41**:175–181.

Index

Index

Index

T - #0938 - 101024 - C288 - 261/194/13 - PB - 9781482225877 - Gloss Lamination